Diagnostic Techniques in Renal Disease

CONTEMPORARY ISSUES IN NEPHROLOGY

VOLUME 25

Series Editor
Jay H. Stein, M.D.

Series Editors, Vols. 1-21
Barry M. Brenner, M.D.
Jay H. Stein, M.D.

Volumes Already Published

Forthcoming Volumes in the Series

Diagnostic Techniques in Renal Disease

Guest Editor

ROBERT G. NARINS, M.D.
Division Head
Division of Nephrology and Hypertension
Henry Ford Hospital
Detroit, Michigan

Series Editor

JAY H. STEIN, M.D.
Professor and Chairman
Department of Medicine
Dan F. Parman Chair in Medicine
University of Texas Medical School at San Antonio
San Antonio, Texas

 CHURCHILL LIVINGSTONE
New York, Edinburgh, London, Melbourne, Tokyo

Library of Congress Cataloging-in-Publication Data

Diagnostic techniques in renal disease / guest editor, Robert G.
  Narins.
    p. cm.—(Contemporary issues in nephrology ; v. 25)
    Includes bibliographical references and index.
    ISBN 0-443-08806-3
    1. Kidneys—Diseases—Diagnosis. I. Narins, Robert G.
  II. Series: Contemporary issues in nephrology ; vol. 25.
    [DNLM: 1. Kidney Diseases—diagnosis. W1 CO769MR v.25 / WJ
  302 D5363]
  RC904.D52 1992
  616.6'1075—dc20
  DNLM/DLC
  for Library of Congress   92-4098
                                                    CIP

Distributed in the United Kingdom by Churchill Livingstone, Robert
Stevenson House, 1–3 Baxter's Place, Leith Walk, Edinburgh EH1
3AF, and by associated companies, branches, and representatives
throughout the world.

Accurate indications, adverse reactions, and dosage schedules for
drugs are provided in this book, but it is possible that they may
change. The reader is urged to review the package information data of
the manufacturers of the medications mentioned.

The Publishers have made every effort to trace the copyright holders
for borrowed material. If they have inadvertently overlooked any, they
will be pleased to make the necessary arrangements at the first opportunity.

Acquisitions Editor: *Avé McCracken*
Copy Editor: *Katharine Leawanna O'Moore*
Production Designer: *Jody L. Ouellette*
Production Supervisor: *Jeanine Furino*

Printed in the United States of America

First published in 1992   7 6 5 4 3 2 1

Diagnostic Techniques in Renal Disease

Guest Editor

ROBERT G. NARINS, M.D.
Division Head
Division of Nephrology and Hypertension
Henry Ford Hospital
Detroit, Michigan

Series Editor

JAY H. STEIN, M.D.
Professor and Chairman
Department of Medicine
Dan F. Parman Chair in Medicine
University of Texas Medical School at San Antonio
San Antonio, Texas

CHURCHILL LIVINGSTONE
New York, Edinburgh, London, Melbourne, Tokyo

Library of Congress Cataloging-in-Publication Data

Diagnostic techniques in renal disease / guest editor, Robert G.
Narins.

    p. cm.—(Contemporary issues in nephrology ; v. 25)
    Includes bibliographical references and index.
    ISBN 0-443-08806-3
    1. Kidneys—Diseases—Diagnosis. I. Narins, Robert G.
II. Series: Contemporary issues in nephrology ; vol. 25.
    [DNLM: 1. Kidney Diseases—diagnosis. W1 CO769MR v.25 / WJ
302 D5363]
    RC904.D52 1992
    616.6′1075—dc20
    DNLM/DLC
    for Library of Congress   92-4098
                                          CIP

Distributed in the United Kingdom by Churchill Livingstone, Robert
Stevenson House, 1–3 Baxter's Place, Leith Walk, Edinburgh EH1
3AF, and by associated companies, branches, and representatives
throughout the world.

Accurate indications, adverse reactions, and dosage schedules for
drugs are provided in this book, but it is possible that they may
change. The reader is urged to review the package information data of
the manufacturers of the medications mentioned.

The Publishers have made every effort to trace the copyright holders
for borrowed material. If they have inadvertently overlooked any, they
will be pleased to make the necessary arrangements at the first opportunity.

Acquisitions Editor: *Avé McCracken*
Copy Editor: *Katharine Leawanna O'Moore*
Production Designer: *Jody L. Ouellette*
Production Supervisor: *Jeanine Furino*

Printed in the United States of America

First published in 1992   7 6 5 4 3 2 1

To Joseph Paul DiMaggio

Even more than his prodigious talents, his dedication,
style, and grace under pressure inspired generations.
A shame he wasn't a Chairman of Medicine.

Contributors

Micheal J. Adcox, M.D.
Senior Fellow, Division of Nephrology, Department of Medicine, University of Washington School of Medicine, Seattle, Washington

M. Donald Blaufox, M.D.
Professor and Chairman, Department of Nuclear Medicine, and Professor, Department of Medicine, Albert Einstein College of Medicine of Yeshiva University and Montefiore Medical Center, Bronx, New York

Joao Chequer Bou-Habib, M.D.
Postdoctoral Fellow, Immunogenetics and Transplantation Laboratory, Department of Surgery, University of California, San Francisco, School of Medicine, San Francisco, California

Bonnie Collins, M.D.
Senior Fellow, Division of Nephrology, Department of Medicine, University of Washington School of Medicine, Seattle, Washington

Francis Dumler, M.D.
Associate Clinical Professor, Department of Medicine, University of Michigan Medical School, Ann Arbor, Michigan; Senior Staff Physician, Division of Nephrology and Hypertension, Department of Medicine, Henry Ford Hospital, Detroit, Michigan

Ronald J. Falk, M.D.
Associate Professor, Division of Nephrology, Department of Medicine, University of North Carolina at Chapel Hill School of Medicine, Chapel Hill, North Carolina

Patricia A. Gabow, M.D.
Professor, Division of Renal Diseases and Hypertension, Department of Medicine, University of Colorado Health Sciences Center; Deputy Manager, Medical Affairs, Denver General Hospital, Denver, Colorado

Marvin R. Garovoy, M.D.
Professor, Departments of Surgery and Medicine, and Director, Immunogenetics and Transplantation Laboratory, Department of Surgery, University of California, San Francisco, School of Medicine, San Francisco, California

Stanley Goldfarb, M.D.
Professor, Department of Medicine, University of Pennsylvania, School of Medicine; Co-chief, Renal Electrolyte Section, Department of Medicine, Hospital of the University of Pennsylvania, Philadelphia, Pennsylvania

Mitchell L. Halperin, M.D.
Professor, Division of Nephrology, Department of Medicine, St. Michael's Hospital, Toronto, Ontario, Canada

J. Charles Jennette, M.D.
Professor, Department of Pathology, and Director, Nephropathology Laboratory, University of North Carolina at Chapel Hill School of Medicine, Chapel Hill, North Carolina

William D. Kaehny, M.D.
Professor, Division of Renal Diseases and Hypertension, Department of Medicine, University of Colorado Health Sciences Center; Assistant Chief, Medical Department of Service, Veterans Affairs Medical Center, Denver, Colorado

Kamel S. Kamel, M.D.
Assistant Professor, Department of Medicine, St. Michael's Hospital, Toronto, Ontario, Canada

Stephen M. Korbet, M.D.
Associate Professor, Division of Nephrology, Department of Medicine, Rush Medical College of Rush University, Chicago, Illinois

Calvin M. Kunin, M.D.
Professor, Department of Internal Medicine, Ohio State University College of Medicine, Columbus, Ohio

Edmund J. Lewis, M.D.
Professor, Division of Nephrology, Department of Medicine, Rush Medical College of Rush University, Chicago, Illinois

Francisco Llach, M.D.
Professor, Division of Nephrology, Department of Medicine, University of California, Los Angeles, UCLA School of Medicine, Los Angeles, California; Chief, Renal Section, Department of Medicine, Wadsworth Veterans Administration Hospital, West Los Angeles, California

Robert G. Narins, M.D.
Division Head, Division of Nephrology and Hypertension, Henry Ford Hospital, Detroit, Michigan

Bijan Nikakhtar, M.D.
Associate Clinical Professor, Division of Nephrology, Department of Medicine, University of California, Los Angeles, UCLA School of Medicine, Los Angeles, California; Staff Physician, Ambulatory Care, Wadsworth Veterans Administration Medical Center, West Los Angeles, California

Rebecca J. Schmidt, D.O.
Fellow, Division of Nephrology and Hypertension, Department of Internal Medicine, Henry Ford Hospital, Detroit, Michigan

Melvin M. Schwartz, M.D.
Professor, Department of Pathology, Rush Medical College of Rush University; Associate Attending Physician, Department of Pathology, Rush Presbyterian Hospital/St. Luke's Medical Center, Chicago, Illinois

Mohammed A. J. Sikder, M.D.
Fellow, Renal Electrolyte Division, Department of Medicine, Hospital of the University of Pennsylvania, Philadelphia, Pennsylvania

Byungse Suh, M.D., Ph.D.
Professor, Department of Medicine, and Associate Professor, Division of Microbiology and Immunology, Section of Infectious Diseases, Department of Internal Medicine, Temple University School of Medicine and Hospital, Philadelphia, Pennsylvania

Bedri Yousif, M.D.
Postdoctoral Fellow, Immunogenetics and Transplantation Laboratory, Department of Surgery, University of California, San Francisco, School of Medicine, San Francisco, California

Richard A. Zager, M.D.
Professor, Division of Nephrology, Department of Medicine, University of Washington, Harborview Medical Center and Fred Hutchinson Cancer Research Center, Seattle, Washington

Preface

A preface? Here I sit, pen in hand, attempting to determine the whys and wherefores of "prefacing." Who reads a preface anyway? I can assure you, there are more people who read the instructions on a shampoo bottle label than who read a preface! I can also assure you that there are more airline passengers who have read the riveting details of how to open and close a seatbelt than have read prefaces from all the books since Gutenberg invented the printing press. I have never read a preface in my life, but nonetheless, *I love prefaces* because they represent several pages I can ignore in a book that is usually too long anyway. Indeed, I could write this preface in some extraterrestrial tongue and only Messrs. Churchill and Livingstone would realize it! So what am I worrying about? The world will "little note nor long remember" what I say here anyway. In the now-famous extraterrestrial words of my grandmother Celia Bircher, I am *machen a tsimmes* (making a fuss over nothing).

For this volume of *Contemporary Issues in Nephrology,* the authors have been selected not only for their profound understanding of the topic, but also for their ability to articulate and simplify the information. They share with you their diagnostic insights on a wide range of nephrologic topics. Where appropriate, practical discussions of the mechanisms, indications, and applications of various diagnostic techniques are stressed. Scholarly reviews of newer assays and fresh insights into the use of older procedures are provided by this outstanding array of authors.

Halperin, Kamel, and I have explored the pathophysiologic basis for the tests of renal electrolytes and water handling. Acid-base and electrolyte assays and studies of osmoregulation are applied to practical clinical settings, with updates on newer applications of pre-existing tests.

Kaehny and Gabow focus their attention on autosomal dominant adult polycystic kidney disease, a disorder accounting for approximately 12 percent of the end stage renal disease in this country. Clinical, invasive, and noninvasive testing—including newer developments in genetic counseling—are reviewed.

The myriad causes of acute renal failure are teased apart and methodically sorted out in a most logical manner by Adcox, Collins, and Zager. The roles of blood, urinary, and newer invasive and noninvasive tests are clearly summarized.

Because dietary, pharmacologic, and metabolic therapies may slow the progression of the nephropathy complicating types I and II diabetes mellitus, its early diagnosis has become critical. Schmidt and Dumler review the disorder's natural history, indicate how to distinguish it from other nephropathies that the diabetic may contract, and stress the importance of microalbuminuria.

Falk and Jennette take the difficult topic of serologic diagnoses in renal disease and digest it, simplify it, and convey it to those of us who are otherwise immunologically incompetent. Their major contributions to the field allow for their authoritative and articulate commentary on this changing and important area.

Yousif, Bou-Habib, and Garovoy classify and sort out the various terms of renal transplantation rejection and review the immunologic and histologic bases for diagnosis. The various tests required for immune monitoring, their indications, and the interpretation of results are deftly presented.

Llach and Nikakhtar have acquired enormous experience with renal osteodystrophy, and they provide a lucid outline of the diagnostic approach to this debilitating and largely preventable disorder. Chemical, radioisotopic, radiologic, and histologic testing are reviewed and presented in a well-organized fashion.

When and how far testing should be carried out in the patient with a kidney stone are critically analyzed by Sikder and Goldfarb. The differential diagnosis of nephrolithiasis and the wedding of testing to the practical management of these patients are artfully presented.

Using carefully selected case material, Schwartz, Korbet, and Lewis illustrate why the renal biopsy continues to be a safe and valuable tool in the nephrologist's diagnostic armamentarium. The importance of histopathology to therapy is stressed.

For years, devotees of nuclear medicine have promised us better living and diagnosing through radiopharmaceuticals. They have dazzled us with their curves, curies, and colors. Blaufox provides an update on the developments in this evolving area.

Finally, Suh, Kunin, and I summarize the various diagnostic approaches to defining, localizing, and following patients with infected urinary tracts. It was enlightening for me to review these tests and concepts and to work with such experienced talents as Drs. Suh and Kunin.

Thusly, I have "prefaced"! The world may not be a better place for this, but at least I used no more paper than could be provided by the branch of a small tree. For those of you who have persisted in reading this preface, I can assure you of a far more informative and entertaining time when you read the text!

Robert G. Narins, M.D.

Contents

1

Use of Urine Electrolytes and Osmolality

Bringing Physiology to the Bedside

Mitchell L. Halperin
Kamel S. Kamel
Robert G. Narins

INTRODUCTION

Our aim is to apply recent advances in the physiology of fluid, electrolyte, and acid–base metabolism to the bedside. Although our focus will be on information that can be obtained from an in-depth interpretation of electrolyte concentrations (sodium [Na^+], potassium [K^+], and chloride[Cl^-]) and osmolality in a spot urine, it is obvious that a proper clinical assessment requires an integrated interpretation of the history, physical examination, and other laboratory data. For the sake of brevity, we emphasize those areas where new advances have been made. Case studies are presented to illustrate new and/or important points.

Before considering individual electrolytes, one point common to all areas needs to be emphasized. Although there are "usual ranges" for solute and water excretion, there are no "normal values." Rather, these values must be interpreted in view of the expected response for that clinical situation. For example, a subject who is water deprived should excrete a urine with the highest possible osmolality (greater than 1,000 mOsm/kg H_2O) and minimum volume, whereas a patient who has taken in a surplus of water should excrete the most dilute urine possible (50 mOsm/kg H_2O) and maximum volume of electrolyte-free water. Thus, failure to find the expected response rather than a deviation from usual values should indicate whether a lesion is present or not.

CONCENTRATIONS OF Na^+ AND Cl^- IN THE URINE

Background

Individuals with a normal effective arterial blood volume (EABV) should excrete all the Na^+ and Cl^- of dietary origin that is in excess of their extrarenal losses (sweat, feces). Excretion of these electrolytes usually ranges from 10 to 300 mmol/d. In contrast, in patients with a low EABV, Na^+, and Cl^- are conserved by the kidneys through a number of physiologic adaptations (for review, see ref. 1); thus, concentrations of Na^+ and Cl^- in the urine should be less that 15 mmol/L, unless oliguria is present.[2] If renal conservation of water exceeds that of salt, the concentration of electrolytes may be greater than anticipated, despite their very diminished content in the urine. In this setting, the concentrations of Na^+ and Cl^- may approach 25 mmol/L and still be in keeping with a low EABV. Thus, the distinction between concentration (millimolar) and content (millimole) must be kept in mind.

Determination of the causes of a number of complicated diseases is often facilitated by measurements of the concentration of Na^+ and Cl^- in the urine (Table 1-1). The values obtained bear importantly on such questions as, Is the extracellular fluid (ECF) volume contracted? and Is the renal response to a contracted ECF volume appropriate? If the ECF volume is contracted and

Table 1-1. Conditions for Which the Concentrations of Na^+ and Cl^- in the Urine Are Important

To detect a contracted effective circulatory volume in a patient with
Metabolic alkalosis
Hyponatremia
Acute renal failure
Edema states
To detect the cause of a contracted effective circulatory volume (see Table 1-2)
To assess the renal response to a contracted extracellular fluid volume, and thereby detect
Renal salt wasting
Low aldosterone bioactivity
Bartter's syndrome
Occult abuse of diuretics or vomiting
Unusual anions in the urine
Excessive excretion of NH_4^+

either Na^+ or Cl^-, but not both, is present in the urine in inappropriately large quantities, the cause of ECF volume contraction should become obvious (Table 1-2).

Key Physiologic Principles

Twenty-seven thousand mmol of Na^+ are normally filtered at the glomerulus. Each major nephron segment reabsorbs approximately two-thirds of its delivered load, thereby allowing less than 1 percent of the filtered load to be eventually excreted. Downstream nephron segments cannot fully accommodate for a very large defect in upstream nephron segments. Nevertheless, they can leave their "impression on the electrolytes excreted (e.g., secretion of K^+ if a defect of reabsorption of Cl^- and Na^+ occurs in the loop of Henle; Fig. 1-1).

The quantity of Na^+ excreted depends on signals related to the EABV. One should not think of a normal value for the ECF volume as being constant one for an individual. For example, the ECF volume is maintained at a higher level in a trained athlete or during pregnancy.[3] Hence, the renal response reflects the EABV in these settings. When this volume is low, the rate of excretion of Na^+ and Cl^- should be less than 10 mmol/d.[4] If the volume of urine is very low (0.5 L/d), the concentration of Na^+ could approximate 20 mmol/L; lower concentrations should be expected in the absence of oliguria. The normal hormonal response to ECF volume contraction provides another indirect guide to the status of the EABV. Increased levels of renin, antidiuretic hormone (ADH), and catecholamines in plasma are, in fact, the "gold standard" for assessing the EABV.[5]

With these principles in mind, we address the use of the concentrations of Na^+ and Cl^- in the urine in clinical conditions for which the EABV is being assessed. In this regard, "spot values" from random urine specimens are superior to 24-hour collections. The spot identifies the renal responses to

Table 1-2. Concentrations of Na^+ and Cl^- in the Urine: Indications for Their Measurement

Differential diagnosis
    Disorders classified by the status of their EABV
        Metabolic alkalosis
        Hyponatremia and hypernatremia
        Acute renal failure
        Edema states
    Disorders characterized by renal salt wasting
        Some interstitial nephritides
        States of low aldosterone bioactivity
        Bartter's syndrome
        Diuretic abuse or surrepititious vomiting
    As a clue to other urinary components
        Unsuspected anions
            Ketones, hippurate, glycolate, formate, etc.
        Ammonium
Therapeutic guideline
    Hyponatremia and hypernatremia: To define the character of replacement solutions
    Metabolic alkalosis: To define need for volume repletion or the need to antagonize mineralocorticoid
    Acute renal failure: To define the need for EABV repletion in prerenal acute renal failure
    Edema states: To guide character and vigor of diuretic therapy

Abbreviation: EABV, effective arterial blood volume.

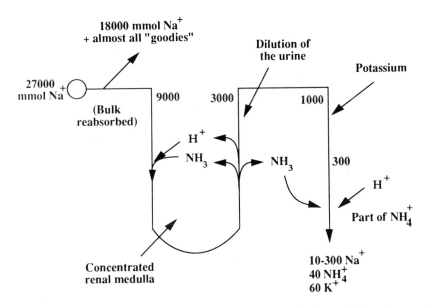

Fig. 1-1. Nephron site where major events occur. "Goodies" are defined as useful substances that are filtered (glucose, amino acids, organic anions, inorganic phosphates, bicarbonate, carnitine, sulfate, etc.).

systemic conditions during the period of renal collection. The 24-hour collection, however, may be viewed as a mixture of many "spot" urines, each of which may have been formed under widely different physiologic conditions. Thus, the integrated 24-hour urine is likely to be less meaningful than the random specimen. To approximate the excretion rate of ions, one can divide the value for Na^+ or Cl^- by that of orinary creatinine because the latter is excreted at a near-constant rate throughout the day.[6] The quantity of creatinine excreted is a function, primarily, of muscle mass with average values for the rate of excretion of 1 mg/min (10μmol/min) in a typical 70-kg adult male.[6] This calculation will of course be flawed when the glomerular filtration rate (GFR) is changing and if creatinine production is abruptly changed, as in rhabdomyolysis.

The Role of Na^+ and Cl^- Concentrations in the
Urine in the Differential Diagnosis of Common
Clinical Conditions

Assessment of the EABV in Patients With Hyponatremia and/or Metabolic Alkalosis

Chung and co-workers[5] reported that the sensitivity and specificity of detecting a low EABV by the physical examination of patients with hyponatremia in the absence of edema is only 50 percent. This clearly underscores the need for more sensitive tools for detecting a mild degree of contraction of the EABV. The diagnosis and rational management of disorders such as hyponatremia and metabolic alkalosis make it important to detect mild degrees of contraction of the EABV. The differential diagnosis of both disorders is conveniently classified in terms of the state of the EABV. Furthermore, normovolemic and hypervolemic forms of these metabolic disturbances receive different therapies. In the hypovolemic form of hyponatremia, reexpansion of the ECF volume could cause an electrolyte-free water diuresis that is due to suppression of release of ADH and increased renal perfusion. If hyponatremia is severe, this might lead to a large water diuresis with very rapid correction of the hyponatremia and the development of central pontine myelinolysis.[7] Once initiated, the water diuresis can be stopped by administering a small quantity of short-acting preparation of ADH.[8]

Pitfalls in the Use of Urine Na^+ and Cl^- to Assess the EABV

A prerequisite for the use of the concentrations of Na^+ and Cl^- in the urine in the assessment of EABV is that renal and adrenal function is intact and that diuretics have not been recently administered.

A proper laboratory assessment of the EABV requires examination of both sodium and chloride concentration.[2] Relying on only the urinary concentration of either Na^+ or Cl^- can lead to errors in the assessment of the EABV, even in the absence of renal or adrenal disease or the use (or abuse) of diuretics. The concentration of Na^+ in the urine might not be low despite a low EABV, if the excretion of Na^+ is obligated by the excretion of a poorly reabsorbable anion such as bicarbonate or ketone anions. In this setting, the hypovolemic stimulus to reabsorb Na^+ allows for the total reclamation of filtered Na^+ and Cl^- from the urine while the Na^+ salts of ketone acids are excreted. Thus, the urinary content of Na^+ will be high while that of Cl^- will be appropriately low. Alternatively, the concentration of Cl^- in the urine might not be low in a patient with a low EABV if the excretion of Cl^- is obligated by the excretion of a cation such as NH_4^+. In this setting with acidosis and hypovolemia, all the filtered Na^+ and some of the filtered Cl^- will be reabsorbed while NH_4^+ and Cl^- will be excreted. Thus, the urine will be devoid of Na^+ but rich in Cl^-. Hence, *both* the concentrations of Na^+ and Cl^- should be determined (Table 1-2).

Cause of Acute Renal Failure

The concentration of Na^+ or Cl^- in the urine represents the ratio of cation or anion to water and hence will be affected by the amount of water reabsorbed by the kidney. This has to be taken into consideration in the patients with oliguria or polyuria. The fractional excretion of Na^+ (FE_{Na}) (equation 1) or Cl^- (FE_{Cl}) provides a means for correcting the concentration of Na^+ or Cl^- in the urine for the amount of water reabsorbed throughout the nephron and relates it to the filtered load of Na^+ or Cl^-.

$$FE_{Na} = \frac{[Na]_{urine}}{[Na]_{plasma}} \times \frac{(creatinine)_{plasma}}{(creatinine)_{urine}} \times 100 \qquad (1)$$

The FE_{Na} provides a better index for differentiating between prerenal and renal causes of acute renal failure than the urinary concentration of Na^+. Although there are exceptions, an FE_{Na} less than 1 percent favors a prerenal cause, while one that is above 1 percent favors a renal cause.[9] Settings of acute parenchymal renal failure with superimposed stimuli for Na^+ retention may manifest an FE_{Na} of less than 1 percent. When acute tubular necrosis complicates the course of patients with preexisting ascites, extensive body burns, or congestive heart failure, a low fractional excretion of electrolytes may occur. In truth, both the FE_{Na} and the FE_{Cl} should be measured to avoid the pitfalls listed previously.[9,10]

Detecting the Cause of a Reduced EABV

When advanced and progressive degrees of azotemia and hypercreatinemia are secondary to prerenal causes, the physical signs and cause of the reduced EABV are usually blatantly apparent. Hypotension, tachycardia, and their postural accentuation are easily elicited, and diminished skin turgor is a common accompaniment. History and hospital records (including diet, intake and output logs, and serial body weights) usually afford decisive information in defining the prerenal nature of the patient's azotemia. In uncomplicated cases, the oliguria, low fractional excretion of Na^+ and Cl^-, and the increased urinary osmolality confirm the diagnosis. In addition to the pitfalls noted in interpreting these urinary findings, certain other clinical caveats should be kept in mind.

When azotomia complicates the course of the diuretic treatment of congestive heart failure, it is not always clear whether overdiuresis or a primary decrease in cardiac function is at fault. The physical findings occasionally may not clearly distinguish these two possible causes even after discontinuing the diuretic. Both conditions may be associated with diminished urine volume and the disappearance of urinary Na^+. In such ambiguous settings, rather than continuing to remove ECF volume or to dangerously challenge with salt solutions, measurement of pulmonary capillary wedge pressure can be the least threatening and most helpful maneuver.

Hypokalemia and metabolic alkalosis are common electrolyte abnormalities in young adults who are concerned with their body image. This is almost always secondary to diuretic abuse or vomiting. In many cases, the diagnosis is made difficult because the patient may deny vomiting or drug abuse. Not uncommonly, an incorrect diagnosis of "Bartter's syndrome" is made, and hence the term *pseudo-Bartter's syndrome* (Table 1-3).

Patients who abuse laxatives tend to have hypokalemia and metabolic acidosis of the normal anion gap type. The concentration of Na^+ in the urine should be less than 15mmol/L, reflecting a low EABV. In contrast, the concentration of Cl^- in the urine may not be low, reflecting the augmented rate of excretion of NH_4^+.[2]

In patients with recent vomiting, the concentration of Na^+ in the urine is usually high, because the excretion of bicarbonate obligates the excretion of Na^+. The concentration of Cl^- in the urine, however, is usually less than

Table 1-3. Urine Electrolytes in the Differential Diagnosis of "Pseudo-Bartter's" Syndrome

	Urine Electrolyte	
Condition	Na	Cl
True Bartter's syndrome	High[a]	High
Pseudo-Bartter's syndromes		
Vomiting		
Recent	High	Low
Remote	Low[b]	Low
Diuretic abuse		
Recent	High	High
Remote	Low	Low
Laxative abuse	Low	High

[a] A value for the urine electrolyte designated as "high" indicates that its concentration is greater than 15 mmol/L.

[b] A designation of "low" indicates a concentration of less than 15 mmol/L.

15 mmol/L. Patients with remote vomiting and a low EABV usually have concentrations of Na^+ and Cl^- in the urine that are less than 15 mmol/L.[11] A different pattern is seen in patients who abuse diuretics. The urine may have abundant Na^+ and Cl^- while the diuretic is acting. When the action of the the diuretic abates, the concentrations of Na^+ and Cl^- in the urine should be less than 15mmol/L.

Patients who have taken diuretics in the recent past may be confused with those who have Bartter's syndrome because they have high concentrations of Na^+ and Cl^- in the urine while the diuretic is acting (Table 1-3). They can be recognized, however, by serial measurements of urine electrolytes because the concentrations of Na^+ and Cl^- in the urine should fluctuate widely in the diuretic abuser, whereas patients with Bartter's syndrome usually have persistent losses of these electrolytes in the urine. Screening the urine for the presence of diuretics is a useful technique. The following case, which is confusing initially, offers important insights into the pathophysiology of these electrolyte abnormalities.

Case Studies

Case 1: The Value of Urine Na^+ and Cl^- in a Patient Suspected of Vomiting or Abusing Diuretics

A 29-year-old woman volunteered to participate in a clinical research project. Hypokalemia and metabolic alkalosis were noted. She was asymptomatic and denied taking medications. She ran 6 to 10 km/d and ate a diet low in salt and high in vegetables. On physical examination, her blood pressure was 90/55 mmHg and heart rate was 62 beats per minute; no significant postural changes were noted in these parameters. The jugular venous column height was 1 cm below the sternal angle, and peripheral edema was not present. Table 1-4 provides a summary of the laboratory data.

Discussion. Taken together, hypokalemia, metabolic alkalosis, and her urine electrolyte pattern suggest, on superficial examination, that recent

Table 1-4. Blood and Urine Chemistries[a]

Parameter	Units	Plasma	Urine
Na^+	mmol/L	144	57
K^+	mmol/L	3.2	50
Cl^-	mmol/L	101	5
HCO_3^-	mmol/L	30	<5
PCO_2	mmHg	45	—
pH		7.44	6
Organic anions	mEq/L	—	103
Creatinine	μmol/L (mg/dl)	52 (0.6)	—
Osmolality	mOsm/kg H_2O	296	600

Abbreviation: PCO_2, partial pressure of carbon dioxide.
[a] For details, see text.

vomiting was the underlying cause of her problem (Table 1-3). She, however, emphatically denied vomiting. Furthermore, her urine contained abundant Na^+ and K^+, but the pH of 6.0 virtually excluded the presence of significant amounts of bicarbonate, thereby making the diagnosis of recent vomiting unlikely. The excretion of Na^+ and K^+ in the urine were obligated by an unusually high rate of excretion of organic anions, presumably related to her unique diet. Thus, superficially, she had the essential features of vomiting that is, Cl^- depletion, a source of bicarbonate. The features resulted from a low-salt, high "alkaline" ash diet, together with excessive loss of NaCl during exercise. The relatively high rates of excretion of Na^+ and K^+ were due to her high rate of excretion of organic anions. This scenario might not be unusual now, as many people are concerned with their body image, exercise more, and eat a diet low in protein and high in vegetables.[12]

USE OF URINE ELECTROLYTES IN PATIENTS WITH METABOLIC ACIDOSIS

Background

Metabolic acidoses are categorized pathogenetically on the basis of the rate of endogenous production of acids. Those disorders characterized by overproduction of acids almost always have an increase in the anion gap of plasma and/or urine (Tables 1-5 and 1-6).[13] In contrast, the acidoses with the usual rate of production of acids are caused by loss of bicarbonate through renal or extrarenal (absorption into the bone or excretion via the stool or gastrointestinal fistula) routes or by retention of the daily acid load resulting from generalized renal failure. When acid production exceeds its renal excretion, retained protons destroy bicarbonate, which in turn is replaced by the anion

---

Table 1-5. Basis for Metabolic Acidosis With an Increased Anion Gap in Plasma

L-Lactic acidosis
    Resulting from hypoxia
    Other causes, mainly low removal of lactate by the liver
Ketoacidosis
    Fasting
    Diabetic
    Alcoholic
D-Lactic acidosis (and other acids of gastrointestinal origin)
    Stasis in gastrointestinal tract ± altered bacteria flora
Intoxicants
    Methanol, ethylene glycol
Renal failure, which yields metabolic acidosis and an elevated anion gap
Cause unclear
    Hyperglycemic, hyperosmolal syndrome

Table 1-6. Pathophysiologic Classification of Metabolic Acidosis

Overproduction of acids
    With accumulation of anions in plasma
        L-Lactic acidosis
        Ketoacidosis
        D-Lactic acidosis
        Intoxicants (methanol, ethylene glycol)
        Others (e.g., hyperglycemic, hyperosmolal syndrome)
    With excretion of anions in the urine
      secretion of anions
            Hippuric acid (toluene abuse)
      Failure to reabsorb anions
            Ketoacidosis + lactic acidosis or ingestion of acetysalicylate
Loss of sodium bicarbonate
    Direct loss
        Gastrointestinal tract (diarrhea, ileus)
        Urine (proximal renal tubular acidosis, acetazolamide)
    Indirect loss
        Consumption of HCl (very rare)
        Low excretion of NH_4^+ (see Table 1-7)

that accompanied these protons (e.g., lactate$^-$, β-hydroxybutyrate$^-$). The value for the anion gap in plasma usually rises ($Na^+ - Cl^- - HCO_3$); in some cases, the urinary excretion of Na^+ plus β-hydroxybutyrate is very high, and the urinary anion gap ($[Na^+ + K^+] - Cl^-$) will also be high.[14]

The chemical effects of mild ketoacidosis provide important insights into the serum and renal effects of acid overproduction. In mild ketoacidosis, equal rates of excretion of NH_4^+ and ketoacid anions allow the level of bicarbonate in plasma and the anion gap to remain constant and normal. If renal synthesis of bicarbonate were to lag behind ketone anion excretion, however, a fall in the concentration of bicarbonate in plasma would result, but the serum ketone levels would not rise due to their clearance by the kidney. Lagging renal synthesis of bicarbonate means that a significant amount of excreted ketone anion must be accompanied in the urine by Na^+ and K^+ and not by NH_4^+. Thus, the urinary anion gap must increase. The ECF volume contracts because Na^+ and K^+ salts of ketoacids are lost with obligate amounts of water. Although body content of Cl^- may not change very much, hyperchloremia occurs because the remaining Cl^- is now distributed in a smaller space. Thus, when the kidney excretes ketoacid anions faster than it resynthesizes bicarbonate (i.e., synthesizes and excretes NH_4^+), a hyperchloremic metabolic acidosis (HCMA) results. Two other clinical examples in which acid overproduction may be associated with a hyperchloremic acidosis follow. When oxidized, methionine, a sulfur-containing amino acid, transiently forms sulfuric acid (H_2SO_4), which converts $NaHCO_3$ to Na_2SO_4. Because the kidney clears the sulfate with water faster than it replenishes lost bicarbonate, HCMA results. Toluene ("glue sniffing") is converted to hippuric acid, which converts Na^+ bicarbonate to

Na^+ hippurate. Because the kidney clears the hippurate with water faster than it replenishes lost bicarbonate, HCMA ensues.[15] In both these settings, the increased urinary anion gap serves an an important clue to the acid overproduction. More commonly, HCMA results when body stores of bicarbonate are replaced by Cl^-. This may follow the direct renal (proximal renal tubular acidosis [RTA]) or gastrointestinal (GI) loss of bicarbonate. This loss of Na^+, bicarbonate, and water causes unchanged body stores of Cl^- to be distributed in a smaller space with resulting hyperchloremia. The associated reduction of EABV also provides renal retention of ingested NaCl, thereby adding to the hyperchloremia. In distal RTA, the pathogenesis of the hyperchloremia is a bit more complex. Normally, acid produced by metabolism (H_2SO_4, $H_2PO_4^-$, organic acids; generally, HX) destroys bicarbonate, converting Na^+ bicarbonate to NaX. Excretion of NH_4X simultaneously rids protons and the anion, X^-, and regenerates bicarbonate, thereby replenishing depleted stores. In distal RTA (see following discussion), failed NH_4^+ excretion causes excretion of Na^+ salts of phosphate, sulfate, and organic anions with appropriate amount of water (Table 1-7). Thus, stores of bicarbonate are depleted, and the loss of "salt water" once again concentrates the ECF volume, leaving unchanged body stores of Cl^-, thereby causing hyperchloremia. Uremic acidosis, in contrast, is also associated with impaired excretion of NH_4^+, but the marked reduction in GFR causes retention of some sulfate, phosphate, and organic anions in body fluids as replacement for bicarbonate, thereby *raising* the anion gap in plasma.

From this pathophysiologic construct, it follows the HCMA can occur if

Table 1-7. Causes for a Low Rate of Excretion of NH_4^+

Low NH_3 in the medullary interstitium
    Low production of NH_4^+
        Usually low GFR (renal failure), hyperkalemia
        Rarely low glutamine or the presence of fatty acid or ketoacid anions in
            very large quantities (TPN)
        Alkaline proximal cell (isolated proximal RTA?)
    Low transfer of NH_4^+ to lumen of proximal tubule
    Low reabsorption of NH_4^+ in the thick ascending limb (hyperkalemia)
    Defect in countercurrent system
        Usually infection, infiltrations, interstitial nephritis, congenital lesions
            (medullary cystic disease), postobstruction
Low net secretion of H^+ into the lumen of the collecting duct
    Pump defect
        Congenital defect, interstitial disease, obstructive disorders
    Failure to stimulate pump
        Lack of aldosterone
        Less lumen-negative transepithelial potential difference
        Alkaline cell (theoretic)
    Back-leak of H^+
        Amphotericin B

Abbreviations: GFR, glomerular filtration rate; RTA, renal tubular acidosis; TPN, total parenteral nutrition.

there is relative or absolute failure of renal ammoniagenesis and excretion of the Na^+ salts of the acid (Table 1-8 and Fig. 1-2). Massive acid loads with poorly metabolized anions would be required to overwhelm normal renal buffer synthesis, or more modest acid loads could yield HCMA when renal ammoniagenesis is limited.

The anion gap in plasma is a convenient, practical measurement for classifying metabolic acidosis although pitfalls in its interpretation exist (see preceding discussion). Nevertheless, an increase in this anion gap in plasma occurs with overproduction or underexcretion of anions (conjugate base of the acid), whereas a normal value for this anion gap occurs with loss of Na^+ bicarbonate, low excretion of NH_4^+, and with high rates of excretion of the conjugate base of the added acid (Tables 1-5 and 1-6).

In ambiguous cases wherein an HCMA might be associated with increased clearance of an overproduced acid anion, the high urinary anion gap will prove decisive. In patients with metabolic acidosis, characterized by a high plasma anion gap, measuring the electrolytes in urine affords little insight into the cause of the disorder. Accordingly, the bulk of the ensuing discussion focuses on normal anion gap metabolic acidoses. In this setting, the critical questions addressed are, Is the rate of excretion of net acid low and if so, why is it low?

The Use of Urine Electrolytes to Detect the Cause of HCMA

Some patients develop HCMA from the loss of alkali through the GI tract or from its sequestration in bone ("hungry bone syndrome"). In these cases, the resulting acidosis stimulates the normal kidney to excrete large amounts of acid, thereby stimulating renal synthesis of replenishing amounts of bicarbonate. Net acid excretion, largely accounted for by urinary NH_4^+, will of course, be increased. Other patients with HCMA are likely to have some form of RTA. Net acid excretion (i.e., NH_4^+ excretion) is relatively or absolutely reduced in all forms of RTA when hypobicarbonatemia is present. Measurement of urinary NH_4^+ levels will distinguish these disorders.

Table 1-8. Causes of Hyperchloremic Metabolic Acidosis

Wide anion gap type of metabolic acidosis presenting as hyperchloremic metabolic acidosis because of hypoalbuminemia, unusual cations (e.g., multiple myeloma), or overestimation of the Cl concentration

HCl or NH_4Cl loading

Sodium bicarbonate loss
    Via the gastrointestinal tract (diarrhea, ileus)
    Via urine (proximal RTA, carbonic anhydrase inhibitor)

Failure of the kidney to generate "new" bicarbonate (low excretion of NH_4^+ as in distal RTA)

Gain of an acid together with the excretion of its conjugate base in the urine along with Na^+ or K^+ (Fig. 1-2)

Abbreviation: RTA, renal tubular acidosis.

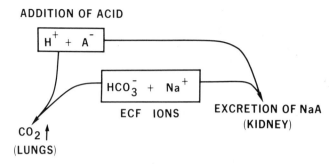

Fig. 1-2. "Indirect" loss of sodium bicarbonate. Na^+ and bicarbonate are present in the body (larger rectangle). There are two components to the loss of Na^+ and bicarbonate: (1) there is production of an acid (H^+) other than carbonic acid (smaller rectangle); and (2) the anion or conjugate base of that acid (A^-) is excreted in the urine with Na^+ or K^+ and not H^+ or $NH_4{}^+$. Thus, there is loss of $NaHCO_3$ from the body. ECF, extracellular fluid.

Certain caveats must be noted regarding the renal response to acidosis before discussing the urinary acid–base parameters. Under normal acid–base conditions, the 30 to 40 mmol of $NH_4{}^+$ excreted represents approximately half of all acid excreted; titratable acid (TA) (largely, $H_2PO_4{}^-$) accounting for the rest. While TA increases only modestly during chronic, severe acidoses, $NH_4{}^+$ excretion can increase to more than 200 mmol/d. Thus, $NH_4{}^+$ is the flexible component of net acid excretion, and while capable of increasing greatly, it takes several days to reach maximal values. It follows then, that to know whether $NH_4{}^+$ excretion is quantitatively appropriate to the acid stimulus, one must know the duration of acidosis.

Assays of Urinary $NH_4{}^+$

Because most clinical laboratories do not routinely measure urinary $NH_4{}^+$, physicians have sought indirect clues of its presence. The urinary pH, anion gap, and osmolal gap are relevant to these issues.

In this setting, the critical questions addressed are, Is the rate of excretion of net acid low and if so, why is it low?

HCMA secondary to the loss of bicarbonate in the urine is recognized by its characteristic bicarbonaturia (urine pH greater than 7.0) during bicarbonate loading, despite a low filtered load of bicarbonate.[16, 17] Patients with HCMA due to the loss of $NaHCO_3$ via the GI tract should have the expected renal response to acidosis, that is, $NH_4{}^+$ excretion levels greater than 200 mmol/day.[18–20] Thus, a measure of the rate of $NH_4{}^+$ excretion should help to identify patients with this disorder as compared to those with distal RTA (a defect characterized by urinary $NH_4{}^+$ levels of less than 50 mmol/d).[21,22]

Key Physiologic Principles

1. A typical Western diet produces acid at the rate of 1 mmol/kg of body weight per day.[23]

2. The titration of H^+ leads to the loss of bicarbonate and the formation of CO_2, which is excreted via the lungs.

3. The kidney has a dual role in acid–base balance. First, it *reclaims* virtually all of the filtered bicarbonate,[24] and second, it *generates* sufficient "new" bicarbonate to replace that lost in buffering endogenous or exogenous acid loads.[25]

4. Regeneration of the bicarbonate deficit requires that net acid be excreted. The rate of excretion of free H^+ is trivial, and the excretion of TA varies to only a modest degree. Renal "new" bicarbonate generation is a function of metabolism of glutamine in the cells of the proximal tubule to yield carboxylate anions and NH_4^+. Further metabolism of the carboxylate anions to neutral end products (CO_2 or glucose) yields bicarbonate that is added to the body.[26] For net gain of bicarbonate to occur, however, NH_4^+ has to be excreted. If not excreted, NH_4^+ will return to the liver, where it is converted to urea, a process that consumes bicarbonate.[27] Therefore, although NH_4^+ excretion by itself does not result in generation of "new" bicarbonate, it provides a quantitative marker for the rate of addition of new bicarbonate to the body by the kidney.

5. A lag period of several days occurs before maximum rates of NH_4^+ excretion are achieved during metabolic acidosis.[26]

6. The excretion of NH_4^+ in the urine requires the following physiologic forces to be in place (for review, see ref. 28):

    a. A high concentration of NH_3 in the medullary interstitium: NH_4^+ that is produced in the proximal tubule is preferentially secreted into the lumen. Reabsorption of NH_4^+ by the thick ascending limb represents the "single effect" for a countercurrent multiplication process that leads to accumulation of NH_3 in the renal medullary interstitium.

    b. Secretion of H^+ in the collecting duct to lower the luminal concentration of NH_3 by converting it to NH_4^+. The diffusion of interstitial NH_3 down its concentration difference from the medullary interstitium into the collecting duct is thereby facilitated.

Normal Values

There are no normal values for the rate of excretion of NH_4^+, just expected ones. In normal persons, the usual rate of excretion of NH_4^+ is 20 to 30 μmol/min (30 to 40 mmol/d). The rate of excretion of NH_4^+ should rise to 100 to 200 μmol/min (150 to 300 mmol/d) during chronic metabolic acidosis if the renal response is normal.[18, 20]

Diagnostic Tests for Patients With Chronic Metabolic Acidosis to Examine the Rate of Excretion of NH_4^+

Unfortunately, a direct assay for the rate of excretion of NH_4^+ is not available on a routine basis in the biochemistry laboratory in most hospitals. An indirect assessment of the rate of NH_4^+ excretion can be achieved using one of the following techniques.

The Urine pH

The urine pH has assumed a central role in the diagnosis of distal RTA (a disease characterized by a low rate of excretion of NH_4^+).[29] An inability to lower urinary pH to less than 5.5 in a patient with chronic metabolic acidosis has been considered the sine qua non for the diagnosis of distal RTA by some investigators.[16, 29–34] The question, however, is, Does the urine pH provide the clinician with unambiguous information about the rate of excretion of NH_4^+? Two interesting but rather conflicting sets of data might help to answer this question.

When an acute acid load is administered, the rate of excretion of NH_4^+ is not immediately raised to a major extent because there is a lag period of days before the full ammoniagenic capacity of the kidney is induced.[26] In this case, the increased secretion of H^+ in the distal nephron is relatively large and is not matched by an equal increase in availability of NH_3 in the collecting duct. Hence, a high concentration of free H^+ or low pH obtains at this stage (equation 2).

$$H^+ \quad + \quad NH_3 \quad \leftrightarrow \quad NH_4^+$$

(high)   (not high)   (modest increase)   (2)

In contrast, during chronic metabolic acidosis, production of NH_4^+ is augmented, and its reabsorption by the loop of Henle plus an active countercurrent system leads to a high concentration of NH_3 in the renal medullary interstitium.[28] The rate of excretion of NH_4^+ will rise manyfold, while the free H^+ concentration in the urine will not be high; indeed, the appropriate urine pH may approximate 6 (Fig. 1-3 and equation 3). Therefore, the urine pH is not a good guide to the amount of NH_4^+ in the urine.[19]

$$H^+ \quad + \quad NH_3 \quad \leftrightarrow \quad NH_4^+$$

(not high)   (very high)   (very high)   (3)

The urine pH is valuable, however, once one has established that a low rate of excretion of NH_4^+ is present (distal RTA). The question then becomes, Is the defect in the excretion of NH_4^+ due to a problem in NH_3 availability or due to a defect in the excretion of H^+ in the distal nephron? A urine pH that is less than 5.3 is in keeping with a major NH_3 defect (Table 1-7), whereas one

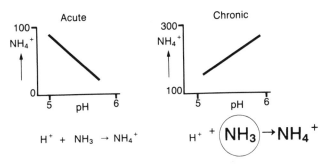

Fig. 1-3. Use of the pH of the urine to detect NH_4^+. In acute acidosis (left side), the rate of excretion of NH_4^+ is higher when the urine pH is lower. The main driving force is an increased rate of secretion of H^+. In chronic asidosis (right side), the main driving force is an increase in NH_3 in the medullary interstitium due to augmented ammoniagenesis. Because ammonia becomes relatively more abundant than H^+, the filtrate becomes more alkaline. Thus, the rate of excretion of NH_4^+ is increased in conjunction with a *higher* pH of the urine. (From Richardson and Halperin,[19] with permission.)

that is close to 6 is in accord with an H^+ defect (Table 1-7). Many patients have mixed disorders, that is, flawed NH_3 synthesis and impaired H^+ secretion.[22]

The Urine Net Charge or Anion Gap

The use of the urine net charge (or anion gap) provides the clinician with a simple and reliable index of the concentration of NH_4^+ in the urine as long as NH_4^+ is being excreted with Cl^-.[35] The urine net charge is calculated using the concentrations of Na^+, K^+, and Cl^- (equations 4 and 5). Because the sum of the milliequivalents of anions and cations in the urine must be equal:

$$Na^+ + K^+ + 2\,Ca^{2+} + 2\,Mg^{2+} + NH_4^+$$
$$= Cl^- + HCO_3^- + H_2PO_4^- + 2\,HPO_4^{2-} + 2\,SO_4^{2-} +$$
organic anions $\qquad\qquad (4)$

On a regular diet, the amount of Ca^{2+} and Mg^{2+} destined for excretion is small, and the excretion of phosphate, sulfate, and organic anion is fairly constant.[36] The difference in rates of excretion of these anions and divalent cations approximates 80 mEq/d. Therefore, in a random urine with pH of less than 6.5, equation 5 will obtain, assuming that dietary intake is relatively normal. This equation also requires that polyuria be absent (i.e., urine volume should not exceed 1.5 L/d).

$$Na^+ + K^+ + NH_4^+ = Cl^- + 80 \qquad\qquad (5)$$

Hence, when a random urine has a "net negative charge" ($Cl^- > Na^+ + K^+$), the excretion of NH_4^+ exceeds 80 mmol/d and therefore, the kidney is not the sole cause for the acidosis. On the other hand, a "net positive charge" in the urine ($Na^+ + K^+ > Cl^-$) in a patient with metabolic acidosis could suggest a major defect in excretion of NH_4^+ and the diagnosis of low NH_4^+ excretion disease (distal RTA).[35] This is not always the case, because NH_4^+ may be excreted with anion other than Cl^-. Additional tests are required in this setting.

The Urinary Osmolal Gap

If NH_4^+ is being excreted with an anion other than Cl^-, the urine net charge would underestimate the rate of excretion of NH_4^+. Under these circumstances, the urinary osmolal gap provides a reliable estimate of the rate of excretion of NH_4^+.[37–39] The osmolal gap is the millimolar difference between the measured urine osmolality and that calculated from the sum of $2(Na^+ + K^+)$ + urea + glucose and reflects the presence of NH_4^+ salts (equation 6). Hence, a value for the urine osmolal gap that exceeds 100 reflects the presence of more than 50 mmol of NH_4^+ per liter of urine.

$$NH_4^+{}_{urine} = 0.5 \text{ (measured}$$
$$\text{osmolality} - [2(Na^+ + K^+) + \text{urea} + \text{glucose}]) \tag{6}$$

Examination of the Urine to Help Identify the Properties of the Anion Excreted

At times, the basis for acid overproduction is not clear from an examination of the plasma anion gap. In this setting, deducing the properties of the conjugate base by examining the renal handling of this anion can provide useful clues. The tool we use is the fractional excretion of anions.[14] The fractional excretion of anions can be estimated as illustrated in equation 7. The concentration of anions in plasma is best estimated from the anion gap (including K^+) and an estimate for the anionic charge on albumin, 4 mEq/L for every 10 g albumin per liter.[40] [a]

$$100 \times [(\text{anion})_{urine}/(\text{anion})_{plasma}]/[(\text{creatinine})_{urine}/$$
$$(\text{creatinine}/_{plasma})] \tag{7}$$

---

[a] Before reviewing the value for the fractional excretion of anions, two notes of caution must be emphasized. First, the value for the anion gap in plasma depends on accurate values for Na^+, K^+, Cl^-, and bicarbonate in plasma. In addition, the contribution of proteins in plasma must be assessed. The net cation equivalence of albumin is 19 mEq/L when the concentration of albumin is 40 g/L.[40] Given the binding of cations such as calcium, a value of 4 mEq/L/10 g of albumin per liter of plasma is a reasonable correction factor. Using this and adjusting for K^+, a reasonable estimate of the concentration of extra anions in plasma can be obtained. The second caution concerns creatinine. Falsely high values may be present when the picric acid method is used if the concentration of acetoacetate is elevated.[41]

The value for the anion concentration in the urine is the difference between the concentration of the major cations, ($Na^+ + K^+ + NH_4^+$) and anions (Cl^-), and are readily measured, whereas that of NH_4^+ can be estimated from the urine osmolal gap (equation 6). If bicarbonate is a major contributor to the urinary anions, it is readily detected because the urinary pH must be greater than or equal to 7.0 when bicarbonaturia is substantial. Because alkali excretion is rare in most cases of severe metabolic acidosis, one would not expect bicarbonate to add much to the urinary anions in this setting. Further, owing to their relatively small quantities in high anion gap metabolic acidosis, phosphaturia, sulfaturia, and the usual organic anions in the urine will not pose a major problem when dealing with the major diagnostic categories (Table 1-6).

We use the fractional excretion of anions as follows. When this value exceeds 100 percent, anion secretion must be occurring in addition to filtration. In this case, we would suspect the overproduction of acids such as hippuric acid, due to glue sniffing (see Case 2). A second major category contains anions that are not filtered or are largely reabsorbed by the kidney. When the anion is not filtered, a macromolecular anion or an anion bound to a macromolecule (e.g., fatty acids bound to albumin) would be suspected. The best example of near-complete reabsorption is L-lactic acid because the fractional excretion of L-lactate is usually less than 10 to 15 percent. The third group of patients consists of those whose fractional excretion of anions is between 20 and 80 percent.[43,44] With this rate of fractional excretion, the usual cause will be ketoacidosis. When values are in the higher range (40 to 80 percent), a mixture of ketoacidosis and lactic acidosis should be suspected[45] (see Case 3).

Case Studies

Case 2: Tools to Detect NH_4^+ and Anions in the Urine

A 23-year-old woman was found lying on a park bench; she was brought to the emergency room. No history was available. The principal findings were confusion, extreme weakness, and contraction of the ECF volume. Laboratory results revealed hypokalemia, metabolic acidosis, and a urinary pH of 6.0 (Table 1-9). The physician in the emergency room relied heavily on the electrolytes and osmolality of the urine to establish a likely basis for this metabolic acidosis with a modest increase in the plasma anion gap. The reasoning was as follows:

1. The most likely cause for the metabolic acidosis was loss of $NaHCO_3$ because the plasma anion gap was not significantly elevated.

2. Given that there was no evidence for loss of $NaHCO_3$ in the urine (urine pH was 6) or the GI tract, and that the urine net charge and pH suggested a low rate of excretion of NH_4^+, a provisional diagnosis of distal RTA was made; hypokalemia is common in this setting.[46] Nevertheless, not all the information was consistent with this diagnosis.

Table 1-9. Metabolic Acidosis: Detection of NH_4^+ in Urine[a]

Parameter	Units	Plasma	Urine
Na^+	mmol/L	139	15
K^+	mmol/L	1.9	17
Cl^-	mmol/L	108	7
HCO_3^-	mmol/L	15	0
Albumin	g/L	40	0
Urea	mmol/L	0.5	5
Creatinine	μmol/L	100	200
pH		7.33	6.0
Glucose	mmol/L	5	0
Osmolality	mOsm/kg H_2O	284	180
Fractional excretion of anions	%		205

[a] For details, see text.

3. The urinary osmolal gap, however, suggested a high rate of excretion of NH_4^+, and the anion excreted with NH_4^+ was not Cl^-. Hence, the diagnosis of distal RTA was discarded as the sole cause of metabolic acidosis. This underscores the fact that the urine anion gap only reflects the excretion of NH_4^+ plus Cl^{-35} and that the pH of the urine is an unreliable way to detect the rate of excretion of NH_4^+.[19]

Conclusion to this point: The basis for the metabolic acidosis was overproduction of an acid with excretion rather than retention of the conjugate base of that acid.

4. The properties of the anion can be deduced from its renal handling (equation 8). The fractional excretion of the anion was 205 percent. Hence, one property of the anion is that it was secreted by the renal tubules.[42]

$$\frac{100 \times ([\text{plasma anion gap (including } K^+) - 16]/[Na^+ + K^+ - Cl]^-]_{\text{urine}})}{[(\text{creatinine})_{\text{urine}}/(\text{creatinine})_{\text{plasma}}]} \quad (8)$$

5. Another clue to the property of the anion is that it probably contained nitrogen. This speculation drew support from the very low rate of appearance of urea (expected rate is 10 to 26 mmol/h, whereas the rate of appearance was less than 5 mmol/h). The physician deduced that the anion excreted was probably hippurate (containing nitrogen from glycine), derived from the metabolism of toluene.[15] A high plasma osmolal gap is not observed with this form of intoxication because toluene is not very soluble in water.

6. The excretion of hippurate at a rate exceeding the rate of excretion of NH_4^+ (normally high, but limited in quantity) leads to metabolic acidosis with a normal plasma anion gap (Fig. 1-2) and contraction of the ECF volume.

7. The hypokalemia was associated with a high transtubular K concentration gradient (TTKG).[47–49] This probably reflects the high level of aldosterone (contraction of the ECF volume) and the increased delivery of Na^+ with hippurate and not Cl^- to the distal nephron.[50]

Case 3: Metabolic Acidosis With an Increased Anion Gap in Plasma

A 66-year-old obese woman presented with non–insulin-dependent diabetes mellitus (NIDDM) of 10 years' duration. Her NIDDM was treated with diet and oral hypoglycemic agents (sulfonylurea and metformin). Gangrene had developed around ulcerated areas on several toes during the past 2 weeks. Because of ascending lymphangitis, antibiotics had been given 10 days previously. Anorexia and nausea progressed, and she had vomited on several occasions over the preceding 2 days. Her current physical examination revealed that she was afebrile, respirations were rapid and deep, and her skin was dusky, cool, and clammy. Although she exhibited signs of a contracted ECF volume, she was not in shock. Of note, bowel sounds were present.

Laboratory results (Table 1-10) revealed metabolic acidosis with an increase in the plasma anion gap, negative plasma ketones, and marked hyperglycemia, with a surprisingly low value for plasma urea. The plasma osmolal gap was elevated despite negative tests for ethanol, methanol, and ethylene glycol.

Because her plasma K^+ concentration was very low despite her deficiency of insulin, a debate ensued as to whether insulin should be given to stop the production of acids. The issues follow:

Renal Failure and Intoxicants. Both renal failure and intoxicants were ruled out by screening tests.

Diabetic Ketoacidosis. If ketoacidosis is present, insulin must be given. Ketoacidosis, however, is unlikely in NIDDM, nevertheless, with infection, diabetic ketoacidosis (DKA) was a distinct possibility. Although the nitroprusside screening test for ketones (i.e., acetoacetate) was negative, ketoacidosis (as B-hydroxybutyric acid) could still be present in the face of lactic acidosis (high $NADH/NAD^+$). Hyperglycemia is in keeping with NIDDM, but it does not indicate whether ketoacidosis was present or not. The source of the glucose did not seem to be diet (history) or liver glycogen (anorexia).

Table 1-10. Metabolic Acidosis: Increased Plasma Anion Gap[a]

Parameter	Units	Plasma	Urine
Na^+	mmol/L	138	36
K^+	mmol/L	4.0	30
Cl^-	mmol/L	106	7
HCO_3^-	mmol/L	10	0
Albumin	g/L	40	0
Urea	mmol/L	11	94
Creatinine	μmol/L	126	2,550
pH		7.28	6.0
Glucose	mmol/L	40	222
Osmolality	mOsm/kg H_2O	362	533
Fractional excretion of anions	%		50

[a] For details, see text.

Thus, there was a large production of glucose. The source of this glucose was not protein because glucose was produced without urea.[51]

L-Lactic Acidosis. This diagnosis is possible because there may be poor delivery of O_2 to tissues on a regional basis owing to the vasculopathy. Another potential contributor to overproduction of lactic acid is stimulation of glycogenolysis is muscle by catecholamines. Glycolysis in muscle also provides the carbon precursor of glucose without nitrogen[b]. A factor that might compromise removal of lactate by the liver is metformin.

D-Lactic Acidosis. Insulin could be advantageous to treat this condition because by limiting the rate of oxidation of fatty acids, more organic acids could be oxidized (Fig.1-4). Factors favoring D-lactic acidosis are the prior use of antibiotics that would change the bacterial flora of the GI tract. The altered flora could lead to the production of unknown osmoles (increased osmolal gap in plasma) and could be a source of glucose without nitrogen[b] (from the metabolism of cellulose in the GI tract). Against this diagnosis is the absence of stasis in the GI tract.

Use of the Fractional Excretion of Anions. Because the fractional excretion of anions was 55 percent in this case (Table 1-10), the provisional diagnosis was ketoacidosis plus L- or D-lactic acidosis. Hence, initial treatment consisted of saline, K^+, water, and insulin. Subsequent lab reports revealed that the L-lactate and β-hydroxybutyrate levels were each 6 mmol/L.

THE CONCENTRATION OF K^+ IN THE URINE IN THE ASSESSMENT OF DISORDERS OF K^+ HOMEOSTASIS

Background

The kidney plays an important role in long-term K^+ homeostasis. For example, in normal individuals rendered hypokalemic by K^+ deprivation, the rate of excretion of K^+ diminished to 10 to 15 mmol/d.[52] In contrast, the rate of excretion should increase in response to an increased intake of K^+; in fact, values as high as 400 mmol/d have been noted.[50,53]

---

[b] *Production of glucose with nitrogen:* Protein is 16 percent nitrogen by weight. Because 100 g of protein yields 60 g (333 mmol) of glucose[51] and 16 g of nitrogen will yield 576 mmol of urea (mol wt nitrogen in urea is 28), the expected ratio of urea to glucose is close to 2:1 during gluconeogenesis. In this case, the rate of excretion of urea was less than that of glucose, and the concentration of urea in plasma was not particularly elevated (Table 1-10). Hence, in the absence of dietary intake, either glycogen in muscle or cellulose in the GI tract are likely sources for the overproduction of glucose.

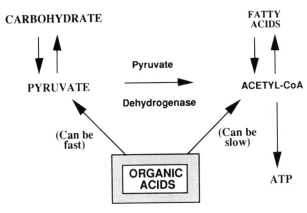

Fig. 1-4. Use of insulin to treat acidosis that is due to accumulation of organic acids. By decreasing the availability of fatty acids as a precursor to synthesize ATP (antilipolytic action of insulin), more organic acids could be oxidized. (From Halperin and Rolleston,[51] with permission.)

Key Physiologic Principles

1. Two control mechanisms, extrarenal and renal, maintain balance for K^+ and its distribution between ECF and ICF.[54]

2. Extrarenal mechanisms include the effective, albeit transient, movement of K^+ in and out of ICF. This is achieved predominantly by the hormones insulin and catecholamines (β_2- stimulation) and perhaps by adrenal mineralocorticoids.[54,55]

3. Long-term homeostasis of K^+ is maintained by regulating renal K^+ excretion. Most of the K^+ that is filtered is reabsorbed by the proximal tubule and the thick ascending limb of the loop of Henle. Most of the K^+ that appears in the urine depends on the function of the principal cells of the cortical distal nephron. Hence, assessment of the renal response to disorders of K^+ homeostasis requires an understanding of the events in this latter segment of the nephron.

4. Two major factors are known to modulate the activity of the K^+ secretory process in the cortical distal nephron: aldosterone[59] and nonabsorbable anions.[50,60–62] Recent evidence from studies in animals and humans suggests that nonabsorbable anions such as sulfate stimulate the secretion of K^+ only when the concentration of Cl^- in the lumen is less than 15 mmol/L. Bicarbonate anions, however, seem to have a unique effect to stimulate the secretion of K^+, even at high concentrations of Cl^- in the lumen.[50]

Assessment of the Renal Response to Disorders of K^+ Homeostasis

The rate of excretion of K^+, although it provides a measure of the overall renal response to disordered K^+ balance, does not differentiate an enhanced excretion of K^+ that is due to an increase in the urine volume from one that is due to an increased concentration of K^+ in the urine.

The concentration of K^+ in the urine is the K^+/H_2O ratio. Therefore, it would be affected to a major degree by the amount of water reabsorbed in the medullary collecting duct and hence does not provide unambiguous information about the activity of the K^+ secretory process in the cortical distal nephron (Table 1-11).

To gain insights into events in the cortical distal nephron, one must obtain an approximation of the concentration of K^+ in that segment of the nephron. Needless to say, this must be done noninvasively, and one must use information that is readily available at the bedside. An approximation of the concentration of K^+ in the terminal collecting duct can be obtained by correcting

Table 1-11. Tests to Examine K^+ Excretion in Patients With Hypokalemia or Hyperkalemia

Test	Advantages	Disadvantages	Expected Values
24-hour K^+ excretion rate or K^+ excretion per unit creatinine	Indicates overall excretion in patients with hypokalemia or hyperkalemia	Does not indicate the mechanism responsible for the defect Takes 24 h or measurement of creatinine in urine Collections are not always accurate	Normal: 60–80 mmol/d or 6–8 mmol/0.1 g creatinine Hypokalemia: <10 mmol/d or 1–1.5 mmol/0.1 g creatinine Hyperkalemia: >150 mmol/d or 10–15 mmol/0.1 g creatinine
Fractional excretion of K^+		Results must be compared with GFR, so it is impractical.	Cannot express a value without knowing the GFR
Random urine [K^+]	Convenience	Influenced by two independent factors: Secretion and water reabsorption in the medulla	Hypokalemia: <20 mmol/d if not due to a renal cause and >20 mmol/d if due to a renal cause Hyperkalemia: No expected values reported

Abbreviation: GFR, glomerular filtration rate.

the concentration of K^+ in the urine for the amount of H_2O reabsorbed in the medullary collecting duct (equation 9 and Fig. 1-5).

$$[(K^+)_{urine}/(Osm)_{urine}/(Osm)_{plasma}] \qquad (9)$$

This concentration of K^+ in the terminal collecting duct can be then related to the concentration of K^+ in the plasma to obtain a semiquantitative as-

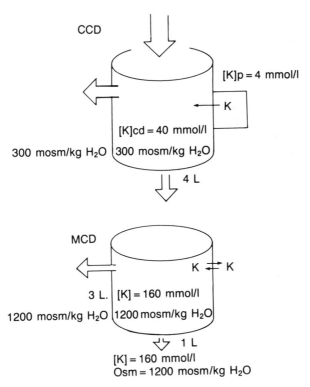

Fig. 1-5. Assessment of the K^+ secretory process. The top barrel represents the cortical collecting duct (CCD) and the bottom one the medullary collecting duct (MCD). Water movement is shown by the thick white arrows and K^+ movement by the thin black one. The concentration of K^+ in the plasma, $[K^+]_p$, is 4 mmol/L in these examples. In the presence of antidiuretic hormone and of a given stimulus for K^+ secretion, the osmolality and the $[K^+]$ at the end of the CCD are 300 mOsm/kg H_2O and 40 mmol/L ($[K^+]cd$), respectively. If 75 percent of the water is reabsorbed in the MCD, the osmolality rises to 1,200 mOsm/kg H_2O, and the urine $[K^+]$ increases by 120 mmol/L, even though there is no net secretion of K^+ in the MCD.

$$TTKG_{CCD} = 40 \text{ mmol/L}/4 \text{ mmol/L} = 10$$

$$TTKG_{MCD} = \frac{160 \text{ mmol/L}}{\dfrac{1200}{300}\text{mOsm/kg } H_2O}$$

sessment of the activity of the K^+ secretory process called the TTKG. The TTKG has been proposed as a simple, noninvasive, semiquantitative reflection of the activity of the K^+ secretory process in the cortical distal nephron that is based on the preceding premises.[47,48,63] The TTKG is calculated as follows, in equation 10:

$$TTKG = ([K^+]_{urine}/(U/P)_{osm})/[K^+]_{plasma}$$

The fractional excretion of K^+ (FE_K) (urine K^+ corrected for ratios of creatinine in urine to plasma instead of using the osmolality ratio), has been proposed as a useful diagnostic tool in hyperkalemia to assess the tubular secretion of K^+.[64] When one examines the formulae for both calculations, the FE_K adjusts for reabsorption of water throughout the nephron, while the TTKG adjusts the concentration of K^+ in the urine for the amount of water reabsorption that is downstream to the terminal cortical collecting duct. Hence, the calculation of the TTKG provides a closer approximation of the concentration of K^+ in the terminal cortical collecting duct (CCD) and more closely represents the pathophysiologic events in this cortical nephron segment. Moreover, using the FE_K the values obtained have to be evaluated with a nomogram related to the GFR, a step that limits its practical value.

Pitfalls With the TTKG

Some pitfalls and limitations to the use of the TTKG should be recognized. First, the urine must be at least isoosmolal (thus, one can assume that the osmolality of the luminal fluid in the terminal CCD is the same as that of plasma). Second, at very high flow rates, the TTKG, if examined in isolation, could create the false impression that secretion of K^+ is defective because there is not enough time for equilibration in the cortical distal nephron. This latter pitfall can be avoided by examining the TTKG in conjugation with an estimate of the rate of excretion of K^+. One must be clear that the TTKG reflects the K^+ secretory process in the terminal CCD and it does not simply reflect the actions of aldosterone.

Clinical Use of the TTKG

The TTKG is used to reflect the role of the cortical distal nephron in the pathogenesis of the disorders of K^+ homeostasis. The expected values for the TTKG, under different stimuli, are as follows: During hypokalemia, the expected value is less than 2; a higher value suggests that the K^+ secretory process is inappropriately stimulated. After KCl loading in normal individuals, the TTKG was 13.1 ± 3.8 when the $[K^+]$ in plasma was 4.3 ± 0.2 mmol/L; therefore, the expected values during hyperkalemia should be greater than 10.[63]

A lower than expected TTKG in a patient with hyperkalemia indicates an inappropriately low rate of secretion of K^+ in the cortical distal nephron (Table 1-12). The clinician can quickly determine if the defect is consistent with hypoaldosteronism rather than a tubular defect by reevaluating the TTKG 3 hours after the administration of 50 μg of the mineralocorticoid, 9α-fludrocortisone. A rise in the TTKG to greater than 7 suggests that the primary cause for hyperkalemia was hypoaldosteronism.[65] This presumptive diagnosis can be confirmed by measuring the levels of aldosterone and renin in the plasma. In contrast, if there is no rise in the TTKG after administration of 9α-fludrocortisone, a tubular defect may be present. One such defect is type II pseudohypoaldosteronism. Schambelan et al.[66] suggested that its basis was a "Cl shunt disorder" in which the cortical distal nephron is believed to be excessively permeable to Cl^-.[50,66,67] These patients reabsorb most of the Na^+ with Cl^- in these segments, that is, electroneutral rather than electrogenic, thus failing to generate the negative transepithelial potential difference required to promote the secretion of K^+ (Fig. 1-6). In these patients one would expect to find a high TTKG if Cl^- is absent from the lumen (prior ECF volume contraction and then delivering Na^+ to the distal

Table 1-12. Causes of Hyperkalemia: Importance of the Rate of Excretion of K^+

Hyperkalemia with a high rate of excretion of K in the urine
　Intake of a high content of K (not the sole cause of hyperkalemia)
　Shift of K from cells
　　Metabolic acidosis with a normal value for the anion gap
　　Low activity of hormones (insulin, β_2-adrenergics and possibly
　　　aldosterone)
　　Cell necrosis (trauma, burns, rhabdomyolysis)
　　Depolarization (exercise, succinylcholine)
　　Drugs (digitalis overdose, β_2-adrenergic blockade)
　　Periodic paralysis (hyperkalemic type)
Hyperkalemia with a low rate of excretion of K in the urine
　Low volume of filtrate delivered to CCD (conditions with a very low GFR)
　Low biologic activity of aldosterone
　　Low levels of aldosterone
　　　Low concentration of renin (disorders of juxtaglomerular apparatus)
　　　　Diseases such as diabetes mellitus or tubulointerstitial diseases
　　　　Drugs (e.g., nonsteroidal antiinflammatory agents, β-adrenergic
　　　　　blockers)
　　　High concentration of renin
　　　　Adrenal gland destruction
　　　　Drugs (angiotensin-converting enzyme inhibitors)
　　Levels of aldosterone are not low
　　　Drugs (aldosterone antagonists, amiloride)
　　　Aldosterone resistance
　　　　Low volume of filtrate or low delivery of Na to the CCD
　　　　Electroneutral versus electrogenic reabsorption of Na^+
　　　　　Chloride shunt disorders
　　　　Decreased flux through the K channel?

Abbreviations: CCD, cortical collecting duct; GFR, glomerular filtration rate.

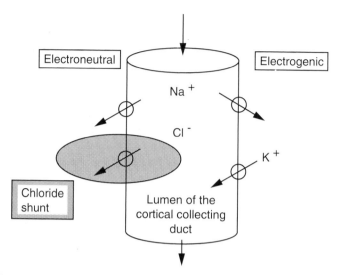

Fig. 1-6. Electrogenic versus electroneutral reabsorption of Na^+. The site of net secretion of K^+ is the principal cell of the cortical distal nephron. Reabsorption of Na^+ occurs via a specific channel down a favorable electrochemical gradient. If this rate is matched by reabsorption of Cl^-, the reabsorpton is electroneutral and does not stimulate secretion of K^+. If reabsorption of Na^+ exceeds that of Cl^-, the reabsorption is electrogenic and stimulates the secretion of K^+.

nephron with another anion, e.g., sulfate) or if the absorption of Cl^- is inhibited (presumably caused by bicarbonaturia). A rise in the TTKG with such maneuvers offers a presumptive evidence for a "Cl shunt" in this nephron segment.[50]

The TTKG is also useful for assessing the potential benefits of treatment. In patients with hypokalemia, for example, a high TTKG indicates an inappropriately active secretion of K^+ that could be blocked by K^+-sparing diuretics (amiloride, spironolactone, or triamterene). In contrast, in a patient with hyperkalemia who has a high TTKG (high K secretory activity), the leverage in therapy will be to increase the flow rate in the late distal nephron (volume repletion diuretics).

Case Studies

Case 4: Hyperkalemia in a Patient Taking Cyclosporine

A 40-year-old man received a renal transplant 6 months before presentation. He was maintained on triple antirejection therapy of prednisone, azathioprine, and cyclosporine. The concentration of plasma creatinine was stable at 110 μmol/L, but hyperkalemia (5.5 mmol/L) was noted on many occasions. He had no history of diabetes mellitus, and he was receiving a calcium channel blocker for hypertension. The results of laboratory investigations are shown in Table 1-13.

Discussion. Our first step in the investigation of hyperkalemia was to rule out pseudohyperkalemia, an elevation of the plasma K^+ concentration occurring after blood is drawn. It is the result of lysis of cells in vitro or local hyperkalemia that is caused by fist-clenching during phlebotomy[68] (Table 1-11). These problems were not present in this patient.

Our next step was to assess the renal response to hyperkalemia. The expected value for the rate of excretion of K^+ with normal kidneys is several hundred millimoles per day. Two major components could be responsible for a low rate of excretion: a low concentration of K^+ in the urine and a low volume of urine. The former factor is evaluated by examining TTKG. In chronic renal failure, hyperkalemia usually does not occur until the creatinine clearance has fallen to less than 10 to 20 ml/min, but this was not the problem in this case (Table 1-13). Because the rate of excretion of K^+ was low and the TTKG was 4, this indicates an inappropriately low rate of secretion of K^+ in the cortical distal nephron.

The next question to answer was, Will the TTKG increase if a physiologic quantity of aldosterone is present? Because a significant time interval would elapse before the results of blood tests returned (aldosterone and renin), a provocative test was performed (a physiologic dose of mineralocorticoids [50 to 200 μg] of 9α-fludrocortisone was administered). Because the TTKG did not rise, a tubular insensitivity to aldosterone was the basis for hyperkalemia. This was confirmed by finding a low level of renin, but a value for aldosterone in the plasma that was in the usual normal range (400 pmol/L).

Tubular insensitivity to aldosterone could be the result of structural damage to the tubules or possibly to an intrinsic defect in the activity of the K^+

Table 1-13. Laboratory Values in Case 4, A Patient With Hyperkalemia[a]

Laboratory Value	Units	Plasma	Urine	TTKG
Na^+	mmol/L	140	60	
K^+	mmol/L	5.5	44	
Cl^-	mmol/L	109	71	
HCO_3^-	mmol/L	21	—	
pH		7.34	5.0	
Creatinine	μmol/L	110	—	
Osmolality	mOsm/kg H_2O	288	585	
TTKG				
before 9α-fludrocortisone				4
after 9α-fludrocortisone				5
after acetazolamide				14

Abbreviation: TTKG, transtubular K concentration gradient.
[a] The level of aldosterone in plasma was high and that of renin was low. For details, see text.

secretory process. The latter may be due to a defect in the Na^+ channel or in the K^+ channel or may be due to a decreased ability to generate a lumen-negative electrochemical gradient in the cortical distal nephron. In the latter lesion, there is electroneutral rather than electrogenic reabsorption of NaCl in the CCD (Fig. 1-5). The net result is expansion of the ECF volume, hypertension, and hyporeninemia. The hyperkalemia leads to low excretion of NH_4^+ (observe the positive value for the urine net charge) and metabolic acidosis with a normal anion gap—all features present in this patient (Table 1-13). To confirm this impression, one would expect to find a high TTKG if Cl^- is absent from the lumen or if its reabsorption is inhibited (possibly caused by bicarbonaturia). When acetazolamide was administered to induce bicarbonaturia, the TTKG rose to 14. This large rise in the TTKG suggests an intact Na^+ channel and also an intact K^+ channel. Taken together with the findings described previously, the hyperkalemia seems to be due to a lesion in the subgroup called type II pseudohypoaldosteronism.[22,66]

Case 5: Hypokalemia in a Patient Without Hypertension

The patient was a 17-year-old ballet dancer. A routine evaluation revealed her to be hypokalemic (2.6 mmol/L). She denied vomiting or the use of diuretics and laxatives. Her blood pressure was 100/60 mmHg, and her heart rate was 80 per minute while recumbent; blood pressure fell to 85/55 mmHg, and the heart rate rose to 110 beats per minute in the upright posture. Her jugular venous pressure was at the sternal angle, and she did not have edema. The results of laboratory investigations are shown in Table 1-14.

Discussion. The first issue to resolve was whether the kidney played a major role in the cause of hypokalemia (Table 1-15 and Fig. 1-7). The expected renal response during hypokalemia is a low rate of excretion of K^+ (less than 15 mmol/d) and a TTKG less than 2. The rate of excretion of K^+

Table 1-14. Laboratory Values in Case 5, a Patient With Hypokalemia[a]

Laboratory Value		Plasma	Urine	TTKG
Na^+	mmol/L	133	47	
K^+	mmol/L	2.6	52	
Cl^-	mmol/L	87	7	
HCO_3^-	mmol/L	33	—	
pH		7.47	7.0	
Creatinine	μmol/L	110	—	
Osmolality	mOsm/kg H_2O	278	555	
TTKG				10

Abbreviation: TTKG, transtubular K concentration gradient.
[a] For details, see text.

Table 1-15. Causes of Hypokalemia: Importance of the Rate of Excretion of K[a]

Hypokalemia with a low rate of excretion of K in the urine
    Diet with an extremely low K content
    Shift of K into cells
        Hormone action
            Insulin (administration of glucose), or β-adrenergics
            Anabolism (e.g., recovery from diabetic ketoacidosis, use of TPN)
            Drugs (e.g., α-adrenergic antagonists, β-adrenergic agonists)
            Periodic paralysis of the hypokalemic type
    Loss of K via gastrointestinal tract
    Former loss of K in urine
        Remote diuretics, laxatives, or vomiting
Hypokalemia with a high rate of excretion of K in the urine
    Increased volume of filtrate delivered to CCD, e.g., diuretics (osmotic,
      pharmacologic)
    Increased mineralocorticoid action (loss of K is greater if bicarbonaturia is
      present)
        With a low ECF volume
            Vomiting, diuretics, laxative abuse, Bartter's syndrome,
                hypomagnesemia
        With hypertension
            Low level of renin
                Exogenous mineralocorticoids
                Drugs with exogenous mineralocorticoid action such as cortisol,
                    progesterone
                Drugs potentiating the action of mineralocorticoids such as
                    licorice
            Endogenous mineralocorticoids
                Primary lesion of adrenal gland (tumor, hyperplasia) releasing
                    aldosterone
                Release of compounds with mineralocorticoid action (e.g., inborn
                    errors)
        With high levels of renin
            Renal artery stenosis, malignant hypertension, tumor or
                hyperplasia of the juxtaglomerular apparatus,
                hypomagnesemia
            Normal levels of renin
             Cushing's syndrome
      Others
        Distal RTA, proximal RTA treated with large quantities of
          bicarbonate
        Amphotericin B

Abbreviations: CCD, cortical collecting duct; ECF, extracellular fluid; RTA, renal tubular acidosis; TPN, total parenteral nutrition.
  [a] This table is designed to complement the approach outlined in Figure 1-7.

exceeded 15 mmol/d, and the TTKG was 10. A stimulated K^+-secretory process was indeed playing a major role in the pathogenesis of hypokalemia.

Having established that there was an increased rate of secretion of K^+ in the cortical distal nephron, one should evaluate factors responsible for this secretion (Table 1-15). The major factor that stimulates this K^+ secretory

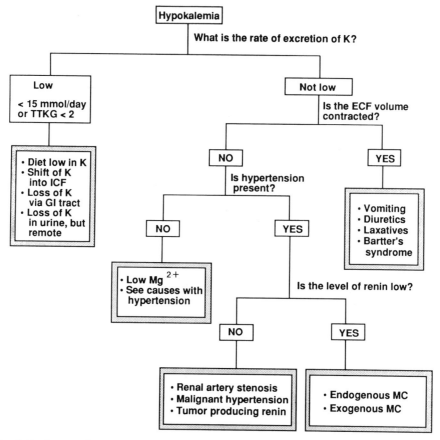

Fig. 1-7. Approach to hypokalemia. The flow chart should be used in conjunction with Table 1-15. The hatched boxes contain the final diagnosis. (For details, see text.) (From Halperin,[84] with permission.)

process is aldosterone. Therefore, the next question focuses on whether there is a physiologic stimulus for the secretion of aldosterone in the absence of hyperkalemia: Is the ECF volume contracted? Clinical signs in this patient pointed to a contracted ECF volume (postural hypotension and tachycardia with low jugular venous pressure). Examination of the concentration of Na^+ and Cl^- in the urine would confirm the clinical impression of a low ECF volume and might also provide important clues to the cause of hypokalemia (Table 1-3). In this case, because the concentration of Cl^- in the urine was very low (and metabolic alkalosis was present), the most common causes of hypokalemia would be vomiting or the intake of diuretics that occurred in the remote past. Because the concentration of Na^+ in the urine was high and the urine had an alkaline pH (7.0), the most likely diagnosis was occult, but recent, vomiting.

OSMOLALITY OF THE URINE

Background

It is often important to measure the urinary osmolality to determine the cause of a number of disease states (Table 1-16). Because urinary osmolality is defined as the number of particles excreted per volume of urine, one needs information on at least two of the three parameters listed in equation 11 to assess this value properly. A similar logic is more familiar when considering acid–base diagnoses. Hence, we discuss the particles in and the volume of the urine independently in the following sections.

$$osmolality = numbers\ of\ particles/volume\ of\ urine \qquad (11)$$

Two points need to be stressed concerning the number of particles excreted and their physiologic properties. First, whereas all particles contribute equally to the osmolality of urine, not all particles are equal "from the point of view of body fluid compartments."[69] Hence, the nature of the particles that are excreted should be considered (vide infra). Second, the number of particles excreted depends on dietary intake and the physiologic response of the kidney. The two major groups of particles in the urine are urea and electrolytes. Urea normally makes up 50 to 60 percent of the particles excreted (Table 1-16). The quantity of urea excreted reflects the amount of protein ingested and the presence or absence of a catabolic state (fever, infection, stress, drugs, GI blood loss, etc.). In general, the fractional excretion of urea should be close to 50 percent unless urine flow rates are very low (less than

---

Table 1-16. Importance of the Urine Osmolality in Clinical States

Test of physiologic function
    Maximum osmolality of urine (1,200 mOsm/kg H_2O)
        Assess renal medullary interstitial function
        Assess action of ADH
    Minimum osmolality of urine (40–50 mOsm/kg H_2O)
        Assess diluting sites of nephron
        Assess if ADH release normally suppresses

Use in differential diagnosis of
    Polyuria
        Osmotic diuresis (usually 400–700 mOsm/kg H_2O)
        Central DI (usually <200 mOsm/kg H_2O
        Nephrogenic DI
            Isoosmolal variety (involve medulla only)
            Hypoosmolal variety (involve cortex ± medulla)
    Hypernatremia

Use in the disorders of
    Potassium homeostasis (to calculate the TTKG)
    Acute renal failure: differential diagnosis

Abbreviations: ADH, antidiuretic hormone; DI, diabetes insipidus; TTKG, transtubular K concentration gradient.

0.5 mL/min) or high (greater than 4 mL/min).[70,71] The excretion of the major electrolytes, Na^+ and K^+, will depend on intake and the capability of the kidney to excrete these cations (see preceding discussion.)

Particles That Do or Do Not Count for Urine Osmolality

When examining the osmolality of the urine in the context of water movement between the lumen of the collecting duct and the medullary interstitium, two factors are paramount. First, the medullary interstitium must contain a higher concentration of particles that are not well reabsorbed from the lumen of the collecting duct. This concentration gradient will favor the reabsorption of water. Second, a high permeability of the luminal membrane of the collecting duct to water permits water to flow into the interstitium. The presence or absence of ADH controls this permeability.

An example of a particle that does not count with respect to reabsorption of water is ethanol because it is largely reabsorbed in parallel with water.[72] This latter point will be illustrated in Case 7; it is only of potential importance in the differential diagnosis of diabetes insipidus.

Particles That Do or Do Not Count With Respect to the ICF–ECF Interface

Water moves across the ICF–ECF interface as dictated by the "effective osmolality" or tonicity of body fluids. These terms refer to the number of particles that are restricted to the ICF or to the ECF. Because particles such as urea and ethanol cross cell membranes at a sufficiently rapid rate, they achieve an equal concentration in the ICF and ECF and can be ignored with respect to factors that influence cell volume. In contrast, the major particles restricted to the ECF are Na^+ and its attendant anions, Cl^- and HCO_3^-, whereas the major intracellular particle is K^+, which is "attracted" by macromolecular anions (intracellular phosphate esters). Hence, one should examine the concentration of Na^+ and K^+ in the urine and plasma rather than the osmolality of these fluids to gain insights into whether the excretion of urine would decrease or increase the ICF and/or ECF volumes.[69] An excellent example of this in nature is the ability of the alligator to excrete Na^+- and K^+-free-water but to do so without the ability to excrete hypoosmolal urine. This task is achieved by excreting NH_4^+ and HCO_3^- in place of Na^+ and Cl^- in the urine. The NH_4^+ and HCO_3^- are derived from macromolecules (proteins) and are excreted in place of urea in times of water excess.[73,74]

Key Physiologic Concepts Regarding Water Excretion

To conserve electrolyte-free water, two major physiologic forces must be in place. First, the osmolality of the renal medulla must be very high. This is a combined function of the active reabsorption of Na^+ and Cl^- in the thick ascending limb of the loop of Henle (the so-called "single effect"), an effective countercurrent mechanism and the specific restrictive permeabilities of the membranes of individual nephron segments in the renal medulla to water, Na^+, and urea.[75,76] The second factor required is the presence of ADH, which opens water channels in the luminal membrane of the late distal convoluted tubule and the collecting duct.[77]

The quantitative importance of the cortex and the medulla of the kidney for conservation of water are illustrated in the following example. Data show that the vast majority of electrolyte-free water is reabsorbed in the cortex under the influence of ADH. Consider a subject excreting 0.5 L of urine with an osmolality of 1,200 mOsm/kg H_2O. The osmolality is 100 at the end of the loop of Henle, 300 at the end of the CCD, and 1,200 mOsm/kg H_2O in the urine (Fig.1-1). Approximately 24 L of fluid exits the loop of Henle in a day. Because the osmolality rises from 100 mOsm/kg H_2O to 300 mOsm/kg H_2O by the end of the CCD under the influence of ADH, two-thirds of this volume of water (16 L) is reabsorbed in the cortex. In addition, perhaps two-thirds of the load of osmoles will be also reabsorbed, leaving 2.7 L of isoosmotic urine to enter the medullary collecting duct. Because the osmolality rises fourfold under the influence of ADH (300 to 1,200 mOsm/kg H_2O), the volume of filtrate declines to one quarter or approximately 0.7 L (reabsorption of only 2 L of water). Again, some solute (and water) is also reabsorbed, resulting in a volume of 0.5L/d.

This physiology has two major implications: First, if the cortex is intact and if ADH is present, the osmolality of the urine should equal that of plasma. Because up to 900 mOsm/d are excreted (Table 1-16), the maximum volume of urine is 3 L/day. In contrast to the preceding, a patient who excretes a urine with an osmolality less than plasma despite plasma hypertonicity must have involvement of the cortical portion of the distal nephron. If, under these conditions, dilute urine continues to be excreted despite the administration of ADH, nephrogenic diabetes insipidus (DI) must be present. However, if the osmolality of the urine rises to or above 300 mOsm/kg H_2O, the disorder is at least partly related to impaired synthesis or release of ADH.

In a patient with hyponatremia, the maximum osmolality of the urine when ADH acts will not be as high as in normal persons. Consider the numbers provided previously for fluid exiting the loop of Henle (24 L and 100 mOsm/kg H_2O). If the osmolality of the plasma is 200 instead of 300 mOsm/kg H_2O, 12 L instead of 16 L of free water will be reabsorbed at osmotic equilibrium in the CCD. Hence, 4 more liters of water will enter the medullary collecting duct per day. Under the influence of ADH, as more of this water is reabsorbed, it will traverse the inner medullary interstitium and "wash out" solute (anything that increases flow in the inner medulla decreases the maximum osmolality in this region). Hence, the maximum osmolality of the urine declines with greater degrees of hyponatremia. This probably helps explain why patients with syndrome of inappropriate secretion of ADH (SIADH) achieve water balance at a given degree of hyponatremia and water intake. Restriction of water intake permits their concentration of Na^+ in plasma (and the osmolality of their urine) to rise.

To excrete free water, Na^+ and Cl^- must be reabsorbed from the filtrate in nephron segments where there is a restricted permeability to water. Although the thick ascending limb of the loop of Henle and the early distal convoluted tubule are the major sites responsible for this function,[78] Na^+ and Cl^- can also be reabsorbed without water in the collecting duct.[79] The importance of these latter sites of action become evident by examining data for minimum osmolality of fluid in the early distal convoluted tubule of the rat[80] (close to 100 mOsm/kg H_2O) versus that of the final urine (30 to 40 mOsm/kg H_2O)[81]

If the minimum osmolality of the urine happens to be 40 mOsm/kg H_2O and 800 mOsm/d of solute are excreted, the volume of urine is 20 L/day. If water permeability rises such that the osmolality of the urine is now 80 mOsm/kg H_2O, the volume of urine is now only 10 L. Thus, if this increase in permeability is attributed to ADH, the most impressive action of ADH (saving 10 L of free water) is exerted at these very low osmolalities of urine. As a corollary, one should not examine the osmolality of the urine relative to the plasma to see if ADH is acting. Rather, this osmolality should be compared to the expected value of the minimum osmolality of the urine. The second point to stress is that the excretion of 20 L of urine with an osmolality of 40 mOsm/kg H_2O requires the availability of 800 mOsm of solute. If a subject drinks beer in large quantities without protein or salt ingestion, there will not be sufficient osmoles to excrete this water load. Accordingly, either Na^+ and/or urea must be excreted, or water will be retained. In effect, both occur in this setting. As Na^+ is excreted, the ECF volume declines, ADH is released, and water is retained. This is the basis of severe hyponatremia in psychogenic polydipsia. Note that the osmolality of the urine might be high at some times (low ECF volume that is due to loss of Na^+) and low at others (normal ECF volume due to excessive retention of water) during the pathophysiology of this disorder.

Normal Values

1. There are *no* normal values for the osmolality of the urine. Rather, there are expected values depending on the clinical situations.

2. Normal persons on a typical Western diet who are deprived of water should excrete urine with a maximum osmolality (1,200 mOsm/kg H_2O) and a minimum volume (0.5 L/d). The value for the maximum osmolality of the urine tends to decrease with age.[82]

3. With a huge water load, the expected osmolality of the urine is less than 50 mOsm/kg H_2O, and the expected volume is close to 1 L/hr. The value for the minimum osmolality of the urine tends to rise with age.[82]

4. Typical values for urine osmolality, volume, and rate of excretion of osmoles are shown in Table 1-17. These values reflect a typical Western diet.

Table 1-17. Average Composition of the Urine

Parameter	Units	Usual Range
Volume	L/d	1–1.5
Urea	mmol/d	300–600
Na^+	mmol/d	100–250
K^+	mmol/d	40–80
Cl^-	mmol/d	100–250
Osmolality	mOsm/kg H_2O	500–900

In the preceding collections, one must be certain that a freshly voided specimen is examined, especially when provocative tests are performed. In some cases, a "second-voided" specimen should be obtained to have urine that most closely reflects the current physiologic conditions.

Pitfalls in Assessing the Osmolality of the Urine

The osmolality of the medullary interstitium is not known. Hence, achieving an osmolality of the urine of 800 mOsm/kg H_2O may represent a defect in water permeability (maximum 1,200 mOsm/kg H_2O on a typical Western diet) or an intrinsic lesion of the renal concentrating mechanism. Possibilities would include restricted permeability to water or a renal medullary interstitium with a less than optimal osmolality.

Many different particles are included in the term *osmolality*. Some particles are restricted to one compartment (e.g., Na^+ to the ECF) and influence water movement, whereas others do not (e.g., urea). A similar situation occurs in the urine. In this case, NH_4^+ and urea are "effective" osmoles that influence movement of water across the membranes of the distal nephron, whereas ethanol is not. This latter point can become important in the differential diagnosis of central diabetes insipidus in alcohol intoxication (Case 7).

By focusing on the osmolality, one can lose sight on the ultimate aim, the excretion of as little water as possible when there is a stimulus to retain water. This point becomes clear when examining events during chronic fasting. Successful adaptation to starvation results in the excretion of urine with the following composition[43,83]: urea, 75 mmol/d; NH_4^+, 125 mmol/d; ketoacid anions, 125 mmol/d; and very few electrolytes. Thus, with other minor components, the rate of excretion of osmoles is 350 mOsm/d. If this patient does not drink water and has the stimulus to conserve water (excrete 0.5 L/d under the influence of ADH), the osmolality of the urine will only be 700 mOsm/kg H_2O. In one sense, this is a defect in electrolyte-free water conservation (maximum osmolality of urine achieved is low). In another sense, however, the subject is only excreting 0.5 L of electrolyte-free water per day, a value comparable to normals. Hence, it is no longer a simple matter to say whether this is an important "defect" or not.

Case Studies

Case 6: What Is Oliguria?

A patient with severe liver disease excreted 0.4 L of urine per day. Was oliguria present? Because of hepatic encephalopathy, the patient consumed a diet containing little protein. Metabolism of this protein resulted in the production of 80 mmol of urea. Owing to a low EABV (hypoalbuminemia), there was a reduced delivery of filtrate to the distal nephron and the excretion of little Na^+ or K^+ in the urine (20 mmol of $Na^+ + K^+ + Cl^-$). There was also little NH_4^+ in the urine because the acid load from the diet was minimal. Hence, the total excretion of osmoles was only 100 mOsm/d. If the osmolality of the medulla were very low (600 mOsm/kg H_2O)[c] and ADH were present, this patient should have excreted 0.167 L/d (100 mOsm at 600 mOsm/kg H_2O). Therefore, although 0.4 L/d represents oliguria when 500 mOsm must be excreted (1,250 mOsm/kg H_2O), this patient actually had "polyuria" in this clinical setting. This conclusion could be reached only by examining urine volume and osmolality in conjunction with the rate of excretion of osmoles.

Case 7: Excretion of Unusual Osmoles

A 36-year-old woman consumed a large quantity of alcohol; no other history was available. The patient was obviously very intoxicated. There were no physical findings to suggest that the volume of her ECF was contracted or expanded. She was noted to have polyuria in the emergency room (0.2 L/h). Of note, hypernatremia was present (152 mmol/L, Table 1-18). Other pertinent laboratory data included a urine osmolality of 287 mOsm/kg H_2O, the absence of glycosuria, and a concentration of glucose and urea in the plasma, which should not be associated with an osmotic diuresis. A drug screen revealed that the concentration of ethanol in the plasma was 119 mmol/L.

Over the next 8 hours, the patient received thiamine and an intravenous infusion of 0.8 L of 5 percent glucose in water. At the end of this period, the osmolality of the urine had increased to 532 mOsm/kg H_2O and the concentration of Na^+ in the plasma had fallen to 140 mmol/L. The concentration of ethanol in the plasma had declined to 51 mmol/L after 8 hours (Table 1-18). Hence, without definitive therapy, polyuria and hypernatremia were no longer a clinical problem.

Discussion. There are three major categories in the differential diagnosis of hypernatremia and polyuria: osmotic diuresis, nephrogenic diabetes insipidus (DI), and central DI (Figs. 1-8 and 1-9).

---

[c] How much of a defect is present when the urine osmolality is 600 mOsm/kg H_2O (normal 1,200 mOsm/kg H_2O)? A superficial analysis would indicate that the urinary concentrating ability is reduced by 50 percent (600/1,200 mOsm/kg H_2O). The osmolality of plasma is 300, however, so the rise in osmolality is 300 mOsm/kg H_2O (600 − 300) compared to an expected value of 900 mOsm/kg H_2O (1,200 − 300). Therefore, the defect is 67 percent (300 versus 900 mOsm/kg H_2O).

Table 1-18. Laboratory Values on Admission and 8 Hours Later[a]

Parameter	Units	Admission	8 h Later
Plasma			
Na$^+$	mmol/L	152	140
Osmolality	mOsm/kg H$_2$O	420	338
Glucose	mmol/L (mg/dl)	8 (144)	9 (162)
Urea	mmol/L (mg/dl)	1 (2.8)	1 (2.8)
Ethanol	mmol/L	119	51
Urine			
Na$^+$	mmol/L	52	139
K$^+$	mmol/L	10	39
Osmolality	mOsm/kg H$_2$O	287	532

[a] Therapy consisted of 0.8 L of 5% glucose in water. For further details, see text.

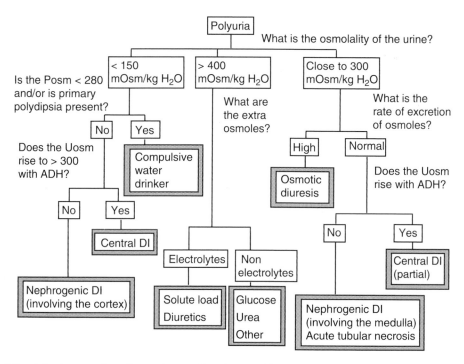

Fig. 1-8. Approach to the patient with polyuria. The options to evaluate are shown in the clear rectangles, and the final diagnostic categories are shown in the rectangles with hatched markings. (ADH, antidiuretic hormone; DI, diabetes insipidus.) (From Halperin and Rolleston,[51] with permission.)

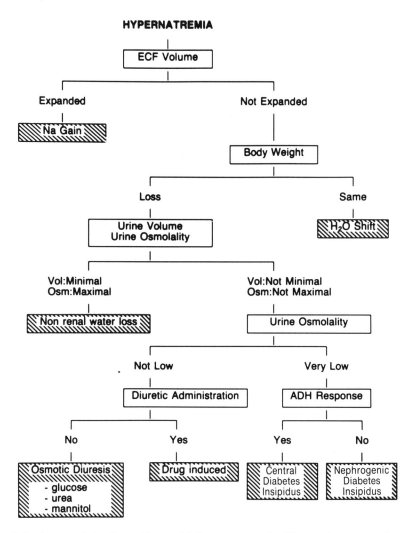

Fig. 1-9. Approach to the patient with hypernatremia. The options to evaluate are shown in the clear rectangles, and the final diagnostic categories are shown in the rectangles with hatched markings. ADH, antidiuretic hormone; ECF, extracellular fluid. (From Halperin[84], with permission.)

Given the history, the lack of findings suggestive of ECF volume contraction, the concentrations of urea and glucose in the plasma that are not associated with an osmotic diuresis (Table 1-18), the absence of glucosuria, and the relatively low value for the osmolality of the urine, an osmotic diuresis is an unlikely diagnosis in this patient. Notwithstanding, the rate of excretion of osmoles was 57 mOsm/h (287 mOsm/kg $H_2O \times 0.2$ L/h), a value consistent with this diagnosis. Ethanol was present in the urine. Ethanol, however, does not cause an osmotic diuresis.[72]

Given the osmolality of the urine (Table 1-18), the diagnosis of nephrogenic DI must be considered. The rate of excretion of osmoles, however, was too high for this diagnosis (56 mOsm/h). Because ethanol was present in the urine, it would elevate both the osmolality of the urine and the rate of excretion of osmoles, thereby confounding their use as diagnostic tools. Hence, we could not rule out a diagnosis of nephrogenic DI at this time, but no drugs or abnormalities that should have caused this disorder were identified.

This patient with ethanol intoxication seemed to have central DI on clinical grounds. The osmolality of the urine, however, was 287 mOsm/kg H_2O, a value that made this diagnosis unlikely. Because the concentration of ethanol in plasma was 119 mmol/L, the urine might have contained an appreciable quantity of alcohol; this might have obscured the presence of a lack of action of ADH.

Because the concentration of ethanol in the urine should have been 167 mmol/L (1.4 times the concentration of ethanol in plasma),[72] one should subtract the estimated contribution of ethanol from the osmolality of the urine. This makes the "nonethanol" osmolality 120 mOsm/kg H_2O (287 − 167 mOsm/kg H_2O) and the rate of excretion of osmoles (other than ethanol) 24 mOsm/h, values more representative of central DI or nephrogenic DI rather than an osmotic diuresis. Because the causes of nephrogenic DI are unlikely to reverse over a short period of time without specific therapy, nephrogenic DI is not the most likely diagnosis. The absence of a past history of central DI, the spontaneous recovery to normonatremia, and the urine osmolality of 532 mOsm/kg H_2O 8 hours later without administration of ADH all point to a transient cause of central DI.

CONCLUSIONS

Our purpose is to provide an update on the use of measurements of urine electrolytes and osmolality in patients with disorders of fluid, electrolytes, and/or acid–base metabolism. It is critical to appreciate that there are no normal values for these parameters, only expected values relative to clinical situations.

To detect a mild to moderate degree of reduction of the "effective" intravascular volume, both the concentrations of Na^+ and Cl^- in urine should be measured. Pitfalls in this assessment are abnormal renal and adrenal function and the presence of diuretics (osmotic or pharmacologic). Insights into the cause of the low "effective" intravascular volume can be deduced by comparing the concentrations of Na^+, K^+, and Cl^- in the urine.

In the differential diagnosis of hyperchloremic metabolic acidosis, the key measurement is the rate of excretion of NH_4^+. Direct measurement of NH_4^+ in the urine is not provided by most clinical laboratories. The urine net charge (anion gap) and the urine osmolal gap may provide reliable estimates of the rate of excretion of NH_4^+. The urine anion gap detects only NH_4^+ that is excreted with Cl^-. If $Na^+ + K^+$ is greater than Cl^- in the urine, the osmolal gap in the urine should be calculated to be sure that the rate of excretion of NH_4^+ is low. The urine osmolal gap detects the presence of any NH_4^+ salt in the urine. Sometimes it is advantageous to examine the rate of excretion of anions other than Cl^- to understand the basis for an overproduction of acids.

To examine the renal response to hypokalemia or hyperkalemia, the two components of excretion of K^+ (the concentration of K^+ in the urine and the urine flow rate) should be examined separately. The former is best evaluated using the TTKG.

The osmolality of the urine is used to assess the action of ADH, and the osmolality of the renal medullary interstitium is used to determine the cause of polyuria and/or hypernatremia. The rate of excretion of osmoles can also be useful to assess the cause of hypernatremia and/or polyuria or to detect a catabolic state.

REFERENCES

1. Oh M, Carroll H: Regulation of extra- and intracellular fluid composition and content. p. 1. In Arieff A, Defronzo R (eds): Fluid Electrolyte and Acid-Base Disorders. Churchill Livingstone, New York, 1985
2. Kamel K, Magner P, Ethier J, Halperin M: Urine electrolytes in the assessment of extracellular fluid volume contraction. Am J Nephrol 9:344, 1989
3. Shrier R: Pathogenesis of sodium and water retention in high output and low output cardiac failure, nephrotic syndrome, cirrhosis and pregnancy. Engl J Med 319:1065, 1988
4. Raymond K, Stein J: Effector limb of volume hemeostasis. Contemp Issues Nephrol 16:33, 1987
5. Chung H, Kluge R, Schrier R, Anderson R: Clinical assessment of extracellular fluid volume in hyponatremia. Am J Med 83:905, 1987
6. Levey A, Perrone R, Madias N: Serum creatinine and renal function. Ann Rev Med 39:465, 1988
7. Oh M, Uribarri J, Barrido D, et al: Case report: the danger of central pontine myelinolysis in hypotonic dehydration and recommendation for treatment. Am J Med Sci 296:41, 1989
8. Halperin M, Goldstein M: Fluid, Electrolyte and Acid-Base Emergencies in Fluid, Electrolyte and Acid-Base Emergencies. WB Saunders, Philadelphia, 1988
9. Espinal C, Gregory A: Differential diagnosis of acute renal failure. Clin Nephrol 13:73, 1980
10. Anderson R, Gabow P, Gross P: Urinary chloride concentration in acute renal failure. Miner Electrolyte Metab 10:92, 1980
11. Kassirer J, Berkman P, Lawrenz D, Schwartz W: The critical role of chloride in the correction of hypokalemic alkalosis in man. Am J Med 38:172, 1965
12. Kamel K, Ethier J, Levine A, Halperin M: Hypokalemia in the "beautiful people." A syndrome which mimics vomiting. Am J Med 88:534, 1990

13. Halperin M, Vasuvattakul S, Bayoumi A: A modified classification of metabolic acidosis: a pathophysiologic approach. Nephron 60:129, 1991
14. Bayoumi A, Vasuvattakul S, Kamel K, Halperin ML: Deducing the cause of metabolic acidosis from the renal handling of the anion. Clin Invest Med 14:A134, 1991
15. Carlisle E, Donnelly S, Vasuvattakul S, et al: Glue-sniffing and distal renal tubular acidosis: sticking to the facts. J Am Soc Nephrol 1:1019, 1991
16. Morris RJ: Renal tubular acidosis. Mechanisms, classification and implications. N Engl J Med 281:1405, 1969
17. Soriano J, Biochis H, Stark H, Edelmann C, Jr: Proximal renal tubular acidosis. A defect in bicarbonate reabsorption with normal urinary acidification. Pediatr Res 1:81, 1967
18. Madison L, Seldin D: Ammonia excretion and renal enzymatic adaptation in human subjects, as disclosed by administration of precursor amino acids. J Clin Invest 37:1615, 1958
19. Richardson R, Halperin M: The urine pH: a potentially misleading diagnostic test in patients with hyperchloremic metabolic acidosis. Am J Kidney Dis 2:140, 1987
20. Simpson D: Control of hydrogen ion homeostasis and renal acidosis. Medicine 50:503, 1971
21. Halperin M, Richardson R, Bear R, et al: Urine ammonium: the key to the diagnosis of distal renal tubular acidosis. Nephron 50:1, 1988
22. Carlisle E, Donnelly S, Halperin M: Renal tubular acidosis (RTA): Recognize The Ammonium defect and pHorget the urine pH. Pediatr Nephrol 5:242, 1991
23. Halperin M, Jungas R: Metabolic production and renal disposal of hydrogen ions. Kidney Int 24:709, 1983
24. Alpern R: Cell mechanisms of proximal tubule acidification. Physiol Rev 70:79, 1990
25. Halperin ML: How much "new" bicarbonate is formed in the distal nephron in the process of net acid excretion? Kidney Int 35:1277, 1989
26. Halperin ML, Kamel K, Ethier J, et al: Biochemistry and physiology of ammonium excretion. p. 2645. In Seldin D, Giebisch, G (eds): The Kidney, Physiology and Pathophysiology. 2nd Ed. Vol. 2. Raven Press, New York, 1991
27. Halperin ML, Jungas RL, Cheema-Dhadli S, Brosnan JT: Disposal of the daily acid load: an integrated function of the liver, lungs, and kidneys. Trends Biol Sci 12:197, 1987
28. Knepper M, Packer R, Good D: Ammonium transport in the kidney. Physiol Rev 69:179, 1989
29. Wrong O, Davies W: The excretion of acid in renal disease. Q J Med 23:259, 1959
30. Soriano J, Edelman C: Renal tubular acidosis. Annu Rev Med 20:363, 1969
31. Reynolds T: Observations on the pathogenesis of renal tubular acidosis. Am J Med 25:503, 1958
32. Kurtzman N: Disorders of distal acidification. Kidney Int 38:720, 1990
33. Kurtzman NA: Renal tubular acidosis: a constellation of syndromes. Hosp Prac 22:173, 1987
34. Batlle D, Grupp M, Gavira M, Kurtzman N: Distal renal tubular acidosis with intact capacity to lower urinary pH. Am J Med 72:751, 1982
35. Goldstein M, Bear R, Richardson R, et al: The urine anion gap: a clinically useful index of ammonium excretion. Am J Med Sci 29:198, 1986

36. Lennon E, Lemann J, Jr, Litzow J: The effects of diet and stool composition on the net external acid balance of normal subjects. J Clin Invest 45:1601, 1966
37. Dyck R, Asthana S, Kalra J, et al: A modification of the urine osmolal gap: an improved method for estimating urine ammonium. Am J Nephrol 10:359, 1990
38. Halperin M, Margolis B, Robinson L, et al: The urine osmolal gap: a clue to estimate urine ammonium in "hybrid" types of metabolic acidosis. Clin Invest Med 11:198, 1989
39. Kamel K, Ethier J, Richardson R, et al: Urine electrolytes and osmolality: when and how to use them. Am J Nephrol 10:89, 1990
40. Van Leeuven A: Net cation equivalency ("base binding power") of the plasma proteins. Acta Med Scand 422:1, 1969
41. Nanji A, Campbell D: Falsely-elevated serum creatinine values in diabetic keto-acidosis—clinical implications. J Biochem 14:91, 1981
42. Smith H, Finfelstein N, Aliminosa L, et al: The renal clearances of substituted hippuric acid derivitives and other aromatic acids in dogs and man. J Clin Invest 24:388, 1945.
43. Sapir DG, Owen OE: Renal conservation of ketone bodies during starvation. Metabolism 24:23, 1975
44. Kamel K, Ethier J, Stinebaugh B, et al: The removal of an inorganic acid load in subjects with ketoacidosis of chronic fasting: the role of the kidney. Kidney Int 37:507, 1990
45. Marliss E, Fox I, Goldstein M, Halperin M: Paradoxical uricosuric effect of lactate during prolonged fasting in man. Clin Res 21:1078, 1973
46. Sebastian A, McSherry E, Morris R Jr: Renal potassium wasting in renal tubular acidosis (RTA): its occurrence in types 1 and 2 RTA despite sustained correction of systemic acidosis. J Clin Invest 50:667, 1971
47. West M, Bendz O, Chen C, et al: Development of a test to evaluate the transtubular potassium concentration gradient in the cortical collecting duct in vivo. Miner Electrolyte Metab 12:226, 1986
48. West M, Marsden P, Richardson R, et al: New clinical approach to evaluate disorders of potassium excretion. Miner Electrolyte Metab 12:234, 1986
49. Ethier J, Kamel K, Kaiser U, Halperin K: Characterizing sub-types of hyporeninemic hypoaldosteronism syndrome (HRHA): use of acetazolamide (ACZ), abstracted. Clin Res 36:518, 1988
50. Carlisle E, Donnelly S, Ethier J, et al: Modulation of the secretion on potassium by accompanying anions in humans. Kidney Int 39:1206, 1991
51. Halperin M, Rolleston F: Biochemical Detective Stories: A Problem Based Approach to Clinical Cases. Neil Patterson Publications, Burlington, North Carolina, 1990
52. Huth E, Squires R, Elkinton J: Experimental potassium depletion in normal human subjects: 2. Renal and hormonal factors in the development of extracellular alkalosis during depletion. J Clin Invest 38:1149, 1959
53. Brunner H, Baer L, Seally J, et al: The influence of potassium administration and of potassium deprivation on plasma renin in normal and hypertensive subjects. J Clin Invest 49:2128, 1970
54. Brown RS: External potassium homeostasis. Kidney Int 30:116, 1986
55. Bia M, DeFronzo R: Extrarenal potassium homeostasis. Am J Physiol 240:F257, 1981
56. Field M, Giebisch G: Hormonal control of renal potassium excretion. Kidney Int 27:379, 1985

57. Wright F: Renal potassium handling. Semin Nephrol 7:174, 1987
58. Stanton B: Renal potassium adaptation: cellular mechanism and morphology. Curr Top Membrane Trans 28:225, 1987
59. O'Neil R: Adrenal steroid regulation of potassium transport. Curr Top Membrane Trans 28:185, 1987
60. Velazquez H, Ellison D, Wright F: Chloride-dependent potassium secretion in early and late renal distal tubules. Am J Physiol 253:F555, 1987
61. Velazquez H, Wright FS, Good DW: Luminal influences on potassium secretion: chloride replacement with sulfate. Am J Physiol 242:F46, 1982
62. Velazquez H, Wright FS, Good DW: Effects of luminal anion composition and acidity on potassium secretion by renal distal tubule. Fed Proc 39:1079, 1980
63. Ethier J, Kamel K, Magner P, et al: Evaluation of the renal response to hypokalemia and hyperkalemia. Am J Kidney Dis 15:309, 1990
64. Battle D, Arruda J, Kurtzman N: Hyperkalemic distal renal tubular acidosis associated with obstructive uropathy. N Engl J Med 304:373, 1981
65. Zettle R, West M, Josse R, et al: Renal potassium handling during states of low aldosterone bioactivity: a method to differentiate renal and non-renal causes. Am J Nephrol 7:360, 1987
66. Schambelan M, Sebastian A, Rector FC Jr: Mineralocorticoid-resistant renal hyperkalemia without salt wasting (type II pseudohypoaldosteronism): role of increased renal chloride reabsorption. Kidney Int 19:716, 1981
67. Take C, Ikeda K, Kurasawa T, Kurokawa K: Increased chloride reabsorption as an inherited renal tubular defect in familial type II pseudohypoaldosteronism. N Engl J Med 324:472, 1991
68. Burl R, Sebastian A, Cheitlin M, et al: Pseudokyperkalemia caused by fist clenching during phlebotomy. N Engl J Med 322:1290, 1990
69. Halperin M, Skorecki K: Interpretation of the urine electrolytes and osmolality in the regulation of body fluid tonicity. Am J Nephrol 6:241, 1986
70. Mcdaugh H, Schmidt-Nielsen B, Doyle E, O'Dell R: Renal tubular regulation of urea excretion in man. J Appl Physiol 13:263, 1958
71. Epstein FH, Kleeman CR, Pursel S, Hendrick A: The effect of feeding protein and urea on the renal concentrating process. J Clin Invest 10:635, 1956
72. Magner P, Ethier J, Kamel K, Halperin M: Interpretation of the urine osmolality: the role of ethanol. Clin Invest Med 14:355, 1991
73. Lemieux G, Craan A, Quenneville A, et al: Metabolic machinery of the alligator kidney. Am J Physiol 247:F686, 1984
74. Coulson RA, Hernandez T: Source and function of urinary ammonia in the alligator. Am J Physiol 197:873, 1959
75. Moore L, Marsh D: How descending limb of Henle's loop permeability affects hypertonic urine formation. Am J Physiol 239:F57, 1980
76. Jamison R, Oliver R: Disorders of urinary concentration and dilution. Am J Med 72:308, 1982
77. Verkman A: Mechanisms and regulation of water permeability in renal epithelia. Am J Physiol 257:C837, 1989
78. Hebert S, Reeves W, Molony D, Andreoli T: The medullary thick limb: function and modulation of the single-effect multiplier. Kidney Int 31:580, 1987
79. Sonnenberg H: Effect of adrenalectomy on medullary collecting-duct function in rats before and during blood volume expansion. Pflügers Arch 368:55, 1977
80. Malnic G, Klose R, Giebisch G: Micropuncture study of distal tubular potassium and sodium transport in rat nephron. Am J Physiol 211:529, 1966

81. Robinson A: Disorders of antidiuretic hormone secretion. Clin Endocrinol Metab 14:55, 1985

82. Rowe J, Shock N, DeFronzo R: The influence of age on urine concentrating ability in man. Nephron 17:279, 1976

83. Owen O, Morgan A, Kemp H, et al: Brain metabolism during fasting. J Clin Invest 46:1589, 1967

84. Halperin ML: The Acid Truth and Basic Facts—with a Sweet Touch, an En-LYTEnment. Ross Mark Medical Publishers, Stirling, Ontario, Canada, 1991

2

Polycystic Kidney Disease

Clinical, Radiologic, and Genetic Approaches to Problems in Diagnosis

William D. Kaehny
Patricia A. Gabow

Mitral Valve Prolapse
Colonic Diverticulosis

WHEN AND HOW TO DIAGNOSE COMPLICATIONS OF ADPKD

Abdominal Pain
Renal and Hepatic Cyst Infections
Urinary Tract Obstruction
Hematuria and Renal Cell Carcinoma

SUMMARY

INTRODUCTION

Clinicians confront a variety of diagnostic decisions in treating families and patients with autosomal dominant polycystic kidney disease (ADPKD). These diagnostic issues fall into three broad categories regarding when and how to diagnose ADPKD, its extrarenal manifestations, and its complications. The answers we offer to these questions are based on a selected review of the literature and our personal experiences in dealing with a large ADPKD population.

DEFINITION, GENETICS, AND EPIDEMIOLOGY

ADPKD is a systemic hereditary disease equally affecting males and females. It is manifested by bilateral multiple renal cysts, hepatic cysts, cardiac valve abnormalities, intracranial aneurysms, colonic diverticulae, and other findings.[1] ADPKD is by definition inherited as an autosomal dominant mendelian disorder that can be caused by at least two different genes. ADPKD1 is located on chromosome 16 and can be detected by gene linkage techniques (see below).[2] The other gene (or genes), termed non-ADPKD1, or ADPKD2, is identified by the absence of gene linkage markers for ADPKD1,[3,4] and its location is currently unknown. Although the products of the mutant genes are not known at present, the diversity of manifestations suggests that the gene product is operative in many cells.

ADPKD appears to have a worldwide distribution, but the frequency of the clinical disorder and the culprit gene may vary in different racial groups. ADPKD appears to be less common in blacks,[5] whereas approximately 1 in 400 to 1 in 1,000 whites have ADPKD, and 90 percent of the affected families appear to carry the ADPKD1 gene.[6]

WHEN TO PURSUE THE DIAGNOSIS OF ADPKD
Asymptomatic Patient With a Family History of ADPKD

The need to diagnose ADPKD arises in one of three settings: a patient with a positive family history, an individual with symptoms compatible with ADPKD, or an individual in whom multiple renal cysts are found by chance on an abdominal imaging procedure.

A family history of ADPKD often is the stimulus that triggers an evaluation for the disorder. In fact, the best clue to the presence of ADPKD in any patient is a family history of the disease. The presence of ADPKD in a parent imparts a 50 percent chance of the disorder to each offspring. Although the presence of a family history is extremely helpful, the absence of such a history does not exclude the diagnosis. Older reports contain lower frequencies of a positive family history than do several recent studies (Table 2-1).

Table 2-1. History of Familial Kidney Disease in ADPKD

Author	Year	Number	Family History of ADPKD		
			Definite	Suspicious	Negative
Higgins[7]	1952	94	34	10	50
Simon and Thompson[8]	1955	366	66	85	215
Ward et al.[9]	1967	53	17	5	31
Total	Pre-1970	513	117	100	296
Percentage	Pre-1970	100	23	19	58
Sahney et al.[10]	1982	22	—	13	9
Iglesias[11]	1983	56	40	—	16
Delaney[12]	1985	53	35	7	11
Total	Post-1980	131	75	20	36
Percentage	Post-1980	100	57	15	27

Abbreviation: ADPKD, autosomal dominant polycystic kidney disease.

The difference between a 42 percent frequency of a positive or suspicious parent for ADPKD before 1970 and a 72 percent frequency of an affected parent after 1980 likely reflects two major influences: a greater awareness of the disorder among physicians since 1980 and more sensitive and readily available methods for diagnosis. Because ADPKD is the most common hereditary disorder in the United States, affecting one-half million people, and 72 percent of patients in this era are aware of a positive family history, the practicing nephrologist is likely to encounter patients whose chief complaint is solely a family history of ADPKD.

What is the appropriate medical response to this issue? In general, non-clinically directed random screening is not considered appropriate care.[13] Therefore, the presence of a positive family history alone should not reflexively prompt a search for the diagnosis. A screening history and physical examination, however, should be performed to obtain information that could trigger definitive studies for ADPKD (Table 2-2).

The most compelling reason for further evaluation in such persons is their desire to know their status. For some, this need to know addresses ongoing concerns about gene status and their future; for others, the need for family planning will be based on their revealed gene status. In a recent study of attitudes regarding diagnosis of ADPKD, 97 percent of family members at risk for ADPKD indicated that they would seek gene testing to define their own status, demonstrating the often strong desire of individuals within ADPKD families to know if they have the disease.[19] Moreover, 30 percent of at-risk subjects in their childbearing years stated that the diagnosis would affect their family planning.[19] These patients should be counseled regarding methods, interpretation, and risks and benefits of various diagnostic approaches as well as the implications of a positive diagnosis before the physi-

Table 2-2. Symptoms and Signs in ADPKD

Study	Number of Subjects	Pain	Gross Hematuria	Palpable Kidneys	Hypertension
Oppenheimer[14]	59	28	21	49	22
Higgins[7]	94	61	39	76	69
Simon and Thompson[8]	357	163	115	285	202
Dalgaard[15]	350	272	158	213	162
Ward et al.[9]	53	25	25	39	33
Iglesias et al.[11]	56	44	16	—	46
Gabow et al.[16]	164	100	51	85	102
Delaney et al.[12]	53	33	26	—	34
Gonzalo et al.[17]	107	—	32	—	72
Milutinovic et al.[18]	140	58	52	—	53
Sum	1,433	784	535	778	815
Population	1,433	1,326	1,433	1,130	1,433
Percentage	100	59.1	37.3	68.8	56.9

Abbreviation: ADPKD, autosomal dominant polycystic kidney disease.

cian proceeds to define the patient's status. The benefits include information for family planning if that is the patient's desire, perhaps a stimulus for the person to be more committed to positive health practices, and better awareness of treatable complications of ADPKD, such as hypertension. The risks entail the psychological burden of a diagnosed disease and the impact of the diagnosis on the acquisition and cost of health and life insurance.

Screening Asymptomatic Children of Parents With ADPKD

Occasionally, it is not the patient himself who presents with a family history of ADPKD and the desire to know his status, but rather the parent requesting this information for his or her offspring. Sujansky's study of attitudes indicated that 88 percent of ADPKD subjects would have their children tested to define their status.[19] This poses a different problem for the physician. Restriction of nonclinically directed random screening of children to the research setting is even more important than it is with adults.[13] Children, like adults, should undergo a history and physical examination to determine if there is a clinical reason for further evaluation (Table 2-2). The parents should be informed of the risks and benefits of early diagnosis. In the absence of a clinical indication, the benefits are unclear, whereas the risks include the psychological burden of the diagnosis on the child and the future impact on insurability. If screening is carried out, a decision should be made in advance as to whether the child is to be informed of his or her ADPKD status. We do not inform children of a positive diagnosis unless the parents specifically request this.

Evaluation of the Symptomatic Patient

Renal Manifestations

Frequently, patients present to a physician with a complaint that is compatible with but not diagnostic of ADPKD. Approximately 70 percent of adult nonazotemic patients with ADPKD are symptomatic.[16] However, a majority of the complaints, albeit compatible with ADPKD, are neither sensitive enough nor specific enough to make the diagnosis. Although ADPKD is a systemic disorder, the presenting complaints often relate to the kidneys and include flank or abdominal pain, hematuria, urinary tract infection, nephrolithiasis, hypertension, or an abdominal mass. In the presence of a family history of ADPKD, certain of these symptoms, such as urinary tract infection, may be more likely to prompt a renal evaluation. For other manifestations, such as nephrolithiasis, evaluation is likely to occur even without a history of ADPKD. In that circumstance, ADPKD may be an unanticipated finding.

The most common symptom of ADPKD is *abdominal, flank, or back pain* (Table 2-2).[20] Women are more likely than men to note abdominal pain.[15] In both genders, the occurrence of pain increases with age with a frequency of about 10 percent in patients 30 years of age and 50 percent in those 50 years of age.[15] Although pain can be a major problem for the patient, it lacks any specific quality that by itself would raise the suspicion of ADPKD in the absence of a family history.

Gross hematuria, a common presenting symptom, is usually alarming enough to patients or to the parent of a child with this complaint to prompt them to seek medical advice. In a synthesis of 10 studies, 37 percent of 1,433 ADPKD patients had at least one episode of gross hematuria (Table 2-2). In fact, this is the presenting complaint in 13 to 23 percent of patients.[12,17,18,20] Although most episodes occur after 25 years of age,[15] 14 to 26 percent of children also have had hematuria.[21,22] Members of ADPKD families who present with gross hematuria require renal evaluation that would likely include ultrasonography or computed tomography (CT) (see below).

Urinary tract infections, including cystitis, pyelonephritis, and cyst infections, are common in ADPKD.[23] Risk factors for infection include female gender, renal insufficiency, and urinary tract instrumentation.[23,24] No prospective studies of urinary tract infections have been conducted of individuals at risk for ADPKD; therefore, no guidelines exist for evaluation of the urinary tract in at-risk subjects who develop infection. It seems reasonable, however, to evaluate any person at risk for ADPKD, both adult and child, who has an upper urinary tract infection. Certainly, any patient with symptoms and signs compatible with an upper urinary tract infection who does not respond to conventional antibiotics requires urinary tract imaging because the differential diagnosis of this syndrome includes an infected cyst.[24] Twenty percent of adult ADPKD patients develop nephrolithiasis,[25] an incidence that is significantly higher than is seen in the general population.[26,27] About half of these patients are symptomatic. As with any patient, the presumption of nephrolithiasis dictates renal imaging studies.

Hypertension is the most common physical finding in ADPKD, occurring in about 69 percent of 1,433 patients during the course of the disease (Table 2-2). Twenty-seven percent of subjects less than 20 years of age are hypertensive.[28] In a group of 68 patients with newly diagnosed ADPKD, 17 (25 percent) had untreated hypertension.[29] Should the isolated finding of hypertension in an at-risk family member trigger an evaluation for ADPKD? Certainly evaluation is indicated if the judgment to treat hypertension (particularly borderline hypertension), the aggressiveness of therapy, or the choice of therapeutic agent would be influenced by the finding of polycystic kidney disease. Our experience indicates that children appear less likely to be treated even when their blood pressure exceeds that for age- and gender-matched children in the general population. Therefore, in children, the documentation of underlying renal disease might prompt the physician to evaluate more carefully the need for therapy. Blood pressure apparently is one of the major determinants of the rate of progressive deterioration of renal function in ADPKD[11]; therefore, hypertension in ADPKD requires greater effort for adequate control than might occur in a patient with essential hypertension.[28] Thus, if the patient and the physician decide not to pursue the diagnosis of ADPKD in an at-risk subject with hypertension, the hypertension should still be aggressively treated and control monitored regularly.

Abdominal masses are a frequent presenting manifestation of ADPKD in both adults and children and obviously require further diagnostic evaluation. Sixty-nine percent of ADPKD patients develop palpable kidneys (Table 2-2). The age at which this finding becomes manifest has a bimodal distribution. Twenty-two to 36 percent of affected neonates and very young children have palpable kidneys,[21,22] while by the age of 54, this figure increases to 50 percent.[15] The high frequency of palpable kidneys in young children reflects their relatively small body mass and the ease with which their abdomens can be examined. Furthermore, an artifact is introduced by the fact that the neonates and very young children who come to investigation for ADPKD are frequently those in whom nephromegaly prompted investigation.

The differential diagnosis of abdominal masses from cystic kidneys in neonates includes ADPKD and autosomal recessive polycystic kidney disease (ARPKD) as well as other noncystic disorders (Table 2-3). The most reliable distinguishing characteristic is the status of the parents. It is noteworthy, however, that 62 percent of parents who had a neonate with ADPKD were unaware that they had the disorder until they were evaluated following the diagnosis in their child.[30] Previously, liver biopsy was used to differentiate ADPKD from ARPKD based on the common occurrence of congenital hepatic fibrosis in ARPKD.[31] Recent reports of congenital hepatic fibrosis in ADPKD render this diagnostic tool less useful.[32,33]

Table 2-3. Comparison of ADPKD and ARPKD

	ADPKD	ARPKD
Occurrence in parents	90%	Extremely rare
Occurrence in offspring	50%	25%
Liver involvement	Late, cysts	Early, fibrosis
Renal failure	Late	Early
Ultrasonography, infants		
Kidney size	Normal to large	Large
Appearance	Discrete cysts	Increased echogenicity
	Good definition	Poor definition

Abbreviations: ADPKD, autosomal dominant polycystic kidney disease; ARPKD, autosomal recessive polycystic kidney disease.

Extrarenal Manifestations

Infrequently, the chief complaint or abnormal finding that leads to the diagnosis of ADPKD is an extrarenal manifestation (Table 2-4). Although the most common extrarenal manifestation of ADPKD is *cystic involvement of the liver,* this is very rarely a presenting manifestation. Of the array of extrarenal disorders, the most likely to present as the initial major manifestation of ADPKD may be a *ruptured intracranial aneurysm.*[34] Because patients with ruptured intracranial aneurysms are not routinely screened for ADPKD, in the absence of a family history, the diagnosis is not likely to be made. However, all patients with an intracranial aneurysm should be questioned regarding their familial histories for aneurysms, renal disease, and ADPKD. Those with a family history of either renal disease or ruptured intracranial aneurysms should be screened for ADPKD.

A number of *cardiac abnormalities* occur in ADPKD,[35] with mitral valve prolapse being most prominent. In a detailed prospective study of 163 ADPKD patients with a mean age of 40 years, 40 percent complained of palpitations, 25 percent of atypical chest pain, 14 percent had a systolic click, 21 percent had the murmur of mitral valve regurgitation, and 26 percent had echocardiographic evidence of mitral valve prolapse.[36] Of interest, 14 percent of 130 family members without renal cysts also had mitral valve prolapse compared to 2 percent of control subjects, suggesting that in some at-risk family members mitral valve prolapse may precede the renal manifestations of ADPKD. Given the frequency of this finding in ADPKD, these clinical complaints and physical findings in an at-risk subject should raise a high level of suspicion that the patient may have ADPKD. If warranted by the clinical complaints and physical findings, echocardiographic confirmation of valvular disease is indicated. We pursue imaging evaluation for ADPKD in those at-risk subjects with evidence of valvular disease.

Ovarian cysts appear to be more common in subjects with ADPKD than in unaffected family members. Physicians should simply be aware of this manifestation and not consider ovarian cysts in this disorder as equivalent to the polycystic ovary syndrome. Historical and physical evidence for ADPKD should be sought out in patients in whom a recent primary diagnosis of

Table 2-4. Prevalence of Extrarenal Manifestations in ADPKD

Disorder	Prevalence Children	Adults (%)
Hepatic cysts	After age 16	Up to 75
Diverticulosis of colon	Not reported	Up to 80
Mitral valve prolapse	Appears increased	25
Intracranial aneurysm	Not reported	10
Inguinal hernia	Appears increased	15
Cystic ovaries	Not reported	40

Abbreviation: ADPKD, autosomal dominant polycystic kidney disease.

ovarian cysts has been made. Further evaluation for ADPKD should be pursued in at-risk patients.

Although it is our opinion that patients presenting with major systemic manifestations of ADPKD should be further evaluated, individual clinical judgment must prevail. However, because intracranial aneurysms cluster in certain ADPKD families[37] and this is a particularly catastrophic consequence of ADPKD, we believe that family members of ADPKD patients with aneurysms present the best case among those presenting with extrarenal manifestations for screening for ADPKD.

Evaluation of Patients With an Incidental Finding of Renal Cysts

The widespread use of abdominal imaging procedures and the high frequency of renal cysts in the general population[38] occasionally require that multiple bilateral simple cysts be distinguished from ADPKD. The differentiation of these two entities usually is not difficult. The most helpful factors include a positive family history, age, and the occurrence of extrarenal manifestations of ADPKD. The frequency of simple renal cysts increases with age, occurring in 0.1 percent of children and 50 percent of people over the age of 50.[38,39] Thus, 70 percent of children in an ADPKD family who have even a single renal cyst are likely to have ADPKD.[21] However, a 70-year-old with one or two renal cysts in an ADPKD family is most likely to have simple cysts. Between these rather straightforward clinical scenarios lie less apparent diagnostic problems. In such instances, the occurrence of extrarenal manifestations such as hepatic cysts is helpful. Moreover, gene linkage analysis can be used in certain of these individuals to clarify the diagnosis (see below).

HOW TO DIAGNOSE ADPKD

There exists an array of diagnostic approaches to ADPKD. The procedure chosen depends on the age of the patient, the certainty with which the patient and the physician need to be assured of the diagnosis, and the presence of specific symptoms that may require renal anatomic definition. Historical data and physical findings can trigger further evaluation for ADPKD, but they provide information that is neither sufficiently specific nor sensitive to permit a definitive diagnosis. Similarly, routine laboratory studies of renal function are not diagnostic of ADPKD. *Impaired renal concentrating ability* occurs in ADPKD before the development of renal insufficiency[40–42] and is sufficiently common in adults that it can be used as a screening tool.[43] To define this defect more clearly and to normalize for the effects of age on concentrating ability, we studied 177 adult subjects with ADPKD and normal renal function and 123 unaffected relatives. Urine osmolality was measured after 12 hours of abstinence from fluid and following 5 units of aqueous vasopressin administered subcutaneously. Ninety-five percent of normotensive, nonazotemic ADPKD subjects were unable to achieve a maximal osmolality (Umax) above the level predicted from the following formula: Umax = 1,086 − 8.3 × age (years). In contrast, only 40 percent of unaffected family members failed to achieve this level. Thus, the number of false-negative tests is small (~5 percent), whereas the number of false-positives is high (40 percent). In combination with blood pressure determination and measurement of the serum creatinine level, this concentration test can provide a simple, inexpensive screening protocol for ADPKD.

Imaging Studies in ADPKD

The most commonly used diagnostic procedures that are both sensitive and specific for defining ADPKD are imaging studies. The imaging studies of choice for defining renal cysts and establishing the diagnosis are ultrasonography and CT. Other procedures such as plain abdominal roentgenography, excretory urography with or without tomography, radionuclide scanning, and arteriography are no longer recommended for establishing the diagnosis of ADPKD. However, the clinician should be aware of the findings of ADPKD that might be detected fortuitously when these procedures are performed for another indication.[44]

On *plain film* of the abdomen the presence of ADPKD is suggested by a large renal outline, present in a majority of patients over 30 years of age. Curvilinear calcification can also occasionally be seen in the cyst walls. *Excretory urography* with tomography demonstrates thinning and angulation of the collecting system and a moth-eaten appearance of the cortex, which is due to the lucency of the cysts. Excretory urography is rarely now used in ADPKD except when the collecting system needs to be outlined to evaluate the possibility of obstructing calculi or ureteric tumors. Although *radionuclide scanning* can detect cysts,[45] it is not more sensitive than ultrasonography or CT and does not demonstrate anatomy. The distinctive displacement of the renal vasculature on renal arteriography permits the diagnosis of ADPKD, but this study is now reserved for circumstances for which renal tumors or renal vascular abnormalities are being considered.

Ultrasonography

Ultrasonography has become the imaging method of choice for ADPKD.[46-48] Real-time and gray scale imaging allows for the detection of cysts smaller than 0.5 cm in diameter.[46] Its safety and ease of use in children, fetuses, and pregnant women and its lack of radiation and contrast exposure are added advantages. The characteristic ultrasonographic findings are enlarged kidneys, present in 82 percent of subjects over age 12 years,[16] and multiple cysts scattered throughout the kidney parenchyma. A recent study by Parfrey demonstrated that 83 percent of subjects who were less than 30 years of age with the ADPKD1 gene had detectable renal cysts by ultrasonography.[28]

Computed Tomography

Computed tomography has the best resolution of the currently available imaging techniques of the kidney parenchyma.[46-50] It can detect cysts or masses smaller than 0.5 cm.[46,50] CT is generally performed following venous injection of contrast, but it appears to have excellent diagnostic sensitivity without contrast and thus can prove valuable in patients in whom use of contrast is hazardous. Of course, CT is much more costly than ultrasonography.

In Levine and Grantham's report of five adults, asymptomatic but at risk for ADPKD and aged 20 to 28 years, CT showed no cysts in one case for which ultrasonography was interpreted as showing four cysts. CT showed multiple, small, widely dispersed cysts in both kidneys of the other four patients, whereas ultrasonography showed many fewer and nephrotomography even fewer.[46]

CT can also detect such renal complications of ADPKD as infection, hemorrhage, renal cell carcinoma, and urinary tract obstruction. Other imaging modalities are less successful in detecting these complications because of the effects of the cysts themselves on renal architecture. A phenomenon noted on noncontrast CT has been the common (about 70 percent) occurrence of high-density cysts.[51,52] The appearance is thought to result from previous cyst hemorrhage with clot retraction and concentration of proteins. These cysts have smooth walls with distinct margins, are homogeneous in appearance, and do not enhance with contrast, thus allowing them to be clearly distinguished from malignancies. Aspiration is not indicated. Unless calcification occurs, follow-up CT studies, show that the high density resolves as the blood clots liquify and are absorbed.[51,52]

Thus, at present, we reserve CT for situations for which ultrasonography is equivocal or requires confirmation or for detection of complications. This decision is based on radiation exposure, cost, and often contrast exposure for CT, which ultrasonography does not require. Furthermore, ultrasonography is almost as accurate and sensitive as CT.

Magnetic Resonance Imaging

Magnetic resonance imaging (MRI) has the advantage of not requiring radiocontrast material. However, MRI systems have poorer spatial resolution and thus may not be as sensitive in detecting very small cysts.[53] The value of MRI may lie in its ability to detect hemorrhage into cysts of more than a few days' duration by virtue of fluid-iron levels within the cysts, a phenomenon not known to occur with renal cell carcinoma.[54] At present, however, MRI has no identified clinical role in the initial diagnosis of ADPKD.

Renal Biopsy

Renal biopsy was performed in 14 asymptomatic patients with ADPKD who had normal excretory urograms (two had enlarged kidneys). Tubular dilatation was seen in three of four who were subsequently shown to have ADPKD, but in only two of ten without known ADPKD.[55] Nonetheless, in the early stages, pathologic findings were neither specific nor sensitive, causing us not to recommend renal biopsy for the diagnosis of ADPKD.

Biopsy may prove helpful, however, in the diagnosis of superimposed renal disorders such as nephrotic syndrome. Excretion of more than 1 mg protein per 1 mg creatinine in a "spot urine" or more than 1 g/24 h should prompt investigation for a cause other than ADPKD. Such patients have had other renal lesions including IgA nephropathy[56] and focal glomerular sclerosis.[57] We recommend renal biopsy only for the usual reasons that would alter the clinical approach. Although we are aware of anecdotes of uncomplicated percutaneous needle biopsies in ADPKD, we believe that open biopsy might be safer despite the need for general anesthesia.

Gene Linkage Analysis

As sensitive and accurate as imaging techniques are, they are limited by the fact that the diagnosis depends totally on the presence of bilateral renal cysts, precluding the ready diagnosis of the gene carrier state before the development of the phenotype. Thus, in the future, the ideal test will directly demonstrate the ADPKD gene(s). This will, of course, ultimately require that we become capable of isolating the abnormal gene(s). If this technique were available, only the individual desiring the information would need be tested, it would be 100 percent accurate, and it could be used at any point in the natural history of the disease, from fetal life onward.

Until these techniques become available, do we have any way to determine genotype? Gene linkage analysis provides us with an indirect way to determine the presence of the culprit gene.[58] This technique is based on the linkage between detectable markers of the gene in question. Because this technique is used when we do not have a direct test for the gene, it is logical to ask how we know the markers are linked to the gene. In fact, one determines which marker segregates or travels with the characteristic phenotype of the culprit gene.

Chromosomal DNA is isolated and cut into pieces by enzymes called *restriction endonucleases*, forming *restriction fragment length polymorphisms* (RFLPs). These pieces of human strands of DNA may contain sequences that are anonymous—that is, they have no known function or product—or they may contain known genes. The chromosome of origin is known for both the anonymous sequences and known genes. These sequences and genes are inherited according to mendelian rules. These RFLPs can have only a few forms or many forms; that is, they can be very polymorphic. The more forms, the more helpful the marker is in terms of linkage studies. For example, if there are only two forms of a marker, *a* and *b*, there are only three potential combinations from parents who each have a chromosome with an *a* and a chromosome with a *b: aa, ab, bb*. If the father's chromosome has *ab* and the mother's has *ab*, an offspring with *ab* could have inherited the *a* or the *b* from either parent. Thus, this family would be uninformative about any disorder that was linked to one of these markers. If this same marker were highly polymorphic, with 10 forms, the chances of unrelated parents having the same form is very unlikely, and the marker probe would be likely to be informative in most families. For example, if a father had a disease and had marker types *c* and *d*, the unaffected mother had marker types *a* and *b*, and every affected offspring inherited type *c* from the father and every unaffected offspring inherited *d* from the father, one would conclude that in this family the disease was segregating with marker *c*. Because the marker types are not determined by the culprit gene, the type will vary between families. That is, in another family, the *a* or *b* or *d* marker type might be inherited with the culprit gene. Thus, the fact that an RFLP is segregated with the disease in many families permits us to say the culprit gene is on the same chromosome near the RFLP. However, one needs to determine the specific marker form of the RFLP associated with the disease for each individual family by having at least two affected subjects in each family. Importantly, these two or more members must have unequivocal evidence of the phenotypic manifestation of the culprit gene, in this case ADPKD.

The investigation of the genetics of ADPKD using these techniques demonstrated a linkage with a probe for an RFLP having many forms, a hypervariable region (3'HVR) of the α-globin locus, placing the ADPKD gene on the short arm of chromosome 16.[2] This provided a method for defining affected individuals before the development of detectable renal cysts (Fig. 2-1). The method is not 100 percent reliable because there is some physical distance on chromosome 16 between the ADPKD gene and the marker, permitting some chance of crossover of the genetic material between chromosomes during meiosis. With the 3'HVR probe, occurrence of a crossover is about 5 percent, making the test 95 percent accurate. Markers have now been identified on either side of the ADPKD gene,[59] making crossovers less likely to cause an error in interpretation, since double crossovers are much less likely

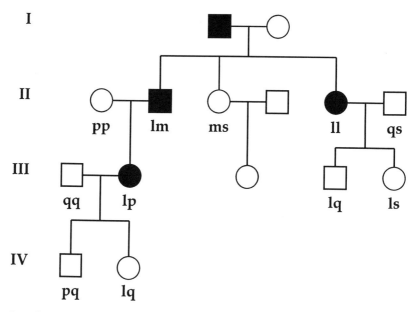

Fig. 2-1. In this figure, circles represent female, squares represent male, and black represents ADPKD. In this family, the marker probe has forms l, m, n, o, p, q, r, and s. The autosomal dominant polycystic kidney disease (ADPKD) gene appears to segregate with the l form, which the male in generation I must have had. Thus, the female in generation IV may be assumed to possess the gene. Unfortunately, the ll female in generation II is homozygous for l and thus the marker is uninformative for her offspring.

than a single crossover. Using these flanking probes, the accuracy is better than 99 percent (Fig. 2-2).

In the first 100 families tested, the linkage to markers on chromosome 16 was confirmed.[60] Subsequently, however, a small number of families has been demonstrated to have an ADPKD gene that is not linked to these markers and hence is not located on the short arm of chromosome 16.[3,4,28,61,62] As discussed previously, the second gene has been labeled either ADPKD2 or non-ADPKD1. The latter nomenclature is meant to convey that there may be multiple other ADPKD genes, ADPKD2, ADPKD3, and so on. Location of the ADPKD2 gene and linkage studies in many families will ultimately clarify this point. Therefore, this finding of a second gene has modestly complicated the use of gene linkage for this disease. In white families (because they are likely to be ADPKD1), even small ones, with no crossover, the diagnostic accuracy of chromosome 16 probes remains high. In non-white families or families with crossovers, more individuals will need to be tested to verify that the family is likely to be ADPKD1, and therefore the current probes can be of value.

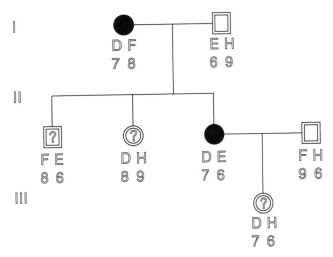

Fig. 2-2. The symbols in this figure are the same as in Figure 2-1. In this family, the two marker genes that flank the autosomal dominant polycystic kidney disease 1 (ADPKD1) gene are determined, one with forms D, E, F, G, and H and the other with forms 6, 7, 8, and 9. Analysis of two affected members demonstrates that the ADPKD1 gene segregates with the markers D and 7. Thus, the third-generation female with D7 and H6 markers has a greater than 95 percent likelihood of having the ADPKD1 gene. Similarly, the second-generation male with F8 and E6 confidently does not have the gene. Of interest is the second-generation female with D8 and H9. She inherited H9 from her father and D8 from her mother. D8 must represent a crossover during meiosis with D from one of her mother's chromosomes and 8 from the other. We cannot tell from this whether the crossover left the ADPKD1 gene with the D part or the 7 part of the chromosome, thus we cannot predict this person's gene status with confidence.

This method is highly accurate and does not require that renal cysts be detectable in the patient as long as the proband has demonstrable disease. Is this the diagnostic test of choice for ADPKD? We believe that gene linkage analysis has still not replaced renal imaging for the following reasons: (1) At least two patients in a family need to have imaging studies to establish the diagnosis and to determine which marker type is segregating with ADPKD. (2) Imaging studies are obviously done only on the patient under question. Gene linkage studies, however, require that other family members be tested. (3) A characteristic ultrasonogram in an ADPKD family member confirms the diagnosis with virtually 100 percent accuracy. (4) Imaging studies provide information about anatomic disease severity that gene typing does not. (5) Renal ultrasonography is considerably less expensive. Gene linkage becomes the test of choice when the need to diagnose ADPKD is clinically important and when renal imaging is either not diagnostic or not likely to be diagnostic. The latter circumstance occurs with prenatal testing.

Prenatal Diagnosis

The prenatal diagnosis of ADPKD can now be made with both imaging and gene linkage techniques in fetuses. Although no prospective studies of at-risk fetuses have been conducted to determine the frequency of detectable renal abnormalities in utero, in a number of reports, ADPKD has been identified in utero with ultrasonography.[21,30,63–71] Fetal kidneys can be visualized as early as 14 to 16 weeks, and two such fetuses have been described with abnormalities compatible with ADPKD.[63,65] However, three other fetuses who underwent serial ultrasonographic studies demonstrated normal kidneys at 16, 21, and 21 weeks only to demonstrate characteristic abnormalities after 30, 36, and 28 weeks.[67,69] In fact, most reports of fetal ADPKD detected with imaging have been after the 24th week. These abnormal kidneys are large and echogenic and may or may not contain renal cysts; the findings are similar in ADPKD and ARPKD.[31] Currently, imaging techniques can only reliably detect ADPKD during the third trimester, but this disorder does not satisfy contemporary guidelines for third-trimester abortion.[72] From the perspective of family counseling, it does appear that an "early onset" of ADPKD may cluster in families. However, an insufficient number of such children have had long-term follow-up to permit definitive conclusions about their outcome. Because of this, the presence of "early onset" should not be used as a guide for deciding whether to terminate a pregnancy (see below).

The same principles and family structure that permit gene linkage techniques to be used in presymptomatic diagnosis apply to its use in the prenatal situation. The only difference is the way the cells for the DNA analysis are obtained. Either amniocentesis or chorionic villus sampling can be used. Chorionic villous sampling is advised because it permits diagnosis in the second trimester.[73] If the female in the third generation in Figure 2-2 is a fetus, the same conclusion is drawn, namely, that the fetus carries the gene for ADPKD1.

Although it appears medically appropriate to inform all parents with an at-risk fetus of the availability of prenatal diagnosis, the physician must appropriately counsel the parents about the interpretation of the results, and the physician must be aware of the complexity of attitudes regarding prenatal diagnosis in this disorder. First, identification that a fetus has a 95 percent chance of being a gene carrier does not predict the natural history of the disorder in such carriers; specifically, the mere presence of the gene does not provide any information regarding age of onset or likelihood of end stage renal disease. Second, it is well to remember that, currently, approximately 50 percent of ADPKD patients are reported to be alive and without end stage renal disease at ages 58 and 73 years in different studies.[28,74] Thus, even without additional improvements in therapy, most patients will live over half a century.

The attitudes regarding prenatal diagnosis in ADPKD are likely to be influenced by the fact that one parent is alive and affected; therefore, in some sense, judgments about the fetus reflect a judgment about the parent. Clearly, this is different from recessive disorders in which neither parent is affected. The study by Sujansky et al. underscores these attitudinal issues. Sixty-five percent of affected individuals in the child-bearing years stated that they would use prenatal diagnosis.[19] However, only 4 percent would definitely terminate a pregnancy for ADPKD, but 25 percent would terminate a pregnancy for an unspecified "very serious medical problem." This suggests that in some sense these affected subjects do not consider this a very serious condition.[19] Substantiating this attitude is the fact that none of our patients have in fact elected to use prenatal diagnosis during a pregnancy. Moreover, despite the availability of gene linkage since 1986, there are only three reports in which it was used to terminate an affected fetus.[63,75,76]

WHEN AND HOW TO DIAGNOSE EXTRARENAL MANIFESTATIONS OF ADPKD

Because it is apparent that ADPKD is a systemic disorder, the logical question is whether every patient with ADPKD should be evaluated for the entire range of extrarenal abnormalities. The answer to this question appears to vary considerably with the patient's age, family history, and clinical circumstances. Although data on children are scarce, current information suggests that extrarenal manifestations are so infrequent in children that evaluation for these manifestations is not warranted. It appears that most of the extrarenal manifestations increase with age, as do the complications related to these abnormalities. In general, therefore, older adults are likely to have the greatest benefit from knowledge of the extrarenal manifestations.

Intracranial Aneurysms

Intracranial aneurysms are not the most frequent extrarenal manifestation, but they are the most dreaded. About 10 to 20 percent of ADPKD patients appear to have aneurysms[77] and about one-half of these rupture.[78] Unfortunately, the mortality after rupture appears to be greater than 50 percent. The clinical questions are who should be studied and with what modality.

Levey et al. concluded that cerebral arteriography was not cost-effective for screening all patients with ADPKD for aneurysms.[77] However, they suggested that a less expensive, less morbid, equally accurate diagnostic technique might change this analysis. Such a technique has not yet emerged. We have used dynamic CT to search for aneurysms. The method is reliably capable of detecting aneurysms greater than 4 to 5 mm in diameter. In two studies, 94 percent of 80 aneurysms greater than 5 mm in diameter were identified.[79,80] In our experience, approximately 15 percent of ADPKD patients studied with this method had an abnormal study, but about one-quarter of the abnormalities were nonpathologic anatomic variants.[81] Thus, this method may have a high false-positive rate. Others have not detected aneurysms in ADPKD patients using CT or MRI. Currently, MRI does not appear to have sufficient sensitivity to be used as a screening tool. However, this modality is rapidly being improved and may eventually prove useful. At present, direct four-vessel arteriography remains the gold standard for detection of intracranial aneurysms.

We have found that intracranial aneurysms rupture with increased frequency when there is a family history of cerebral hemorrhage.[37] No other risk factor has been related to rupture of intracranial aneurysms. However, subjects whose profession or avocation would put them or others at exceedingly high risk in the event of a rupture also should be considered to have a risk factor. Some would be greatly incapacitated by even mild residual damage from a hemorrhage.

Thus, we recommend that dynamic CT be performed in ADPKD patients with symptoms of aneurysms, in those patients over 21 years of age in whom there is a family history of aneurysm, and in patients with occupational or avocational risks. Patients with suspicious or indeterminate CT studies should undergo direct four-vessel arteriography. In those with aneurysms exceeding 10 mm in diameter, we advise prophylactic clipping. Smaller aneurysms may be followed with yearly tomographic studies.

Hepatic Cysts

Hepatic cysts are the most common extrarenal manifestation of ADPKD. They increase with age and with increasing severity of the structural and functional renal abnormality.[82] Of note, massive hepatic cystic disease as well as complications of hepatic cysts are largely restricted to women.[82-84] Pregnancy significantly influences the severity of hepatic cystic involvement, underscoring the role for female steroid hormones in modifying the severity of this manifestation.[82] Therefore, we do not routinely recommend evaluating the liver for cysts in men, but do tend to recommend this in women who have had children, are planning pregnancy, or are contemplating the use of female steroid hormones. Although data specifically addressing the relationship between use of female steroid hormones and hepatic cystic disease are lacking, significant hepatic cystic disease should stimulate the physician to consider carefully the use of such hormones and to counsel the patients regarding the potential effects of pregnancy.

Mitral Valve Prolapse

Mitral valve prolapse is the second most common extrarenal manifestation.[36] Patients should undergo echocardiography only if they have cardiac signs or symptoms that would prompt intervention, if they experience a central nervous system event that is compatible with an embolic event, or if the murmur of mitral valve regurgitation is detected even without symptoms. Antibiotic prophylaxis needs to be considered.

Colonic Diverticulosis

Diverticular disease of the colon appears to be a very common abnormality in ADPKD patients with end stage renal failure.[85] Because of the apparently high morbidity and mortality of this extrarenal manifestation in the transplanted patient, some transplant surgeons suggest barium enemas in all ADPKD patients before transplantation.[86–88] Although no prophylactic surgery is recommended for this finding, it does alert the transplant team to the patient's potential for an acute abdominal event. Currently, no prospective studies provide guidelines for screening for this manifestation in the asymptomatic patient.

WHEN AND HOW TO DIAGNOSE COMPLICATIONS OF ADPKD

We see no need for routine follow-up imaging studies of the kidneys once the diagnosis of ADPKD has been established. However, the systemic nature of ADPKD puts many organ systems at risk for complications. These complications are approached in the same way that they would in patients without ADPKD. This group of complications includes rupture of an intracranial aneurysm, sequelae of mitral valve prolapse, diverticulitis or perforated diverticulum, and consequences of inguinal hernias. However, five problems may require a somewhat more specialized approach: chronic and acute abdominal pain, sepsis, urinary tract obstruction, gross hematuria, and renal cell carcinoma. Unfortunately, there is a paucity of scientific information to support the best approaches.

Abdominal Pain

In a few patients disabled by pain or sheer abdominal mass of the cysts, both surgical cyst decompression and percutaneous cyst decompression have produced significant pain relief without further impairing renal function.[89–91] The surgical approach offers the opportunity to decompress numerous cysts; the percutaneous approach permits only a few large cysts to be decompressed and as currently performed has only a temporary effect in most patients as a result of fluid reaccumulation within the cyst. The efficacy and safety of alcohol sclerosis to prevent reaccumulation of fluid in ADPKD as done with simple cysts remains to be examined further.[90]

Just as renal cysts can cause disability, so can massive hepatomegaly in a few instances, particularly in women. In this setting, percutaneous decompression of large cysts can be helpful.[92] The same caveats apply as in renal cysts. Surgical cyst fenestration and partial hepatectomy have also been used with success.[93,94] Surgical cyst decompression for both the liver and kidney should be reserved for severely disabled patients and should be performed by surgeons with experience in this procedure.

The specialized differential diagnosis of severe abdominal pain in the ADPKD patient includes acute hemorrhage, rupture, or infection of a renal or hepatic cyst; obstruction of the urinary tract by a stone; diverticulitis or perforation of a diverticulum; and incarcerated or strangulated inguinal hernia.

Renal and Hepatic Cyst Infections

Flank or abdominal pain accompanied by leukocytosis, fever, and increased sedimentation rate should raise the question of infection of a renal or hepatic cyst. History and physical examination will help localize the pain and point toward a cause. Acute pyelonephritis and renal parenchymal infection are often accompanied by positive blood cultures and white blood cell casts and respond to the antibiotics commonly used for urinary tract infections.[24] Cyst infections, although accompanied by fever, often are not marked by positive blood cultures, striking pyuria, or white blood cell casts.

Because larger cysts are no longer in continuity with the renal tubule,[95] their infection is blood borne or derives from local spread. The urine will not reflect this type of infection unless the infected cyst ruptures into the urinary tract, at which time pain is often relieved. Renal tenderness and failure to respond to standard antibiotic treatment should raise the possibility of cyst infection. If the patient fails to improve after about 72 hours of treatment with cyst-penetrating antibiotics or worsens, we perform CT without and then with contrast material. If this fails to show signs of localized infection such as thickening and stranding of perinephric fascia and cyst wall thickening, then an indium-111 (^{111}In)–labeled leukocyte scan may help define an abscess or cyst infection.[96] Radiolabeled gallium scanning has not been successful in our experience or in that of others.[24] Percutaneous cyst puncture of a suspicious-appearing cyst can confirm the diagnosis of cyst infection and identify the organism responsible and can provide drainage.[97] In general, however, the approach is not drainage but treatment with the antibiotics that penetrate cysts exceptionally well.[24,98]

Hepatic cyst infection may occur. The same diagnostic approach as for renal cyst infection may be taken. The best outcome, however, has been in patients with percutaneous or surgical cyst drainage and antibiotic therapy.[84]

Urinary Tract Obstruction

The increased frequency of renal calculi in ADPKD[25] increases the risk of obstruction. Ultrasonography is not recommended as the first choice to diagnose upper urinary tract obstruction in subjects with well-developed cysts. Rather, CT with contrast will provide definition of the upper urinary tract from overlying and surrounding cystic renal parenchyma. Depending on the GFR, excretory urography or retrograde pyelography can identify the level of ureteral obstruction. Lithotripsy has been used without apparent complication and with success in removing calcium stones in ADPKD.[99]

Hematuria and Renal Cell Carcinoma

Gross hematuria that lasts more than several days, is accompanied by significant prolonged pain, or occurs for the first time in patients over age 50 requires further investigation. CT appears to be the most appropriate imaging study in this circumstance in that newly hemorrhagic cysts are easily identified and may require no further intervention in a young patient and renal calculi are usually well visualized. If gross hematuria first occurs in the older patient, the question of renal and bladder malignancy arises. Renal cell carcinoma occurs in patients with ADPKD before the end stage.[100,101] Some believe that it is more common in ADPKD[23] and that ADPKD shares the biologic features of neoplasia.[102] A review of the Mayo Clinic autopsy and surgical collection of 87 cases revealed neoplastic proliferations in 24 percent of patients. However, only 2 of 87 (2.3 percent) were malignant (renal cell carcinoma in one and transitional cell carcinoma in the other).[103] In addition to gross hematuria, a changing pattern of renal pain, unilateral renal enlargement, and systemic symptoms and signs of malignancy should induce the clinician to look for a neoplasm. CT detects renal masses as small as 0.5 cm in diameter[50] and is the imaging modality of choice. Renal arteriography may be useful to detect neoplastic vascular patterns.

SUMMARY

Thus, diagnostic decision making in ADPKD entails the assessment and utility of the methods for making an initial diagnosis and the indications for the evaluation of extrarenal manifestations and for diagnosing and managing complications. Although we have new diagnostic tools in our armamentarium, we must use them wisely in the context of total patient care. At each diagnostic decision point, clinical judgment must be exercised, weighing the risks and the benefits. At decision points at which the disease or its manifestations may be first revealed, counseling the patient regarding outcomes and interpretation of information is imperative. In this counseling, the physician must be aware of and sensitive to the attitudes that accompany ADPKD. These guidelines should assist all of us in the care of patients with this most common hereditary disorder.

REFERENCES

1. Gabow PA: Autosomal dominant polycystic kidney disease—more than a renal disease. Am J Kidney Dis 16:403, 1990
2. Reeders ST, Breuning MH, Davies KE et al: A highly polymorphic DNA marker linked to adult polycystic kidney disease on chromosome 16. Nature 317:542, 1985
3. Kimberling WJ, Fain PR, Kenyon JB et al: Linkage heterogeneity of autosomal dominant polycystic kidney disease. N Engl J Med 319:913, 1988
4. Romeo G, Devoto M, Costa G et al: A second genetic locus for autosomal dominant polycystic kidney disease. Lancet 2:8, 1988
5. Yium JJ, Martinez Maldonado M et al: Autosomal dominant polycystic kidney disease in blacks, sickle-cell trait, clinical and genetic studies, abstracted. Sixth International Interdisciplinary Conference on Hypertension in Blacks: Health and Disease in Multicultural Societies: A Focus on Miscegenation. Salvador, Bahia, Brazil, 1991
6. Kimberling WJ, Pieke SA, Kenyon JB, Gabow PA: An estimate of the proportion of families with autosomal dominant polycystic kidney disease unlinked to chromosome 16, abstracted. Kidney Int 37:249, 1990
7. Higgins CC: Bilateral polycystic kidney disease: review of ninety-four cases. Arch Surg 65:318, 1952
8. Simon HB, Thompson GJ: Congenital renal polycystic disease: a clinical and therapeutic study of three hundred sixty-six cases. JAMA 159:657, 1955
9. Ward JN, Draper JW, Lavengood RW, Jr: A clinical review of polycystic kidney disease in 53 patients. J Urol 98:48, 1967
10. Sahney S, Weiss L, Levin NW: Genetic counseling in adult polycystic kidney disease. Am J Med Genet 11:461, 1982
11. Iglesias CG, Torres VE, Offord KP et al: Epidemiology of adult polycystic kidney disease, Olmstead County, Minnesota: 1935–1980. Am J Kidney Dis 2:630, 1983
12. Delaney VB, Adler S, Bruns FJ et al: Autosomal dominant polycystic kidney disease: presentation, complications, and prognosis. Am J Kidney Dis 5:104, 1985
13. Gabow PA, Grantham JJ, Bennett W et al: Gene testing in autosomal dominant polycystic kidney disease: results of National Kidney Foundation workshop. Am J Kidney Dis 13:85, 1989
14. Oppenheimer GD: Polycystic disease of the kidney. Ann Surg 100:1136, 1934
15. Dalgaard OZ: Bilateral polycystic disease of the kidneys: a follow-up of two hundred and eighty-four patients and their families. Acta Med Scand [Suppl] 328:1, 1957
16. Gabow PA, Iklé DW, Holmes JH: Polycystic kidney disease: prospective analysis of nonazotemic patients and family members. Ann Intern Med 101:238, 1984
17. Gonzalo A, Rivera M, Quereda C, Ortuno J: Clinical features and prognosis of adult polycystic kidney disease. Am J Nephrol 10:470, 1990
18. Milutinovic J, Fialkow PJ, Agodoa LY et al: Clinical manifestations of autosomal dominant polycystic kidney disease in patients older than 50 years. Am J Kidney Dis 15:237, 1990
19. Sujansky E, Kreutzer SB, Johnson AM et al: Attitudes of at-risk and affected individuals regarding presymptomatic testing for autosomal dominant polycystic kidney disease. Am J Med Genet 35:510, 1990

20. Zeier M, Geberth S, Ritz E et al: Adult dominant polycystic kidney disease—clinical problems. Nephron 49:177, 1988
21. Sedman A, Bell P, Manco-Johnson M et al: Autosomal dominant polycystic kidney disease in childhood: a longitudinal study. Kidney Int 31:1000, 1987
22. Kaariainen H, Koskimies O, Norio R: Dominant and recessive polycystic kidney disease in children: evaluation of clinical features and laboratory data. Pediatr Nephrol 2:296, 1988
23. Gardner KD, Jr, Evan AP: Cystic kidneys: an enigma evolves. Am J Kidney Dis 3:403, 1984
24. Schwab SJ, Bander SJ, Klahr S: Renal infection in autosomal dominant polycystic kidney disease. Am J Med 82:714, 1987
25. Torres VE, Erickson SB, Smith LH et al: The association of nephrolithiasis and autosomal dominant polycystic kidney disease. Am J Kidney Dis 11:318, 1988
26. Johnson CM, Wilson DM, O'Fallon WM et al: Renal stone epidemiology: a 25-year study in Rochester, Minnesota. Kidney Int 16:624, 1979
27. Hiatt RA, Dales LG, Friedman GD, Hunkeler EM: Frequency of urolithiasis in a prepaid medical care program. Am J Epidemiol 115:255, 1982
28. Parfrey PS, Bear JC, Morgan J et al: The diagnosis and prognosis of autosomal dominant polycystic kidney disease. N Engl J Med 323:1085, 1990
29. Ravine D, Walker RG, Gibson RN et al: Treatable complications in undiagnosed cases of autosomal dominant polycystic kidney disease. Lancet 337:127, 1991
30. Pretorius DH, Lee ME, Manco-Johnson ML et al: Diagnosis of autosomal dominant polycystic disease in utero and in the young infant. J Ultrasound Med 6:249, 1987
31. Cole BR, Conley SB, Stapleton FB: Polycystic kidney disease in the first year of life. J Pediatr 111:693, 1987
32. Cobben JM, Breuning MH, Schoots C et al: Congenital hepatic fibrosis in autosomal-dominant polycystic kidney disease. Kidney Int 38:880, 1990
33. Matsuda O, Ideura T, Shinoda T et al: Polycystic kidney of autosomal dominant inheritance, polycystic liver and congenital hepatic fibrosis in a single kindred. Am J Nephrol 10:237, 1990
34. Gabow PA, Schrier RW: Pathophysiology of adult polycystic kidney disease. Adv Nephrol 18:19, 1989
35. Leier CV, Baker PB, Kilman JW, Wooley CF: Cardiovascular abnormalities associated with adult polycystic kidney disease. Ann Intern Med 100:683, 1984
36. Hossack KF, Leddy CL, Johnson AM et al: Echocardiographic findings in autosomal dominant polycystic kidney disease. N Engl J Med 319:907, 1988
37. Kaehny W, Bell P, Earnest M et al: Family clustering of intracranial aneurysms in autosomal dominant polycystic kidney disease, abstracted. Kidney Int 31:204, 1987
38. Tada S, Yamagishi J, Kobayashi H et al: The incidence of simple renal cyst by computed tomography. Clin Radiol 34:437, 1983
39. Mir S, Rapola J, Koskimies O: Renal cysts in pediatric autopsy material. Nephron 33:189, 1983
40. Martinez-Maldonado M, Yium JJ, Eknoyan G, Suki WN: Adult polycystic kidney disease: studies of the defect in urine concentration. Kidney Int 2:107, 1972
41. D'Angelo A, Mioni G, Ossi E et al: Alterations in renal tubular sodium and water transport in polycystic kidney disease. Clin Nephrol 3:99, 1975

42. Preuss H, Geoly K, Johnson M et al: Tubular function in adult polycystic kidney disease. Nephron 24:198, 1979
43. Gabow PA, Kaehny WD, Johnson AM et al: The clinical utility of renal concentrating capacity in polycystic kidney disease. Kidney Int 35:675, 1989
44. Mellins HZ: Radiologic diagnosis. p. 19. In Grantham JJ, Gardner KD (eds): Problems in Diagnosis and Management of Polycystic Kidney Disease. PKR Foundation, Kansas City, 1985
45. Milutinovic J, Fialkow PJ, Phillips LA et al: Autosomal dominant polycystic kidney disease: early diagnosis and data for genetic counselling. Lancet 1:1203, 1980
46. Levine E, Grantham JJ: The role of computed tomography in the evaluation of adult polycystic kidney disease. Am J Kidney Dis 1:99, 1981
47. Lawson TL, McClennan BL, Shirkhoda A: Adult polycystic kidney disease: ultrasonographic and computed tomographic appearance. JCU 6:297, 1978
48. Rosenfield AT, Lipson MH, Wolf B et al: Ultrasonography and nephrotomography in the presymptomatic diagnosis of dominantly inherited (adult-onset) polycystic kidney disease. Radiology 135:423, 1980
49. Segal AJ, Spataro RF: Computed tomography of adult polycystic disease. J Comput Assist Tomogr 6:777, 1982
50. Warshauer DM, McCarthy SM, Street L et al: Detection of renal masses: sensitivities and specificities of excretory urography/linear tomography, US, and CT. Radiology 169:363, 1988
51. Levine E, Grantham JJ: High-density renal cysts in autosomal dominant polycystic kidney disease demonstrated by CT. Radiology 154:477, 1985
52. Meziane MA, Fishman EK, Goldman SM et al: Computed tomography of high density renal cysts in adult polycystic kidney disease. J Comput Assist Tomogr 10:767, 1986
53. Leung AW-L, Bydder GM, Steiner RE et al: Magnetic resonance imaging of the kidneys. AJR 143:1215, 1984
54. Hilpert PL, Friedman AC, Radecki PD et al: MRI of hemorrhagic renal cysts in polycystic kidney disease. AJR 146:1167, 1986
55. Milutinovic J, Agodoa LY, Cutler RE, Striker GE: Autosomal dominant polycystic kidney disease: early diagnosis and consideration of pathogenesis. Am J Clin Pathol 73:740, 1980
56. Panisello JM, Martinez-Vea A, Garcia C et al: IgA nephropathy and polycystic kidney disease. Am J Nephrol 8:477, 1988
57. Murphy G, Tzamaloukas AH, Listrom MB et al: Nephrotic syndrome and rapid renal failure in autosomal dominant polycystic kidney disease. Am J Nephrol 10:69, 1990
58. Bachner L, Kaplan J-C: Molecular genetics and polycystic kidney diseases. Adv Nephrol 18:3, 1989
59. Breuning MH, Reeders ST, Brunner H et al: Improved early diagnosis of adult polycystic kidney disease with flanking DNA markers. Lancet 2:1359, 1987
60. Reeders ST, Germino GG, Gillespie GAJ: Recent advances in the genetics of renal cystic disease. Mol Biol Med 6:81, 1989
61. Dawson DB, Torres VE, Charboneau JW, Thibodeau SN: Detection of a family with autosomal dominant polycystic kidney disease loosely linked to DNA markers from 16p, abstracted. Kidney Int 35:203, 1989
62. Brissenden JE, Roscoe JM, Silverman M: Linkage heterogeneity for autosomal dominant polycystic kidney disease studied by DNA and chromosomal analysis, abstracted. Kidney Int 37:247, 1990

63. Ceccherini I, Lituania M, Cordone MS et al: Autosomal dominant polycystic kidney disease: prenatal diagnosis by DNA analysis and sonography at 14 weeks. Prenat Diagn 9:751, 1989

64. Cohen HL, Haller JO: Diagnostic sonography of the fetal genitourinary tract. Urol Radiol 9:88, 1987

65. Fryns JP, Vandenberghe K, Moerman F: Mid-trimester ultrasonographic diagnosis of early manifesting "adult" form of polycystic kidney disease, letter. Hum Genet 74:461, 1986

66. Gal A, Wirth B, Kaariainen H et al: Childhood manifestation of autosomal dominant polycystic kidney disease: no evidence for genetic heterogeneity. Clin Genet 35:13, 1989

67. Journel H, Guyot C, Barc RM et al: Unexpected ultrasonographic prenatal diagnosis of autosomal dominant polycystic kidney disease. Prenat Diagn 9:663, 1989

68. Kaariainen H: Polycystic kidney disease in children: a genetic and epidemiological study of 82 Finnish patients. J Med Genet 24:474, 1987

69. Main D, Mennuti MT, Cornfeld D, Coleman B: Prenatal diagnosis of adult polycystic kidney disease, letter. Lancet 2:337, 1983

70. Zerres K, Weiss H, Bulla M, Roth B: Prenatal diagnosis of an early manifestation of autosomal dominant adult-type polycystic kidney disease, letter. Lancet 2:988, 1982

71. Zerres K, Hansmann M, Knopfle G, Stephan M: Prenatal diagnosis of genetically determined early manifestation of autosomal dominant polycystic kidney disease? Hum Genet 71:368, 1985

72. Chervenak FA, Farley MA, Walters LR et al: When is termination of pregnancy during the third trimester morally justifiable? N Engl J Med 310:501, 1984

73. Gabow PA, Wilkins-Haug L: Prediction of the likelihood of polycystic kidney disease in the fetus when a parent has autosomal dominant polycystic kidney disease. In Andreucci VE, Fine LG (eds): International Yearbook of Nephrology 1992. Kluwer Academic Publishers, Boston, in press

74. Churchill DN, Bear JC, Morgan J et al: Prognosis of adult onset polycystic kidney disease re-evaluated. Kidney Int 26:190, 1984

75. Reeders ST, Gal A, Propping P et al: Prenatal diagnosis of autosomal dominant polycystic kidney disease with a DNA probe. Lancet 2:6, 1986

76. Novelli G, Frontali M, Baldini D et al: Prenatal diagnosis of adult polycystic kidney disease with DNA markers on chromosome 16 and the genetic heterogeneity problem. Prenat Diagn 9:759, 1989

77. Levey AS, Pauker SG, Kassirer JP: Occult intracranial aneurysms in polycystic kidney disease: when is cerebral arteriography indicated? N Engl J Med 308:986, 1983

78. Weir B: Intracranial aneurysms and subarachnoid hemorrhage: an overview. p. 1308. In Wilkins RH, Rengachary SS (eds): Neurosurgery. McGraw-Hill, St. Louis, 1985

79. Schmid UD, Steiger HJ, Huber P: Accuracy of high resolution computed tomography in direct diagnosis of cerebral aneurysms. Neuroradiology 29:152, 1987

80. Torres VE, Wiebers DO, Forbes GS: Cranial computed tomography and magnetic resonance imaging in autosomal dominant polycystic kidney disease. J Am Soc Nephrol 1:84, 1990

81. Kaehny WD, Chapman AB, Stears JC et al: Prospective imaging study of asymptomatic intracranial aneurysms in polycystic kidney disease, abstracted. Kidney Int 37:249, 1990

82. Gabow PA, Johnson AM, Kaehny WD et al: Risk factors for the development of hepatic cysts in autosomal dominant polycystic kidney disease. Hepatology 11:1033, 1990

83. Everson GT, Scherzinger A, Berger-Leff N et al: Polycystic liver disease: quantitation of parenchymal and cyst volumes from computed tomography images and clinical correlates of hepatic cysts. Hepatology 8:1627, 1988

84. Telenti A, Torres VE, Gross JB, Jr et al: Hepatic cyst infection in autosomal dominant polycystic kidney disease. Mayo Clin Proc 65:933, 1990

85. Scheff RT, Zuckerman G, Harter H et al: Diverticular disease in patients with chronic renal failure due to polycystic kidney disease. Ann Intern Med 92:202, 1980

86. Carson SD, Krom RAF, Uchida K et al: Colon perforation after kidney transplantation. Ann Surg 188:109, 1978

87. Guice K, Rattazzi LC, Marchioro TL: Colon perforation in renal transplant patients. Am J Surg 138:43, 1979

88. Hadjiyannakis EJ, Smellie WAB, Evans DB, Calne RY: Gastrointestinal complications after renal transplantation. Lancet 2:781, 1971

89. Bennett WM, Elzinga L, Golper TA, Barry JM: Reduction of cyst volume for symptomatic management of autosomal dominant polycystic kidney disease. J Urol 137:620, 1987

90. Garcia MG, Bru C, Campistol JM et al: Effect of reduction of cystic volume by percutaneous cystic puncture on the renal function in polycystic kidney disease, letter. Nephron 56:459, 1990

91. Frang D, Czvalinga I, Polyak L: A new approach to the treatment of polycystic kidneys. Int Urol Nephrol 20:13, 1988

92. Ergun H, Wolf BH, Hissong SL: Obstructive jaundice caused by polycystic liver disease. Radiology 136:435, 1980

93. Howard RJ, Hanson RF, Delaney JP: Jaundice associated with polycystic liver disease: relief by surgical decompression of the cysts. Arch Surg 111:816, 1976

94. van Erpecum KJ, Janssens AR, Terpstra JL, Tjon A Tham RTO: Highly symptomatic adult polycystic disease of the liver. J Hepatology 5:109, 1987

95. Grantham JJ, Geiser JL, Evan AP: Cyst formation and growth in autosomal dominant polycystic kidney disease. Kidney Int 31:1145, 1987

96. Bretan PN, Jr, Price DC, McClure RD: Localization of abscess in adult polycystic kidney by indium-111 leukocyte scan. Urology 32:169, 1988

97. Chapman AB, Thickman D, Gabow PA: Percutaneous cyst puncture in the treatment of cyst infection in autosomal dominant polycystic kidney disease. Am J Kidney Dis 16:252, 1990

98. Sklar AH, Caruana RJ, Lammers JE, Strauser GD: Renal infections in autosomal dominant polycystic kidney disease. Am J Kidney Dis 10:81, 1987

99. Williamson BRJ, Paling MR, Lippert MC, Jenkins AD: Computerized tomographic appearance of renal cysts after extracorporeal shock wave lithotripsy. South Med J 83:287, 1990

100. McFarland WL, Wallace S, Johnson DE: Renal carcinoma and polycystic disease. J Urol 107:530, 1972

101. Roberts PF: Bilateral renal carcinoma associated with polycystic kidneys. Br Med J 3:273, 1973

102. Grantham JJ: Polycystic kidney disease: neoplasia in disguise. Am J Kidney Dis 15:110, 1990

103. Gregoire JR, Torres VE, Holley KE, Farrow GM: Renal epithelial hyperplastic and neoplastic proliferation in autosomal dominant polycystic kidney disease. Am J Kidney Dis 9:27, 1987

3

The Differential Diagnosis of Acute Renal Failure

Micheal J. Adcox
Bonnie Collins
Richard A. Zager

Aminoglycoside Nephrotoxicity
Radiocontrast-Induced ARF
ARF in Multiple Myeloma
Postischemic ATN

OTHER ACUTE PARENCHYMAL RENAL DISEASES
Acute Glomerulonephritis
Acute Interstitial Nephritis
Drug-Induced AIN
NSAID-Induced AIN
AIN in Systemic Diseases
Systemic Infection-Associated AIN
Acute Renal Vascular Disease
Acute Renal Arterial Thrombosis and Thromboembolism
Bilateral Cortical Necrosis
The Microvasculopathies
Renal Vein Thrombosis

URINARY TRACT OBSTRUCTION
Urine Assessments
Serum Chemistries
Radiologic Procedures
Intrarenal Obstruction

SUMMARY

INTRODUCTION

Acute renal failure (ARF) is a term used to describe a sudden decrease in renal function that is of sufficient magnitude and duration that progressive increments in the blood urea nitrogen (BUN) and plasma creatinine (Cr) concentrations result. It is a syndrome, not a specific disease. Thus, its presence mandates a careful differential diagnostic approach, encompassing historical, physical, and laboratory assessments. That 4 to 5 percent of patients admitted to medical-surgical services develop ARF[1] and that the therapy of its possible causes differ greatly underscore the importance of an accurate diagnostic assessment.

Traditionally, ARF has been broadly subdivided into prerenal (hemodynamic), postrenal (obstruction), and intrinsic (parenchymal) causes. Although this approach is a useful one and will be used to help organize this review, it must be recalled that numerous diseases, reflecting very different pathophysiologic mechanisms, can fall within each of these classifications (Fig. 3-1). Thus, correct assignment of a patient to a particular category is only a first step toward obtaining the diagnosis. The potential causes of acute and chronic renal failure (CRF) are equally broad, and the former often complicates the latter. Therefore, the diagnostic approach to the ARF patient can, indeed, be a challenging mental exercise.

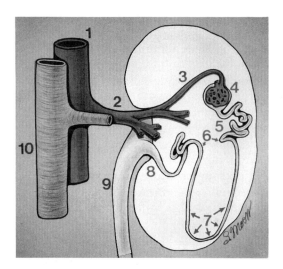

Fig. 3-1. Differential diagnostic overview of acute renal failure; 10 types of lesions should be considered: (*1*) hemodynamic factors leading to prerenal azotemia; (*2*) renal arterial occlusion; (*3*) intrarenal vasculopathies; (*4*) acute glomerulonephritis; (*5, 6*) acute tubular necrosis: most nephrotoxins involve the proximal tubular epithelium (*5*), whereas ischemia may induce injury to both proximal and medullary thick ascending limb segments (*6*); (*7*) acute interstitial nephritis; (*8*) intratubular obstruction; (*9*) extrarenal obstruction; and (*10*) renal venous thrombosis.

GENERAL CONSIDERATIONS

Acute Versus Chronic Renal Failure

In some instances, the first issue that needs to be addressed is whether a patient does, in fact, have ARF, rather than a previously undiagnosed chronic renal disease. Most often, this differential diagnosis is readily accomplished either because (1) the ARF developed in the hospital; (2) the recent history suggests an ARF-precipitating event (e.g., trauma, shock); or (3) a history of CRF exists. In some individuals, however, none of these historical features are present, and ARF must be differentiated from CRF. A careful history searching for chronic diseases that can produce renal failure (e.g., diabetes), a remote history of abnormal laboratory results, or symptoms suggestive of an insidious rather than an acute illness may be helpful. Oliguria and/or daily increments in the BUN and Cr concentrations almost always indicate ARF because they imply virtually no renal function.

If the preceding considerations fail to differentiate ARF from CRF, laboratory and roentgenographic assessments are needed. An abdominal ultrasound is, in general, the most useful test because small kidneys (less than 9 to 10 cm) strongly indicate CRF, while at the same time exclude urinary tract obstruction. Although normal or large kidneys generally imply ARF, this is not 100 percent reliable, because some CRF patients can maintain normal renal dimensions, despite an insidious loss of renal function. Severe anemia has been used as another index of chronicity. Many ARF patients, however, have a recent history of blood loss, or they have underlying illnesses that produce anemia (e.g., malignancies). Thus, a *normal* hemoglobin concentration may be more helpful than anemia because the former is unlikely with advanced CRF. Renal osteodystrophy, as observed by radiograph (e.g., erosion of distal portions of the clavicles) clearly indicates CRF. However, bone changes observed on radiographs usually are absent in CRF patients at the time of their presentation, mitigating their diagnostic value. Hypocalcemia, hyperphosphatemia, and hyperuricemia are usually present in CRF patients. These findings, however, can quickly develop during ARF; thus, their presence has little diagnostic significance. The history, documentation of normal kidney size, and the presence of oliguria and/or rapidly advancing azotemia are the most reliable indices of ARF. On some occasions, however, only a renal biopsy can make this differentiation.

ARF in the Setting of Chronic Renal Disease

Even when a history of chronic nephropathy exists, it is important to consider the possibility of an acute, superimposed disease process if the observed BUN and Cr concentrations are inconsistent with previous determinations. Indeed, patients with chronic renal disease may be predisposed to develop ARF. For example, intravascular volume depletion (prerenal azotemia) may occur in such patients because of excessive diuretic use, and/or nausea and vomiting coupled with an inability to generate a sodium-free urine. Nonsteroidal antiinflammatory drugs (NSAIDs) and converting enzyme inhibitors (CEI) can have their greatest hemodynamic (and hence, functional) impact in renal disease patients (see following discussion). Preexistent renal insufficiency may predispose to acute tubular necrosis (ATN). For example, chronic renal disease is a major risk factor for radiocontrast-induced ARF (see following), and failure to appropriately reduce the dose of nephrotoxic agents (e.g., aminoglycosides) for a given decrement in renal function, may produce nephrotoxicity. Because patients with chronic nephropathies often receive a multiplicity of therapeutic agents, allergic interstitial nephritis may develop. Finally, some chronic nephropathies undergo acute exacerbations (e.g., systemic lupus erythematosis [SLE], immunoglobulin A [IgA] nephropathy), they may predispose to complications (e.g., renal vein thromobosis resulting from nephrotic syndrome), or they may produce apparent de novo ATN.[2] Thus, the presence of chronic renal disease does not negate the need for a careful diagnostic approach if an unexpected decrement in renal function occurs. Unfortunately, this can be a difficult process because the urinary findings at such times represent a composite of both the chronic and acute disease processes. Thus, these tests need to be considered in the context of baseline laboratory assessments and in light of the history and clinical examination.

Urine Flow Rate

ARF has been subdivided into anuric, oliguric, and nonoliguric subtypes, based on 24-hour urine volumes. Anuria has been defined as a volume of 0 to 50 ml/24 h, whereas less than 400 to 500 ml/24 h is considered oliguria. The latter reflects the volume of urine needed to excrete the average daily osmolar load (~600 mOsm), assuming maximum urinary concentration (1,200 mOsm/L). Thus, oliguria in the face of impaired urinary concentration must denote renal failure (assuming normal solute intake), as defined by positive solute balance. The differential diagnostic value of the urinary output is quite limited. Total anuria has been considered to be highly suggestive of renal vascular catastrophes (e.g., bilateral renal artery thrombosis, cortical necrosis), urinary tract obstruction, and profound crescentic (rapidly progressive) glomerulonephritis (RPGN) and to rule out a diagnosis of prerenal azotemia or ATN. However, during the early phase of severe ATN, absolute anuria can, on occasion, be observed; RPGN more often than not has a nonoliguric presentation; and even bilateral cortical necrosis can have variable urine outputs. For these reasons, urinary output, per se, may not be terribly helpful as a diagnostic assessment.

PRERENAL AZOTEMIA/HEMODYNAMIC ARF

The term *prerenal azotemia (PRA)* refers to those forms of renal insufficiency or ARF that reflect a primary disturbance in renal hemodynamics, rather than parenchymal kidney damage. PRA is most often triggered by a decrease in cardiac output (e.g., resulting from heart failure, intravascular volume depletion) or to noncardiac-mediated increments in renal vascular resistance (e.g., sepsis, advanced liver disease). The cause of the increased renal vascular tone in each of these states may include augmented renal sympathetic activity, circulating catecholamines, angiotensin II, antidiuretic hormone (ADH), altered atrial natriuretic peptide release, platelet-activating factor, and possibly, disturbances in endothelial-derived mediators of arteriolar vascular resistance (e.g., references 3 to 5). The cascade of factors operative in each prerenal state and how they are evoked are beyond the scope of this discussion. However, the final result is an increase in afferent arteriolar resistance, a decrease in glomerular capillary pressure, and hence, a decline in the glomerular filtration rate (GFR). A compensatory increase in efferent arteriolar resistance, largely mediated by angiotensin II and norepinephrine, serves to stabilize GFR by helping to maintain glomerular capillary pressure.[6–9] However, an increase in the filtration fraction results, causing both a decrease in postglomerular capillary hydrostatic pressure and an increase in capillary oncotic pressure, thereby rendering proximal tubules highly sodium retentive.[10] These physical factors, plus several of the previously mentioned hormonal influences (e.g., angiotensin II-mediated aldosterone release, ADH, increased sympathetic tone),[11] combine to produce the avid antinatriuresis that is the hallmark of the prerenal state.

The widespread use of NSAIDs, converting enzyme inhibitors, and the increasing role of cyclosporine A as an immunosuppressive agent expands the etiologic list of factors that can induce a hemodynamic form of ARF. The first two classes of drugs will be briefly commented on later.

Diagnosis of PRA

Most typically, PRA presents as oliguric ARF in the setting of severe cardiac or hepatic disease, sepsis, or intravascular volume depletion (see Table 3-1). Since 1980, however, it has been generally accepted that a nonoliguric (or polyuric) presentation is also possible.[12–15] The nonoliguric PRA is most commonly seen in advanced liver disease. Stimulated proximal salt retention coupled with failure to maintain a concentrated medullary interstitium are likely explanations. The diminished delivery of sodium to the loop of Henle and, perhaps, altered vasa recta blood flow could be the pathogenetic causes. Because most of these patients are, in general, quite ill, other causes for ARF, particularly ATN, need to be considered. The clinical setting, the history just before the onset of the renal insufficiency, and the physical examination, are most helpful in this regard. Certainly, a decline in renal function at a time of worsening heart failure, increasing ascites, or weight loss would suggest a prerenal state. Physical signs of extracellular volume depletion (e.g., orthostatic blood pressure and pulse changes, poor skin turgor), congestive heart failure (e.g., gallops, rales, edema), or decom-

Table 3-1. Causes of Prerenal Acute Renal Failure

Intravascular volume depletion
  Renal losses: diuretics, sodium wasting disorders
  Gastrointestinal losses: vomiting, diarrhea, fistulas
  Cutaneous losses: burns, bullous diseases

Cardiopulmonary disease
  Congestive heart failure, cardiac tamponade, right-sided heart failure/poor left atrial filling (pulmonary hypertension, positive end-expiratory pressure [PEEP])

Redistribution of extracellular fluid
  Cirrhosis, sepsis, nephrotic syndrome, peritonitis, ileus, crush syndrome

Drug-induced alterations in renal hemodynamics
  Nonsteroidal antiinflammatory drugs (NSAIDS)
  Converting enzyme inhibitors (CEIs)
  Cyclosporine A

pensated cirrhosis/portal hypertension (e.g., increasing jaundice, ascites) strengthen this assessment. However, that none of these are proof of PRA and that not even a cardiac output determination by Swan Ganz catheter permits firm conclusions about renal hemodynamics (e.g., reference 13) underscores the need for laboratory data to support a presumptive clinical diagnosis of a prerenal state.

Urine Sodium Assessments

As mentioned previously, the most characteristic laboratory finding in PRA is avid sodium retention, as reflected by the *urine sodium concentration* (U_{Na}; less than 20 mEq/L), the *fractional sodium excretion** (Fe_{Na}; less than 1 percent), or the *renal failure index†* (RFI; less than 1).[1,16–22] Because the two most common forms of ARF are PRA and ATN, and because the latter typically presents with a U_{Na}, Fe_{Na}, and RFI of greater than 40 mEq/L, greater than 1 percent and greater than 1, respectively, the U_{Na} has great utility in differentiating these two conditions (discussed further in section on ATN). Several important caveats, however, must be considered before extrapolating from avid sodium retention to a diagnosis of PRA: (1) As discussed later, some ATN patients, particularly those with nonoliguric ATN, may present with a low U_{Na} concentration. (2) Diuretics, acute volume challenges, and renal vasodilator therapy may transiently raise the U_{Na} into the ATN range. (However, such therapeutic interventions should not preclude performing a U_{Na} assessment, because a low value, if found, provides even more compelling evidence for PRA). (3) Disorders other than PRA (and ATN) may, on occasion, cause sodium avidity, most typically, fulminant glomerulonephritis and short-lived urinary tract obstruction. (4) If a prerenal state is

---

* $Fe_{Na} = (U_{Na}/S_{Na} \div U_{cr}/S_{cr}) \times 100\%$.
† $RFI = (U_{Na} \div U_{cr}/S_{cr}) \times 100$ where U = urine, S = serum, cr = creatinine.

superimposed on a chronic renal disease, a low U_{Na} concentration may not develop, as a result of preexistent tubular dysfunction. Because chronic renal insufficiency is a common backdrop for the development of ARF,[23] this possibility must be kept in mind.

Urinalysis

The urine is generally *concentrated* (U_{osm} greater than 500; assuming no diuretic use),[21] reflecting, in part, high circulating levels of ADH. Because parenchymal disease is absent, proteinuria and casts are typically absent. Trace to 1^+ proteinuria may be observed (less than 500 mg/24 h), which is due to alterations in glomerular hemodynamics and a concentrated urine. Muddy brown ATN casts (see following discussion) are characteristically absent.[24] However, in an occasional prerenal patient, sparse "ATN"-like casts can be observed, presumably reflecting subclinical ischemic renal damage induced by a profound prerenal state.

Serum Chemistries

A *high BUN/Cr ratio* has long been considered a marker for PRA.[25] Typically, with parenchymal ARF, the BUN and Scr rise proportionately, yielding an approximate 10:1 ratio. With PRA, however, the BUN classically rises out of proportion to the Cr such that the BUN/Cr ratio generally exceeds 15 or 20:1.[26] This finding is due to a preferential depression in the clearance of urea relative to that of Cr, and is a result of the vasoconstrictive state. In our view, the underlying mechanism for this phenomenon remains incompletely understood, but high circulating ADH levels and low urine flow rates, which facilitate urea but not Cr reabsorption from tubules, are generally held responsible. Obviously, tissue hypercatabolism (e.g., steroid therapy), protein loading (e.g., amino acid hyperalimination), and gastrointestinal bleeding may invalidate this diagnostic clue by driving up the BUN, independent of a depression in its renal clearance. In our experience, another useful serum chemistry guide to the presence of PRA is a normal *serum bicarbonate concentration* in the face of substantial azotemia. Unlike parenchymal ARF, in which the serum bicarbonate typically falls by approximately 1 mEq/L/d, in the prerenal patient, the serum bicarbonate concentration is frequently normal, or elevated, which is due to an intact tubular acidifying mechanism and/or a concomitant metabolic alkalosis (e.g., is due to diuretic use, vomiting, nasogastric suction). If the latter factors are operative, hypokalemia and hyponatremia may be concomitant findings.

Response to Therapy

Ready reversibility is a key feature of PRA, assuming that the underlying cause can be corrected. Indeed, the final diagnosis of PRA is often a retrospective one, made after a particular intervention reverses or improves the ARF. Sometimes "treatment" is undertaken primarily as a diagnostic test (e.g., an intravenous volume challenge for presumptive volume depletion). This type of test should be undertaken carefully, because if volume depletion does not exist, but rather, the ARF is parenchymal in origin, pulmonary edema may result.

Special Forms of Prerenal Azotemia/ Hemodynamic ARF

Hepatorenal Syndrome

The term *hepatorenal syndrome (HRS)* refers to a prerenal form of ARF that occurs in approximately 10 percent of patients with terminal hepatic disease, most commonly Laennec's cirrhosis.[27-34] Proposed mechanisms for the increased renal vascular resistance have been reviewed elsewhere.[35] The resulting ARF mimics in virtually every respect other forms of prerenal ARF: extreme sodium avidity (less than 10 to 20 mEq/L) is almost universal; oliguria invariably occurs before the terminal phase of the disease; the urine is usually highly concentrated (greater than 500 mOsm/L); and the urine sediment is typically benign but in the presence of jaundice may show finely and coarsely granular pigmented casts (see following discussion). The major difference from classic PRA is that HRS has an extremely low potential for reversibility, the latter being essentially confined to those patients who have a spontaneous improvement in hepatic function, undergo successful LeVeen shunting,[36,37] or are subjected to hepatic transplantation.[38]

Although the preceding considerations suggest that the diagnosis of HRS is straightforward, this is often not the case for the following reasons: (1) It is essentially impossible to differentiate reversible ("classic") PRA from HRS on the basis of history, physical examination, and laboratory assessments alone. Of note, these individuals are prone to develop intravascular volume depletion from diuretics (used to treat ascites), diarrhea (e.g., from lactulose therapy), or from worsening ascites (e.g., spontaneous bacterial peritonitis). Thus, an intravenous volume challenge is usually required to rule out unsuspected intravascular volume depletion.[24] Such hemodynamic measures as pulmonary capillary wedge pressures should be followed to assess the adequacy of the fluid challenge. (2) Severe hepatic disease represents a major risk factor for both nephrotoxic and ischemic ATN.[39-42] Coupled with the facts that some HRS patients excrete "ATN-like" casts (which is due to jaundice, discussed later), and that some ATN patients demonstrate sodium avidity, the separation of ATN from HRS can become virtually impossible. (3) Hematuria and red blood cell casts are not uncommon in patients with severe hepatic disease. Although this is usually due to cirrhosis-associated immunoglobulin A (IgA) nephropathy,[43-45] generally a benign disorder, it raises the possibility of ARF from acute glomerulonephritis. (4) Papillary necrosis occurs in approximately 10 percent of patients with alcoholic cirrhosis.[46] Thus, urinary tract obstruction as a cause of ARF needs to be considered.

Given the preceding considerations, a diagnosis of HRS clearly remains one of exclusion. With the appropriate clinical setting (terminal liver failure); characteristic urinary findings (particularly extremely low U_{Na} concentrations on multiple testings); a lack of nephrotoxic drug exposure or hypotensive events; and a failure to respond to a trial of intravascular volume expansion, a diagnosis of HRS can be made with a high degree of confidence. Atypical features must be viewed with caution, however, because a multiplicity of causes of ARF exist in these critically ill patients.

Nonsteroidal Antiinflammatory Drug-Induced ARF

In selected populations, NSAID therapy can precipitate ARF.[47–51] Those at greatest risk include patients with congestive heart failure, intravascular volume depletion, severe cirrhosis, and chronic renal disease. Excluding the latter, the common underlying thread in these individuals are an activated renin–angiotensin system and increased renal adrenergic activity. These factors cause renal vasoconstriction, but renal failure does not necessarily result, because norepinephrine and angiotensin II increase renal vasodilatory prostaglandin synthesis, thereby stabilizing renal blood flow and hence, GFR. The use of NSAIDs in this setting blocks this prostaglandin-mediated compensation, producing a hemodynamic form of oliguric or nonoliguric ARF. This generally occurs within a few days of initiating NSAID therapy. The diagnosis of this form of ARF is usually simple, principally requiring a history of NSAID use in the appropriate clinical setting. Urinary sodium assessments are frequently consistent with a prerenal state, and the sediment is generally benign. Hyperkalemia out of proportion to the ARF is a clue to NSAID-induced ARF,[52–54] reflecting the loss of PGE_2-mediated renin release, thereby inducing a transient hypoaldosteronemic state.[54] The ARF resolves within several days after stopping the offending agent, thereby confirming the original diagnosis. It is important, however, to recognize that NSAIDs can also produce ARF by inducing allergic interstitial nephritis, with or without a concomitant nephrotic syndrome.[55,56] This represents an idiosyncratic reaction and, thus, does not depend on an underlying high renin state. Thus, the occurrence of ARF following NSAID use in an otherwise healthy individual, and/or the presence of heavy proteinuria, strongly suggest that AIN, and not a hemodynamic form of ARF, exists.

Converting Enzyme Inhibitor-Mediated ARF

Like any other class of antihypertensive agents, CEIs can cause a transient decline in renal function that is due to a decrease in renal perfusion pressure. This is most likely to occur in those patients with high renin states (e.g., congestive heart failure, renal artery stenosis, malignant hypertension).[57] CEIs can also cause a hemodynamic form of acute renal insufficiency/ARF without any discernible impact on systemic hemodynamics.[58,59] Typically, this occurs in the presence of bilateral renal artery stenosis or unilateral stenosis of a solitary kidney (e.g., a renal transplant). Because glomerular capillary hydrostatic pressure, and hence GFR, in such kidneys are supported by angiotensin II (A_{II})-mediated efferent arteriolar vasoconstriction, a blockade of A_{II} production can nullify this compensation, inducing ARF in approximately 25 percent of such patients[60] (Fig. 3-2). The diagnosis is usually obvious, assuming one has a history of CEI therapy. Concomitant hyperkalemia (which is due to decreased A_{II}-mediated aldosterone release) further suggests the diagnosis.[57] If CEI-induced ARF occurs in the absence of known renal arterial disease, a search for the latter should subsequently be undertaken. Although poorly documented, CEI-induced ARF has also been ascribed to allergic interstitial nephritis.[57,61] Thus, a decline in GFR with CEI therapy should not necessarily be equated with a perturbation in renal hemodynamics.

Cyclosporine A-Induced Acute Renal Insufficiency

Cyclosporine A (CSA) is associated with several forms of renal insufficiency including an acute hemodynamic (prerenal) form of ARF, an acute thrombotic microangiopathy, and a chronic tubulointerstitial nephropathy.[62–64] The former is by far the most common nephropathy induced by CSA and must be considered in the differential diagnosis of ARF in patients receiving this agent.

The mechanism by which CSA induces afferent arteriolar vasoconstriction is incompletely understood but may involve exaggerated thromboxane A_2[62] and possibly endothelin[63] activity. The diagnosis of CSA-induced ARF is generally a retrospective one, requiring documentation that renal insufficiency reverses on reducing or withdrawing CSA therapy. High plasma/whole blood CSA levels are consistent with the diagnosis but by no means prove it because elevated levels may occur despite normal renal function and

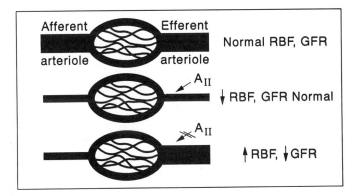

Fig. 3-2. Converting enzyme inhibitor-induced acute renal failure (ARF). The schematic presents an overview of the hemodynamic changes leading to a functional form of ARF (see text).

therapeutic levels may occur despite CSA-induced ARF. A benign urine sediment helps to exclude ATN. It is critical and often difficult to distinguish between acute renal transplant rejection and acute CSA nephrotoxicity because the therapies for each are so diametrically opposed. A renal biopsy is often helpful in this setting. Unfortunately, rejection and ATN may both be patchy in distribution, and there are no pathognomic findings for CSA-induced hemodynamic renal insufficiency. Thus, a "therapeutic" trial of withholding CSA may still be needed. Urine sodium assessments are of little value in differentiating acute rejection from CSA nephrotoxicity because sodium avidity may be seen in either state. In contrast, with ATN a high urine sodium (greater than 40 mEq/L) is expected.

For the sake of completeness, it should be recalled that CSA can predispose to or exacerbate post-transplant ischemic ATN[62] and, on rare occasions, may induce an acute thrombotic microangiopathy.[63] In these cases, a renal biopsy can be quite helpful by differentiating these forms of CSA-related ARF from the more common hemodynamic type of renal insufficiency.

ACUTE TUBULAR NECROSIS AND OTHER ACUTE PARENCHYMAL RENAL DISEASES

Acute Tubular Necrosis

The term *ATN* is used to connote those forms of ARF that are believed to have as their pathophysiologic basis necrosis of proximal and/or distal tubular epithelial cells. The extent of the necrosis is both patchy and sparse, affecting a small minority of the tubular cell population.[65] Thus, it is the *consequences* of that necrosis (tubular obstruction, backleak, and secondary hemodynamic changes),[63] rather than the necrosis, per se, which produce filtration failure. ATN is broadly subdivided into ischemic and nephrotoxic causes. The latter classification can be subdivided, according to whether the toxins have either an exogenous or endogenous origin (Table 3-2). Although the whole organ and cellular pathophysiology of specific forms of ischemic and toxic renal injury have been extensively studied in the laboratory, in clinical practice, it is likely that many, if not a majority,[67] of cases of ATN have a multifactorial basis. Thus, what is called "ischemic" or "nephrotoxic" ATN often reflects the physician's bias as to what was the predominant offender. Because the tubules retain the capacity for repair, the term *ATN* denotes reversibility, assuming the underlying causes and complications of the precipitating diseases can be reversed. Thus, if end stage renal failure results from "ATN", the initial diagnosis should be questioned.

ATN is by far the most common cause of parenchymal ARF (in our experience accounting for approximately 90 percent of cases). The most frequent causes are listed in Table 3-2, with about two-thirds being "ischemic" and one-third being "nephrotoxic" in origin.[67] However, making a specific etiologic diagnosis is often difficult because multiple insults usually exist[67]; it is

Table 3-2. Causes of Acute Tubular Necrosis

Ischemia
Nephrotoxins
Exogenous toxins
Aminoglycosides, radiocontrast agents, cisplatin, amphotericin B, ethylene glycol, CCl_4, trichloroethylene, lithium, mercury, cadmium, high-dose osmotic agents (sucrose, dextran, mannitol), methotrexate (tubular obstruction)
Endogenous toxins
Myoglobin, hemoglobin, light chains, ?endotoxin, hypercalcemia, uric acid/ hyperphosphatemia (tumor cell lysis syndrome)

impossible to determine when, or if, renal ischemia has occurred (because a fall in blood pressure and renal ischemia are not synonymous); and because nephrotoxic drug exposure need not imply nephrotoxic renal damage.

Unfortunately, there are no absolutely reliable markers for ATN. Thus, its diagnosis rests on (1) documentation of a known precipitating event that temporally correlates with the onset of renal insufficiency; (2) finding supportive laboratory data (particularly from urinalyses and urine chemistry studies); and (3) excluding, as fully as possible, other pathophysiologic states that can produce ARF. Typically, severe ATN causes a 1- to 2-mg/dl/d increment in the serum Cr concentration. Using this information, it is usually possible to accurately date its onset. Once done, a careful review of the patient's history, or hospital chart, over the 24 hours before the onset of renal failure frequently uncovers a likely precipitating event (e.g., hypotension, sepsis, radiocontrast administration, surgery). A more expanded historical review, covering 1 week before the onset of ARF, may reveal nephrotoxic drug exposure, which frequently produces a rather insidious onset of renal failure. In approximately 10 percent of patients, however, no clear precipitating cause of ATN is identified.[68] Thus, one must rely either on the laboratory data to make a presumptive diagnosis or, if indicated, perform a renal biopsy.

Diagnostic Tests

The urine sediment, assessments of renal sodium avidity (U_{Na}, Fe_{Na}, RFI), and a determination of urinary concentrating ability (specific gravity, urinary osmolality, urine/serum Cr ratios) have long been, and remain, the most used laboratory tests to help confirm a diagnosis of ATN. As discussed previously, their major utility is in differentiating ATN from PRA, the two most frequent causes of ARF. Before discussing each test, it is important to recognize that the results obtained in ATN patients may vary considerably, depending on whether the patient has an oliguric or nonoliguric presentation, on the nature of the precipitating event, and on whether specific therapies have already been introduced. These points, where appropriate, will be considered in the following discussion.

Urine Sediment Analysis

The most characteristic urinary sediment finding is the presence of large numbers of deeply pigmented "muddy brown" granular ("ATN") casts. These are believed to be composed of necrotic tubular cell debris and are observed in all forms of ATN, irrespective of cause. In oliguric ATN, they are present in approximately 80 percent of patients at the time of initial consultation[24] and they may continue to be excreted over the course of the disease. In nonoliguric ATN, these casts are observed in approximately 50 to 70 percent of cases,[24] the slightly lower frequency probably reflecting less severe tubular injury, a sampling "error" (the best preserved nephrons are excreting the most urine), and a dilutional effect. Besides ATN, only severe jaundice frequently produces this sediment finding,[41] possibly because filtered bile salts exert a detergent-like effect on the proximal tubular brush border, inducing cast formation in the absence of cell necrosis. Thus, the presence of characteristic ATN casts may be observed in severe liver failure, possibly complicating the diagnosis of hepatorenal syndrome. In addition to muddy brown granular casts, large numbers of renal tubular cells are typically observed. In the absence of special stains, it may be difficult to differentiate tubular cells from neutrophils, given their comparable sizes. Therefore, special attention must be paid to nuclear morphology (if definable) because a mononuclear appearance supports a tubular origin. Microhematuria is common in ATN patients. However, this most often reflects lower urinary tract bleeding due to bladder catheterization, rather than being reflective of ATN. Urinary red blood cell (RBC) morphology (Wright's stain) will distinguish lower tract from intrarenal bleeding (see following discussion). Heavy proteinuria (3 to 4+ by "dipstick"; greater than or equal to 300 mg/dL) is highly uncharacteristic of ATN and suggests the presence of acute or chronic glomerular disease, particularly if RBC casts are observed.

Urinary Sodium Content

For approximately 40 years, it has been recognized that ATN patients have high U_{Na} concentrations.[69,70] Using this observation, Waugh and Welt[16,17] suggested that a random U_{Na} could help distinguish PRA from ATN. Since then, it has been widely accepted that a U_{Na} of greater than 40 or less than 20 mEq/L are indicative of ATN and PRA, respectively. However, because most studies have found that a substantial number of patients fall within the intermediate range (20 to 40 mEq/L), the Fe_{Na} and RFI have been applied to improve the U_{Na}'s diagnostic accuracy. Based on several studies,[18–22] it has been concluded that the Fe_{Na} and RFI have 90 percent specificity and sensitivity for differentiating oliguric ATN from PRA.[1] Several important caveats, however, must be borne in mind: (1) During the earliest phase of ischemic ATN, low urinary sodium profiles may be observed, because ischemic renal injury must first pass through a severe "prerenal" phase. (2) A therapeutic trial of diuretics, vasodilators, and volume expansion in PRA patients may raise the U_{Na}, Fe_{Na}, and RFIs into the ATN range. (3) Urinary sodium assessments are less reliable when applied to nonoliguric than oliguric ATN patients. For example, Levinsky and Alexander reported that only 32 percent of nonoliguric ATN patients had initial U_{Na} concentrations of greater than 25 mEq/L, while 12 percent had values of less than 10 mEq/L.[24] Using the Fe_{Na}, Miller et al. found that approximately 15 percent of nonoliguric ATN patients had values of less than 1%.[21] In our unpublished experience, approximately 50 percent of nonoliguric ATN patients have a U_{Na} of less than 20 mEq/L at the time of initial consultation. The reason for this avid sodium retention in the setting of presumed tubular damage remains unknown. (4) Radiocontrast-induced ARF is commonly associated with a low U_{Na} and/or Fe_{Na}, even with *an oliguric presentation.*[71-74] That approximately 12 percent of hospital-acquired ATN is secondary to radiocontrast administration[75] underscores the importance of this observation.

Urinary Concentrating Ability

Because concentrating ability is typically lost in ATN but preserved in PRA, assessments of this kidney function have been used to help make this differentiation. Urinary osmolality (U_{osm}), rather than specific gravity, has most often been used, because the osmolality is a far more accurate test. One prospective study indicated that although U_{osm} of greater than 500 or less than 350 is highly suggestive of PRA and ATN, respectively, only 60 to 70% sensitivity is achieved because of a large number of intermediate values (350 to 500 mOsm/L).[21] A different approach has been to compare urinary to plasma osmolalities (U/P osm), thereby correcting for the fact that all body fluid tonicities rise in renal failure as a result of solute retention. A U/P osm ratio of ~1 is reportedly characteristic of ATN, while values greater than or equal to 1.3 are typically found in PRA.[76,77] The U/P creatinine ratio[20,69] reflects the same type of approach and has been more widely applied: values of less than 20 and greater than 40 are typical of ATN and PRA, respectively. However, approximately 20 percent of patients fall within the intermediate range, making this determination less reliable than U_{Na} assessments.

Diagnostic Clues to Specific Forms of ATN

The preceding discussion has focused on diagnostic features of ATN, in general. Following supplemental information pertaining to some specific and particularly common forms of ATN is presented. In general, the clinical presentation represents a composite of both general features and specific ATN features.

Rhabdomyolysis (Myoglobinuric)-Induced ATN

Rhabdomyolysis-induced ATN results from either traumatic or nontraumatic muscle damage. The most common causes include crush injuries, strenuous exercise, grand mal seizures, prolonged coma (resulting in ischemic necrosis of dependent muscles), hyperpyrexia, alcoholism (particularly if complicated by hypokalemia and hypophosphatemia), and McArdle's syndrome.[78-80] In recent years, cocaine use has become a common cause.[81-84] The diagnosis is usually obvious in trauma patients: oliguria is typical (initially reflecting intravascular volume depletion plus renal damage), massive creatine kinase (CK) elevations occur (more than 20,000 units/ml),[80] and during the early stages, myoglobinuria is apparent (red or dark brown orthotolidine-positive urine in the absence of erythrocytes). Although myoglobin is, under normal circumstances, readily filtered, in the presence of ATN, the marked depression in GFR may produce transient myoglobinemia. (Thus, "pink serum" does not necessarily indicate intravascular hemolysis.) Once the myoglobin has been cleared from the circulation, myoglobinuria is no longer apparent. Hence, its absence does not exclude the diagnosis of rhabdomyolysis-induced ATN if the patient is seen several days after the traumatic event. In contrast, massive CK elevations are, in general, quite persistent, possibly lasting for weeks. In addition to myoglobin and CK, damaged muscles may also release large amounts of potassium, phosphate, purines, and creatine into the circulation. Thus, hyperkalemia, hyperphosphatemia, hyperuricemia (from purine metabolism), and a disproportionate elevation of the serum creatinine for the length of renal failure can result.[78,84-87] However, these findings are by no means invariable.[79] With nontraumatic rhabdomyolysis, the diagnosis of myoglobinuric ATN may be more difficult to make unless gross myoglobinuria is observed. Muscle pain may be absent, a precipitating cause may not be readily apparent, and hyperkalemia and hyperphosphatemia are less likely to be observed, especially in alcoholic patients, who frequently have concomitant potassium and phosphate deficits. Thus, the cornerstone of diagnosis in these patients remains a marked and persistent CK elevation[85-87] (in our experience, virtually always greater than 20,000 units/ml), coupled with an absence of other obvious causes of ARF. Typical ATN urinary findings, in addition to myoglobinuria, are observed. However, at the time of presentation, avid sodium avidity can be seen, which is due to associated intravascular volume depletion, caused by muscle "third" spacing.[80] With volume expansion, more typical urinary sodium profiles result.

Aminoglycoside Nephrotoxicity

Classically, aminoglycoside nephrotoxicity is diagnosed when an insidious onset of azotemia occurs after 7 to 10 days of drug therapy.[88] In this circumstance, nonoliguria is the rule. However, well-known risk factors such as intravascular volume depletion, hypotension/shock, hypokalemia, hepatic insufficiency, and perhaps advanced age and renal insufficiency[88] may compress this time course considerably, possibly producing oliguric ARF. For example, even a single dose of gentamicin can cause severe experimental ARF if administered in the presence of endotoxemia or shock.[89,90] That some patients may first manifest ARF a few days *after* aminoglycosides have been stopped underscores the fact that time frame alone is not an accurate diagnostic guide. Serum aminoglycoside levels provide little diagnostic information. Because these drugs are almost perfect markers of GFR, trough levels predominantly reflect dosage and renal function and not drug toxicity per se. That tubular cell aminoglycoside levels are often 100-fold or more higher than are serum concentrations indicates that the latter do not accurately reflect the tubular drug burden and, hence, toxicity. Thus, the diagnosis of aminoglycoside toxicity is almost always presumptive, based on typical ATN findings in the absence of other known precipitating factors. Although aminoglycosides can produce early changes in tubular function (e.g., a concentrating defect, glycosuria, aminoaciduria, potassium and magnesium wasting, enzymuria),[91–93] these potential markers have not found differential diagnostic application.

Radiocontrast-Induced ARF

Virtually every radiographic procedure using systemic contrast administration has been reported to cause ARF. Despite initial hope that nonionic contrast would avoid this complication, this does not appear to be the case.[94,95] Intravenous pyelography and arteriography are the most common radiographic procedures to induce ARF, undoubtedly as a result of their frequency. Intravascular volume depletion[96] and renal insufficiency, particularly that which is due to diabetes,[97] are the two most prominent risk factors. The clinical diagnosis is straightforward, because the onset or (worsening) of azotemia is noted 24 to 48 hours after contrast administration. Most often, nonoliguria is present and the renal insufficiency is both mild and short lived. Prolonged oliguric ARF, however, is also possible, particularly in patients with preexisting risk factors. The urine sediment generally reveals "ATN" casts. However, the U_{Na} and Fe_{Na} are uncharacteristically low (less than 20 mEq and less than 1%, respectively) in approximately 30 percent of patients,[71–74] whether or not oliguria exists. Occasionally, heavy proteinuria is detected: This typically reflects underlying renal disease (e.g., diabetes). However, transient heavy proteinuria may also result from intrarenal contrast injection.[98] A persistant nephrogram may be observed for 24 to 72 hours following contrast administration.[99–101] However, this is not a specific finding for contrast-induced nephrotoxicity because it can be observed in any ATN patient who receives a radiocontrast agent.

ARF in Multiple Myeloma

Approximately 10 percent of patients with multiple myeloma develop ARF at some time during the course of this disease, and it may be the initial presentation.[102,103] Not only do these individuals develop typical forms of nephrotoxic and ischemic ARF, they may also be predisposed to them because of monoclonal light chain (Bence Jones protein) excretion. Light chains, either because of intrinsic nephrotoxic properties or their proclivity to precipitate within tubular lumina, forming casts, can be either a significant risk factor for ATN or cause de novo ARF (acute cast nephropathy).[103] Frequently, the ARF exacerbates the course of chronic myeloma kidney. Hypercalcemia, volume depletion, and dehydration, and possibly radiocontrast administration, are predisposing factors. The diagnosis of myeloma-associated ARF is predicated on a diagnosis of the underlying disease. If this has not been established, documentation of light chain excretion at the time of initial urine assessment for ARF can yield this information. The simplest screen is to compare the urinary "dipstick" and sulfosalicylic acid (SSA) tests for proteinuria. The latter detects virtually all proteins, whereas the former is relatively albumin specific. Thus, a positive SSA reaction with a negative dipstick implies increased nonalbumin protein excretion, most commonly resulting from light chains if gross myohemoglobinuria are absent. Urine protein immunoelectrophoresis is used to confirm that increased monoclonal light chain excretion is indeed present. Other clues to the presence of multiple myeloma are hypercalcemia, the Fanconi syndrome, and a low anion gap (resulting from a cationic IgG paraprotein).[103] If therapy hinges on a definitive diagnosis of acute myeloma kidney (e.g., initiation of plasmapheresis, chemotherapy), a renal biopsy should be undertaken to confirm intrarenal monoclonal light chain deposition.

Postischemic ATN

The classic diagnostic feature of postischemic ATN is the onset of ARF in the immediate aftermath of a hypotensive event. In many patients, however, the fall in blood pressure is quite modest and short lived. Experimental evidence suggests that the type of shock, and not just the blood pressure, per se, is an important determinant of whether renal ischemia develops. In general, hemorrhagic shock is much less well tolerated than is cardiogenic shock, despite comparable blood pressure reductions.[104,105] However, that virtually no experimental studies have been able to induce postischemic ATN by shock alone raises serious questions as to what causes the clinical postischemic ATN syndrome.[106] A multifactorial cause is likely, but many of the components remain to be defined. The clinical presentation is that of a prototypic ATN, as described. Either oliguric or nonoliguric presentations are possible, the latter having a better prognosis.

OTHER ACUTE PARENCHYMAL RENAL DISEASES

Acute Glomerulonephritis

The glomerulonephridities (GNs) are an extremely heterogeneous group of disorders that typically present with slowly progressive azotemia, rather than ARF. When ARF does result, it is usually due to one of the following three situations: (1) an acute exacerbation of a chronic glomerulopathy; (2) a superimposed, nonglomerular insult; or (3) a de novo acute proliferative or crescentic glomerulonephritis.[107–109] Virtually every chronic nephropathy has been reported to transform into ARF,[109] crescent formation being the usual histologic correlate. Although this most typically occurs with chronic proliferative nephropathies (e.g., SLE, membranoproliferative GN, IgA nephropathy) it can rarely occur in nonproliferative disorders as well, e.g., membranous nephropathy.[110,111] Nonglomerular complications of a chronic glomerular disease that can induce ARF include ischemic and nephrotoxic ATN, allergic interstitial nephritis (e.g., caused by thiazide diuretics),[112] renal vein thrombosis in the setting of nephrotic syndrome (discussed later), and possibly severe hypoalbuminemia, particularly in minimal change disease.[109] Finally, although de novo acute GN can occur, particularly in children, this represents a relatively uncommon cause of ARF in adults (approximately 5 percent of cases).[109] In contrast, acute exacerbations of chronic nephropathies, as discussed, account for approximately 15 to 20 percent of adult ARF cases.[23] These percentages should be borne in mind as one proceeds with a differential diagnostic assessment.

The glomerular diseases that evoke a de novo ARF fall into two general histologic categories: (1) a diffuse proliferative, or exudative GN, of which poststreptococcal GN is a prototype, and (2) crescentic (or rapidly progressive) GN (more than 50 percent of glomeruli involved). This is a somewhat arbitrary division because these histologic lesions are often mixed, particularly in those patients with ARF. The extent of crescent formation correlates with both the severity of the renal insufficiency and the frequency with which irreversible renal failure develops. If one classifies these diseases according to their glomerular immunofluorescence findings, three clinically useful patterns emerge[107]: (1) granular immune deposits; (2) antiglomerular basement membrane-mediated disease (linear immunofluorescence); and (3) GN with pauci-immune or no immune deposits (see Fig. 3-3). Specific disorders falling within each category are presented in Table 3-3.

Obviously, once this information has been gleaned from a renal biopsy, the cause of the ARF is identified. Thus, the clinical and laboratory assessments that lead to this procedure need to be addressed. A *clinical history* suggestive of any of the diseases listed in Table 3-3 may suggest a diagnosis of AGN in an ARF patient. A history of slowly declining urine output, avid sodium retention (peripheral and pulmonary edema, hypertension), and hematuria strongly suggest an acute nephritic syndrome. However, the cornerstone for making a presumptive diagnosis of AGN remains the urinalysis. *Proteinuria* is virtually always present and by qualitative assessment is usually greater than or equal to 2+ to 4+ in degree. Although the nephrotic syndrome does not typically result (because the rapid loss of GFR precludes prolonged, heavy proteinuria), approximately 10 to 30 percent of patients will have greater than 3 g of proteinuria in a 24-hour collection.[113–115] In an oliguric patient, a qualitative "dipstick" protein assessment or a urine protein/urine creatinine ratio[116] may better reflect the loss of glomerular protein permselectivity than does a timed protein excretion rate. The value of documenting heavy albuminuria in a patient with ARF is underscored by the fact that only AGN and NSAID-induced AIN (discussed later) typically produce this result.

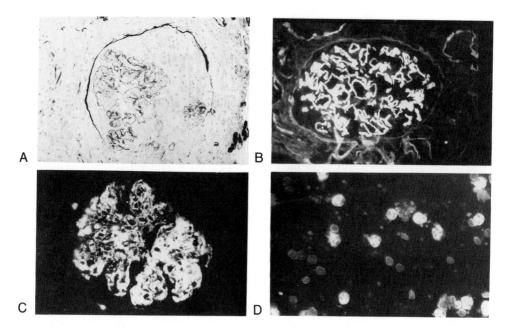

Fig. 3-3. An immunofluorescence categorization of rapidly progressive glomer-onephritis (RPGN). (**A**) Light microscopic evidence of a cellular crescent, the histo-logic hallmark of RPGN. (**B**) Linear imunofluorescence (IgG) in anti-GBM nephritis. (**C**) Granular immune deposits. (**D**) There was an absence of glomerular deposits, but the patient's serum had high titers of antineutrophil cytoplasmic antibody (ANCA; depicted).

Obviously, the diagnostic value of proteinuria is negated if ARF develops in a patient with underlying chronic glomerular disease.

RBC casts are highly specific for AGN but are much less reliably docu-mented than is proteinuria. Delay in examination or the presence of an alkaline urine, which dissolves casts, may contribute to a negative result. Thus, a freshly voided, concentrated, and acid urine will facilitate RBC cast

Table 3-3. Classification of the Acute Glomerulonephritides According to Their Immunofluorescence Patterns

I. Granular immune deposits

    Collagen vascular diseases: SLE, Henoch-Schöenlein purpura, mixed cryoglobulinemia

    Infectious/postinfectious: poststreptococcal GN, endocarditis, shunt nephritis

    Primary renal disease: IgA nephropathy, membranoproliferative GN, idiopathic RPGN with immune deposits

II. Anti-GBM GN: Goodpasture's syndrome, idiopathic anti-GBM nephritis

III. Pauci-immune RPGN: Wegener's granulomatosis, microscopic polyarteritis nodosa, idiopathic pauci-immune RPGN

Abbreviations: GBM, glomerular basement membrane; GN, glomerulonephritis; RPGN, rapidly progressive glomerulonephritis; SLE, systemic lupus erythematosus.

identification. If a delay in examination is necessary, a few drops of 10 percent formalin added to a urine aliquot, or preferably to the urine pellet, will help preserve formed elements. In our experience, reliance on a clinical laboratory for RBC cast identification virtually ensures a negative result. In those patients with absent RBC casts, *urinary RBC morphology* may have utility. Crenated or dysmorphic RBCs appear to arise from glomerular bleeding,[117–119] which is possibly due to intraluminal enzymatic activity on the RBC membrane.[120] In contrast, lower urinary tract bleeding is associated with RBCs with similar morphology to that on a peripheral blood smear. Using automated RBC analyzers, attempts have been made to differentiate glomerular from nonglomerular bleeding on the basis of mean corpuscular volumes (MCVs), with microcytes suggesting the former diagnosis.[121] However, these techniques have not yet proven highly successful, which is due in part to non-RBC particulate matter in the urinary sediment. Urinary sodium and osmolality assessments are highly variable. While indices suggestive of a prerenal state (low sodium, high osmolality) may be found, particularly in oliguric patients, more often, these tests fall within the ATN range.

Thus, other than the urinalysis, and possibly, the clinical setting, there are, at present, no reliable ways to noninvasively diagnose AGN. In the anuric patient, even the urinalysis will not be available, and hence, the *renal biopsy* is essential. As noted, immunofluorescence patterns are of great differential diagnostic value. Once known, selected serologic tests can help to elucidate specific diagnoses.[109] In brief, hypocomplementemia is typically seen in SLE, poststreptococcal GN, shunt nephritis, bacterial endocarditis, mixed cryoglobulinemia, and membranoproliferative GN (all examples of category I, granular immune deposit diseases; Table 3-3). Further tests, including ANAs, cryoglobulin assays, antistreptococcal serologies, and blood cultures help differentiate these disorders. For category II, the presence of circulating anti-glomerular basement membrane antibodies, as assessed by radioimmunoassay, enzyme-linked immunosorbent assay (ELISA), indirect immunofluorescence, or Western blot, help substantiate the renal biopsy findings of linear immunofluorescence. The serologic diagnosis of a pauciimmune RPGN (which can occur as an isolated renal syndrome or as part of a systemic vasculitis, e.g., Wegener's granulomatosis), has been revolutionized in recent years by the discovery of circulating *antineutrophilic cytoplasmic antibodies (ANCA)* detected by indirect immunofluorescence (see preceding discussion).[122,123] The presence of high ANCA titers is highly specific for category III diseases, and serial quantitative assessments may be useful for following their activity.[124]

Acute Interstitial Nephritis

Acute interstitial nephritis (AIN) is a term that denotes a group of diseases characterized by interstitial inflammation (cellular infiltrates, edema) and that presents as either nonoliguric or oliguric ARF. The glomeruli and blood vessels are not involved, thereby differentiating AIN from the glomerulo-pathies and vasculopathies, which also may show prominent interstitial changes. Three broad categories of AIN have been identified: (1) allergic AIN caused by drug hypersensitivity; (2) AIN manifesting as part of a multisystem disease; and (3) infectious AIN. In the United States and Europe, the first category accounts for the vast majority of cases. In the Far East, however, the third category can be prominent. The real incidence of each is not known because a definitive diagnosis requires a renal biopsy. Drug-induced AIN has been reported to account for 0.8 to 8.3 percent of all ARF cases in the United States and Western Europe.[125,126] In our experience, 0.8 percent is a closer approximation. Despite its relative infrequency, AIN almost always must be included in the differential diagnosis of ARF because over 70 drugs have been implicated in its induction.[127] Following, the three categories of AIN are discussed separately.

Drug-Induced AIN

Despite the plethora of agents reported to induce AIN, the most common and best documented are the pencillins and penicillin derivatives, cephalosporins, sulfonamides, antituberculous agents, allopurinol, phenytoin, and NSAIDs. With the exception of NSAIDs (discussed later), a rather uniform presentation exists. After either several days or weeks of drug exposure, renal insufficiency or oliguric ARF is noted. Because this represents a hypersensitivity reaction, it is not dose dependent, and other allergic manifestations—most notably fever, rash, and/or eosinophilia—are typically present.[125–133] The frequency of these three findings, at least in the case of methicillin-induced AIN, are approximately 70 to 100 percent, 30 to 50 percent, and 80 percent, respectively.[131–133] However, the entire triad, is found in less than 50 percent of cases. In the absence of oliguria or severe ARF, it is generally the extrarenal symptoms that first bring patients to medical attention. Additional clinical signs and symptoms may include arthralgias, flank pain (caused by renal edema with stretching of the renal capsule), and gross hematuria, the latter noted in approximately 10 percent of patients.[127] In hospitalized patients, drug-induced AIN most commonly presents as an unexpected rise in the BUN and serum creatinine concentrations.

A diagnosis of drug-induced AIN can be extremely difficult to make without a renal biopsy. Fever, rash, and/or eosinophilia during therapy with an implicated drug strongly suggest AIN, but the absence of these by no means excludes the diagnosis. Documenting eosinophiluria may be helpful, with one recent study suggesting 91 percent sensitivity.[134] This test, however, is not specific for AIN, because eosinophiluria can also occur with other diseases (e.g., prostatitis, acute glomerulonephritis),[134] the percentage of eosinophils that constitutes a positive result has not been rigorously defined (1 to 10 percent), and either a special stain (Hansel's) must be used or the Wright's stain needs to be applied to an alkalinized urine sample. Probably the greatest utility of the urinalysis in approaching a patient with suspected AIN is in helping to rule out other parenchymal renal diseases. ATN casts are typically absent; only mild, or no, proteinuria is observed; and although microhematuria is common, RBC casts are not observed. The Fe_{Na} and U_{osm} are consistent with an intrarenal, not a prerenal, state. Laboratory tests suggestive of allergic reactions do not have proven utility: IgE levels are inconsistently elevated, circulating antibodies to the drugs are inconstant, and the lymphocyte blast transformation and migration tests have not found wide clinical application. Renal ultrasonography is helpful by excluding urinary tract obstruction and by documenting increased kidney size, thereby indicating acute inflammation. Increased renal uptake of gallium citrate Ga 67 (^{67}Ga) has been reported in AIN,[125,135] but a lack of specificity limits its diagnostic application. A decision to perform a renal biopsy must be highly individualized. Factors to be considered include whether the suspected drug can be safely stopped and whether or not steroid therapy will be undertaken if the diagnosis is confirmed.

NSAID-Induced AIN

AIN is an extremely uncommon complication of NSAID use (less than 1 case per 5,300 patient treatment years).[136] However, that 40 million Americans use these agents on a regular basis underscores the importance of this potential complication. The propionic acid derivatives have been the most commonly implicated preparations. Presenting symptoms are usually those of oliguria and edema. In contrast to other forms of allergic AIN, NSAID-induced disease uncommonly produces fever, rash, and eosinophilia or eosinophiluria (less than 5 to 20 percent); the ARF may occur only after months, not days or weeks, of therapy; and nephrotic range proteinuria is typically observed (85 percent of cases).[127] On occasion, the ARF or the nephrotic syndrome occur independently. Renal biopsy is required to make the diagnosis. It typically reveals mononuclear cell interstitial infiltrates, edema, and normal glomerular architecture, consistent with a minimal change lesion. The biopsy is especially important in those patients with heavy proteinuria and ARF since it excludes acute proliferative and crescentic GN in patients who coincidentally are taking NSAIDs. The presence of RBC casts would strongly suggest this latter possibility.

AIN in Systemic Diseases

For the sake of completeness, it should be recalled that AIN can complicate several multisystem diseases, including SLE, Sjögren's syndrome, sarcoidosis, and Wegener's granulomatosis.[127,133] Infiltration by lymphomas and leukemias can also, on rare occasion, cause ARF.[133] Other than renal biopsy, these states have no specific diagnostic markers. Rather, a knowledge of the underlying disease prompts their consideration if ARF develops.

Systemic Infection-Associated AIN

ARF in the setting of sepsis most commonly reflects a prerenal state or hypotension-induced ischemic ATN. However, some infectious diseases characteristically cause an AIN. The best known examples are leptospirosis and Hantaan virus infections (hemorrhagic fever with renal syndrome); the latter is a common cause of ARF in the Far East [137] but has also occurred in Europe.[138] Toxoplasmosis, infectious mononucleosis, brucellosis, syphilis, mycoplasma pneumonia, Rocky Mountain Spotted fever, and Legionnaire's disease may also cause AIN.[127] The key to diagnosis is identifying the underlying infection, recognizing that AIN can occur, and excluding complicating factors, such as shock and volume depletion, which can independently induce ARF.

Acute Renal Vascular Disease

Acute Renal Arterial Thrombosis and Thromboembolism

ARF frequently develops in clinical situations known to produce acute renal arterial thrombosis (trauma, dissecting aneurysms) and thromboembolism (cardiac disease). Acute vascular occlusion, per se, however, remains an uncommon cause of ARF. Thus, other complications of these underlying diseases are more likely to be responsible. For example, the most common cause of acute renal arterial thrombosis is blunt abdominal trauma from car accidents.[139] However, because acute renal thrombosis is usually a unilateral, not a bilateral process, other causes of ARF in this setting need to be entertained, such as urinary tract obstruction by blood clots, ischemic ATN caused by hemorrhage from a ruptured spleen, or a unilateral arterial occlusion with contralateral ATN. Dissections of the abdominal aorta and/or renal arteries can also produce unilateral and, less commonly, bilateral renal arterial occlusion.[140] However, because underlying renal vascular disease frequently exists in these patients, baseline renal function may have been maintained by a solitary kidney, and thus, a unilateral thrombosis can produce severe ARF.

Emboli of sufficient size to occlude major renal arteries generally have a cardiac origin.[141–144] Underlying atrial fibrillation, a recent myocardial infarction, rheumatic valvular disease, prosthetic valves, and endocarditis are the most common predisposing factors. More often than not, however, renal dysfunction in these settings reflects either prerenal azotemia (e.g., resulting from heart failure or overdiuresis) or, in the case of endocarditis, acute glomerulonephritis. Nevertheless, if signs or symptoms of acute renal thromboembolism exist, this possibility should be excluded because this diagnosis has major therapeutic implications, not only for the kidney, but also for the underlying cardiac disease. For example, recurrent embolization is one indication for heart valve replacement.

The clinical signs and symptoms of renal artery thrombosis and thromboembolism are much the same, the major difference being the clinical settings in which they occur. Acute abdominal or flank pain, often coupled with nausea and vomiting, are the usual presenting symptoms. In 25 percent of cases, however, pain may be absent.[143] Most patients develop microscopic, but usually not gross, hematuria. Fever and leukocytosis often occur, particularly 1 to 3 days following the acute event. Elevations in serum lactic dehydrogenase (LDH) are almost universal (reflecting renal infarction), and increments in the serum glutamic oxaloacetic transaminase (SGOT), serum glutamic pyruvic transaminase (SGPT), and alkaline phosphatase may also occur.[143–145] Creatine kinase-MB band elevations are not characteristic of renal infarction and, if found, suggest a recent myocardial infarction as a possible embolic source.

A definitive diagnosis of acute renal arterial occlusion requires abdominal aortography and/or renal arteriography. Other radiographic procedures, such as ultrasonography,[146,147] intravenous pyelography, computed abdominal tomography,[148] isotopic flow studies,[149,150] and possibly, magnetic resonance imaging (MRI) can provide suggestive, but rarely definitive, diagnostic information. Thus, their performance may delay diagnosis. If emergent surgical intervention is contemplated to preserve renal integrity, arteriography should be considered as the first, and only, test to avoid delay. If surgery is not deemed appropriate, then nonarteriographic approaches may suffice. However, because these tests are best at detecting focal or unilateral changes, they may not be useful in diagnosing the cause of ARF.

Bilateral Cortical Necrosis

Bilateral cortical necrosis (BCN) is an uncommon form of ARF, account accounting for 2 percent or less of cases.[151,152] It is characterized pathologically by necrosis of all renal cortical structures, extending from a 1- to 2-mm rim of normal subcapsular tissue to the cortical–medullary junction. That the necrotic process is confluent, involving glomeruli as well as the vasculature, distinguishes it from ATN, which causes patchy necrosis, spares nontubular elements, and often shows preferential outer medullary involvement.[65] The inciting pathologic event is believed to be acute thrombosis of interlobular arteries, afferent arterioles, and possibly, glomerular capillaries.[153] The arcuate vessels are spared, and this is believed responsible for the preservation of medullary structures. Approximately two-thirds of cases occur in the setting of obstetric complications,[153] most prominently abruptio placentae, particularly in multiparous women over the age of 30. A prior history of toxemia may be a predisposing factor. The remaining one-third of cases occur in the setting of hypovolemic or septic shock, particularly if complicated by disseminated intravascular coagulation (DIC). Pancreatitis, trauma, burns, aortic aneurysm dissection, diabetic ketoacidosis, snake bites, and arsenic poisoning have all been reported as precipitating, or associated, conditions.[153] In neonates and infants, profound diarrhea with intravascular volume depletion is a common underlying state.[153]

The most characteristic presentation of BCN is that of oligoanuria. Initially, it can be difficult, if not impossible, to differentiate BCN from ATN, particularly because the latter is far more common and because these two conditions often occur in identical situations. Factors favoring BCN are protracted anuria, concomitant DIC, thrombotic involvement of extrarenal tissues, most common in nonobstetric cases[153] (e.g., patchy cutaneous and hepatic necrosis, pancreatitis, gastrointestinal ischemia), and the clinical setting in which it occurs (e.g., abruptio placenta). Although original reports of BCN stressed the differential diagnostic value of anuria, it is important to recognize that incomplete BCN can occur, with a sparing of some cortical tissue. Thus, an oliguric, or even a nonoliguric, presentation is possible. That ATN can, on occasion, pass through an anuric phase further emphasizes that urine output alone does not reliably differentiate ATN from BCN.

If available, urine generally shows mild to moderate proteinuria, micro- or macroscopic hematuria, and possibly RBC casts.[153] The latter, reflective of glomerular necrosis, can be a helpful clue to the presence of BCN, because ATN, the other leading diagnosis, does not produce this sediment finding. Given the presence of necrotic tubules, urinary sodium and U_{osm} assessments would be expected to mimic those of ATN. However, this issue has not been scrutinized in the literature.

A definitive diagnosis of BCN can only be made by demonstrating confluent areas of necrosis on renal biopsy. This procedure, however, is generally not performed during the initial phase of the disease, owing to frequent dire medical circumstances, including DIC. Thus, the diagnosis is usually a presumptive one at the time of initial evaluation. Renal angiography[154] can provide useful diagnostic information because there is a characteristic absence of interlobular arterial filling and a nonexistent, or extremely faint and mottled, cortical nephrogram. The extent of this nephrogram may have some prognostic value because it generally indicates the amount of nonnecrotic tissue. The value of this information, however, must be weighed against the risk of contrast administration, which can injure remaining nephrons. Isotopic flow studies and renograms provide little practical information because they do not reliably differentiate BCN from the low blood flow state that is characteristic ATN. Renal cortical calcification, although considered a hallmark of BCN, is actually quite rare, is relatively nonspecific, and occurs too late to have much differential diagnostic value.[153] Unfortunately, time commonly makes the final diagnosis of BCN. It has been reported that only 1 in 16 patients ultimately become dialysis independent; this may require up to 4 months to occur, and if it does, GFR recovers to only about 25 percent of normal.[153] In contrast, virtually all ATN patients who recover from their extrarenal diseases become dialysis independent within less than 2 months.[23]

The Microvasculopathies

Renal microvascular diseases can be divided into three histopathologic categories: (1) the thrombotic microangiopathies (hyaline thrombi of small arcuate and interlobular arteries, arterioles, and glomeruli with arterial/arteriolar intimal proliferation and perivascular fibrosis); (2) necrotizing vasculidities; and (3) atheroembolic renal disease. Specific causes falling within each of these categories are presented in Table 3-4. These diseases are

Table 3-4. Acute Vascular Disease-Induced ARF

Renal Arterial occlusion
Thrombosis (trauma), aortic/renal artery dissection, embolism (cardiac origin)
Medium to small vessel disease
Atheroembolic renal disease, bilateral cortical necrosis, classic polyarteritis nodosa
Small vessel/glomerular diseases
Necrotizing vasculitis
Leukocytoclastic vasculitis, hypocomplementemic vasculitis, mixed essential cryoglobulinemia
Thrombotic vasculidities
Hemolytic uremic syndrome, thrombotic thrombocytopenic purpura, malignant hypertension, scleroderma, hyperacute renal transplant rejection
Renal vein thrombosis

Abbreviations: ARF, acute renal failure.

characterized by multisystem organ involvement, a major clue to their diagnosis. Renal failure generally results from progressive ischemic renal injury. Diseases in categories 1 and 2 can also cause direct glomerular involvement. If so, hematuria, RBC casts, and proteinuria are usually apparent. Each of the categories are briefly discussed in the following sections.

Thrombotic Microangiopathies. Each of the diseases within the category thrombotic microangiopathy has the propensity to induce microangiopathic hemolytic anemia (MHA), a reflection of diffuse microvascular damage that leads to traumatic RBC disruption. This process is most marked in the hemolytic uremic syndrome (HUS) and thrombotic thrombocytopenic purpura (TTP), but it can also be observed with malignant hypertension and scleroderma. Diagnoses of malignant hypertension and scleroderma are usually obvious on clinical grounds. ARF in scleroderma patients is uncommon (5 to 15 percent).[109] When it does occur, it is usually on a backdrop of chronic extrarenal disease, which is then punctuated by acute, malignant hypertension-associated ARF.[155–158] However, rapidly progressive renal failure in the absence of malignant hypertension also has been noted.[155,157,159] HUS-TTP represents a disease spectrum ranging from MHA with renal involvement (HUS)[160,161] to a pentad of findings that includes fever, neurologic changes, renal disease, MHA, and thrombocytopenia (TTP).[162,163] Thrombocytopenia is found at some point in almost all HUS-TTP patients, but at any given time, it may be absent. In addition to the nervous system and renal involvement, hepatomegaly, splenomegaly, pancreatitis, gastrointestinal disease (bleeding), hypertension, petechiae, and ecchymoses can be observed. HUS is typically an illness with an abrupt onset, predominantly manifesting with MHA and renal involvement. Precipitating events include verotoxin-producing *Escherichia coli*-0157 enteritis,[164] the postpartum state, oral contraceptives, and cyclosporine A.[109] In contrast, TTP typically produces the full clinical pentad, usually has an insidious onset, and often runs a chronic course. The cornerstone for diagnosing HUS-TTP is documentation of MHA in a patient with typical organ involvement. Schistocytes on peripheral blood smear and the biochemical markers thereof (increased LDH, depressed haptoglobin, slight bilirubin elevations) in conjunction with thrombocytopenia virtually ensure the diagnosis in a patient with a consistent clinical presentation. Thus, renal biopsies are not typically performed, except in unusual cases.

Necrotizing Vasculidities. The necrotizing vasculidities encompass a broad spectrum of disorders,[109] outlined in Table 3-4. Obviously, a complete diagnostic approach to these diseases is beyond the scope of this discussion. However, a few pertinent issues will be raised. First, these diseases are characterized by multisystem involvement, a key to their diagnosis. Second, small arterial disease, as induced by classic polyarteritis nodosa, may cause progressive renal insufficiency or ARF in the absence of direct glomerular capillary involvement. Thus, characteristic findings of necrotizing glomerulitis (RBC casts, proteinuria) may be absent. Third, if the vasculitis is, indeed, confined to medium-sized vessels, a percutaneous renal biopsy will rarely yield the diagnosis. Thus, renal arteriography, possibly coupled with mesenteric arteriography, is the preferred diagnostic procedure. Fourth, if glomerular involvement is present (as manifested by RBC casts) a percutaneous renal biopsy will confirm that involvement, but a specific diagnosis may still not be obtained. This is because several leading causes of renal vasculitis induce nonspecific glomerular involvement (e.g., microscopic polyarteritis, Wegener's granulomatosis, idiopathic pauciimmune RPGN; i.e., diseases marked by high-serum ANCA titers). Thus, differentiating among these diseases will be necessary. However, the biopsy is still of help because it will exclude several small vessel vasculidities that have characteristic immunofluorescence findings (e.g., Henoch Schöenlein purpura, SLE, mixed essential cryoglobulinemia).

Microscopic Renal Atheroembolic Disease. Atheroembolic renal disease typically presents as acute or subacute renal failure in patients over the age of 50 who have severe atherosclerotic disease of the aorta and, possibly, other major vessels.[165–169] It is most often precipitated by aortic trauma, e.g., angiography, or during aortic surgery. However, spontaneous atheroembolism can also occur.[168] Released microscopic atheromatous plaques shower renal and extrarenal vascular beds, lodging in vessels of 150 to 200 μm in diameter. This initial event can induce immediate renal insufficiency (often masquerading as radiocontrast toxicity following arteriography), but more often, this acute phase is clinically inapparent. Over the ensuing days to weeks, the involved renal vessels (arcuates, interlobular arteries) develop progressive intimal proliferation with macrophage, giant cell, and sometimes, eosinophil infiltration. This process causes ongoing renal ischemia and hence, renal failure.

The diagnosis of atheroembolic ARF is generally obvious if a history of aortography/aortic trauma exists. The presence of extrarenal signs and symptoms of embolization (e.g., cutaneous infarcts in lower extremities, gastrointestinal bleeding, pancreatitis, livido reticularis, and reddened, elevated plaque-like lesions) also point to the diagnosis. With spontaneous atheroembolism, however, the cause of the renal failure is much less obvious and the multisystem involvement may suggest a vasculitis. Laboratory findings include hypocomplementemia, an elevated erythrocyte sedimentation rate, transient eosinophilia, and possibly thrombocytopenia.[165,169–171] Documentation of abdominal and femoral artery bruits, indicative of severe atherosclerotic disease, also suggests the diagnosis. There are no definitive urinalysis or urine chemistry changes. A certain diagnosis can only be made by biopsy of involved tissues. If lower extremity skin or muscles are involved, these are preferable sites, obviating the need for renal biopsy. If the latter is to be performed, an open procedure should be considered because the characteristic vascular lesions may be missed by needle biopsy. The decision to perform an open renal biopsy must be weighed carefully because no specific therapies are available for this disease and because the patients are frequently high-risk surgical candidates, given their advanced age and severe underlying vascular disease.

Renal Vein Thrombosis

Renal vein thrombosis (RVT) in adults is most commonly a chronic, insidious process that arises in the setting of the nephrotic syndrome[172,173] and frequently presents with a pulmonary embolus.[174,175] However, an acute thrombosis can also occur, particularly in infants, manifesting with flank pain and hematuria. ARF will result if the thrombosis is bilateral.[176] The most common underlying causes are the nephrotic syndrome, other hypercoaguable states, abdominal trauma (usually in concert with renal artery thrombosis), tumor, and dehydration in infancy. The differential diagnosis includes acute renal arterial thrombosis/thromboembolism, pyelonephritis, papillary necrosis, and urinary tract obstruction. In the presence of ARF, these conditions must be either bilateral, must occur in a solitary kidney, or must be associated with some contralateral acute complication. A definitive diagnosis of acute RVT generally requires inferior venacavography/renal venography.[177,178] An abdominal ultrasound may be quite helpful by documenting a characteristic increase in kidney size, the absence of urinary tract obstruction, and possibly the presence of vena caval or renal venous clot. Duplex Doppler, coupled with ultrasonography,[179,180] can be very helpful by documenting decreased or absent renal venous flow. Intravenous pyelography may yield useful diagnostic information, e.g., notching of ureters that is due to collateral circulation.[181–183] However, in the setting of ARF, nonvisualization is frequently found, and radiocontrast administration poses the risk of additional renal injury. Thus, either noninvasive (ultrasound/duplex Doppler) methods or a definitive venographic study are preferred.

URINARY TRACT OBSTRUCTION

Urinary tract obstruction accounts for approximately 6 percent of ARF cases.[23] It has a plethora of potential causes, ranging from the very common to the obscure; it can involve single or multiple sites within the urinary tract; and a myriad of presentations are possible, ranging from no symptomatology to acute or chronic renal failure. An overview of this expansive field is beyond the scope of this discussion, and excellent clinical and pathophysiologic reviews are available.[184,185] Thus, we will confine ourselves to a consideration of obstructive uropathy/nephropathy as a cause of ARF, focusing on diagnostic considerations.

Because of marked variability in causes, duration, and location of urinary tract obstruction, no uniform clinical presentation exists. Although the history may give valuable clues to the presence of obstructive uropathy, it is not uncommon for patients to offer virtually no symptoms referable to the urinary tract. This is particularly true when chronic, incomplete obstruction exists. Thus, it is important to recognize that a lack of symptoms by no means excludes obstruction, even when induced by lower urinary tract disease. However, in the presence of symptoms (e.g., hesitancy, intermittency, dribbling, polyuria, nocturia, bladder fullness, hematuria, dysuria, or pelvic and/or abdominal pain), the possibility of obstructive uropathy should be entertained. Physical signs may include a palpable bladder (with more than 500 ml of residual urine), prostatic enlargement, an abnormal gynecologic examination, or possibly, enlarged kidney(s). Depending on its duration, signs and symptoms of renal failure may also be present.

Urine Assessments

Anuria, oliguria, polyuria, or fluctuations between them are all possible, depending on the degree of obstruction. Hematuria is frequent, particularly when the obstruction is induced by a lesion within, rather than outside, the urinary tract. It is generally microscopic, but gross hematuria can also occur. Pyuria and bacteriuria suggest superimposed infection, a complication most commonly seen when chronic, incomplete obstruction exists. Minimal to mild proteinuria is the rule, reflecting an absence of glomerular damage. There are no characteristic urinary casts, although granular, hyaline, waxy, or rarely, white blood cell casts can be present. Urinary sodium and osmolality assessments yield variable results. Classically, the U_{Na} is high (greater than 40 mEq/L), and the urine concentration approximates isotonicity (U_{osm} less than 500), mimicking the findings of ATN. With short-lived obstruction, however, sodium avidity and a concentrated urine may be observed,[186] possibly reflecting the renal vasoconstriction that may occur early (within minutes to hours) in the course of this disease.[187] In our experience, a low U_{Na} may persist for several days if secondary pyelonephritis with complicating gram-negative bacteremia occurs. This probably represents a renal hemodynamic response to sepsis, but it underscores the point that sodium avidity does not preclude the possibility of obstruction-induced ARF.

Serum Chemistries

The serum chemistries will predominantly reflect the existence of ARF. However, it is worthwhile to scrutinize the acid-base status to assess whether a mixed high anion gap and normal anion gap acidosis exists. Chronic, incomplete urinary tract obstruction can induce a type 4 renal tubular acidosis, with or without hyperkalemia.[188] Thus, urinary tract obstruction is suggested if a mixed metabolic acidosis is observed and/or if the serum potassium concentration is increased out of proportion to the degree of ARF. As with PRA, the BUN/creatinine ratio may exceed 10:1, which has been attributed to a slowing of urinary flow, which allows for urea back-diffusion across tubules and dilated collecting system. In our experience, however this finding is less commonly observed with obstruction than with PRA. Thus, its existence should prompt a careful assessment of intravascular volume status, particularly because partial obstruction can produce a sodium wasting state.

Radiologic Procedures

Although the history and laboratory assessments can give clues to the presence of obstructive uropathy, this remains a radiologic diagnosis. Indeed, even in the total absence of obstructive signs and symptoms, obstruction must be excluded if the cause of ARF is at all in doubt. Flat-plate examination of the abdomen or nephrotomography may, on occasion, be helpful if enlarged kidney(s) or renal/ureteric stones are observed. These examinations, however, are by no means definitive, and hence, other techniques for visualizing the urinary tract are essential. *Intravenous pyelography* (IVP) traditionally has been the principal diagnostic procedure for excluding obstructive uropathy.[185] However, delayed films (12 to 24 hours) are often necessary to visualize the collecting system and in the presence of severe or long-standing renal failure, such a finding may not develop as a result of inadequate renal function. Furthermore, administration of contrast poses the risk of superimposed nephrotoxic renal injury. *Renal ultrasonography* therefore has become the screening procedure of choice for urinary tract obstruction-induced ARF (Fig. 3-4). The procedure is rapid, requires no radiocontrast material, and has a reported accuracy of 90 percent or more.[189–194] Like all tests, however, it has its limitations. Obesity may preclude an adequate examination, an 8 to 26 percent false-positive rate, which is due to the detection of small increases in renal pelvic volume, has been reported,[189,192] and retroperitoneal fibrosis, or superimposed PRA or ATN, may preclude collecting system dilatation. Last, a major limitation of ultrasonography is that although obstruction can generally be detected, the

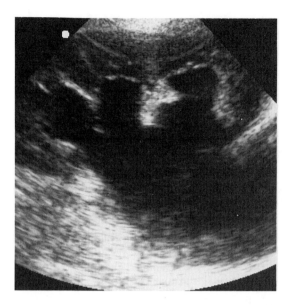

Fig. 3-4. Ultrasound scan of urinary tract obstruction. Massive dilation of the renal pelvis is observed.

cause of that obstruction is usually not revealed. If a dilated ureter is observed, this at least localizes the obstruction to the lower urinary tract.

If obstruction is strongly suspected but the ultrasound is negative, it is worthwhile to either repeat the procedure 1 or 2 days later (allowing time for dilatation to develop) or to proceed with more definitive diagnostic techniques. Abdominal CT can be particularly helpful in this regard.[195] Collecting system dilatation (Fig. 3-5) is routinely observed without contrast administration; retroperitoneal causes of obstruction, such as tumor, are readily defined; and stones are visualized, whether radiopaque or radiolucent in nature. Although a dilated ureter localizes obstruction to the lower urinary tract, the precise level is generally not defined unless a stone or mass lesion is evident. By administering intravenous contrast, this information, as well as a better definition of renal anatomy and function, can be obtained. However, two points should be recalled: (1) contrast may mask the presence of a stone and thus, a nonenhanced CT should be performed first; and (2) there is the ever present risk of contrast-induced renal damage.

Retrograde or antegrade pyelography are other approaches for definitively excluding urinary tract obstruction. These should be considered if the diagnosis and/or site of obstruction have not already been clearly defined. Antegrade pyelography permits pelvic brushings to be obtained for cytology, while a retrograde study allows direct visualization and biopsy of prostatic and bladder lesions. Although both techniques incur small surgical risks, they may permit both diagnosis and therapy at the same time. For example,

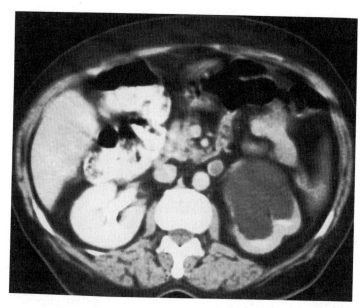

Fig. 3-5. Abdominal computed tomography scan. Massive right hydronephrosis is apparent (no contrast).

nephrostomy tube placement will alleviate unilateral obstruction, lower ureteral stones can be removed during a retrograde procedure, and ureteral stints can be placed. Obviously, the decision to perform invasive pyelography, rather than CT, and the route by which the former is undertaken need to be assessed on a case by case basis.

Radionuclide scanning has been reported to be 90 percent sensitive in detecting urinary tract obstruction.[196] However, it suffers from a lack of specificity, and like IVPs, inadequate visualization can occur with severe renal dysfunction. Thus, these techniques should not be relied on for diagnosis. In contrast, *MRI* may be very useful. However, the great expense and lack of ready availability preclude its use as a routine diagnostic test.

Intrarenal Obstruction

For the sake of completeness, it should be recalled that urinary tract obstruction at the tubular level can also occur. This can result from high-dose methotrexate therapy in the absence of urinary alkalinization and hydration,[197] during high-dose acyclovir treatment,[198,199] and with the tumor cell lysis syndrome.[200–202] The first two are thought to be due to intratubular drug precipitation, while the latter is probably caused, at least in part, by intraluminal uric acid and inorganic phosphate precipitation. Other examples of ARF in which intraluminal precipitation of filtrable substances occur include ethylene glycol intoxication, acute myeloma nephropathy (light chain precipitation), and myohemoglobinuria. In these latter cases, however, intratubular obstruction is almost certainly not the only operative mechanism because direct cytotoxicity from these compounds or their derivatives can occur.

The diagnosis of these forms of ARF is suggested by the clinical setting (e.g., high-dose chemotherapy) or, in the case of multiple myeloma or ethylene glycol intoxication, by specific laboratory tests. Radiographic procedures are of little, if any, value, because intratubular obstruction precludes collecting system dilatation.

SUMMARY

ARF represents a syndrome, not a specific disease, that spans the entire spectrum of renal pathophysiologic disorders. Although it is generally viewed as being prerenal, intrarenal, or postrenal in cause, it is clear that multiple disorders, involving different pathophysiologic mechanisms, fall into each of these three categories. Because ARF, unlike chronic renal failure, is usually reversible, and because treatments vary according to cause, a careful consideration of all diagnostic possibilities in any given patient is imperative. The first step is to ascertain whether the renal failure is truly acute in nature. This is generally simple to do, based on historical grounds and, if necessary, on ultrasonic assessment of kidney size. The latter will also exclude extrarenal urinary tract obstruction in 90 percent or more of cases. A diagnosis of PRA should then be entertained. A presumptive diagnosis can usually be made on the basis of the history and simple physical assessments. Coupled with consistent laboratory findings, most notably a low U_{Na} and normal urine sediment, a relatively secure diagnosis of PRA can be made in most patients. If PRA is excluded, intrarenal causes of ARF are then considered. In approximately 80 to 90 percent of such patients, ATN will be responsible. By knowing the time of onset, plausible precipitating events can usually be identified. The presence of characteristic urine findings (muddy brown granular casts and a high U_{Na}), help to substantiate the diagnosis. An atypical presentation or uncharacteristic laboratory results should raise the possibility of other parenchymal causes of ARF, principally vasculopathies, AGN, and AIN. A vasculopathy is suggested by the presence of an ill-defined multisystem disorder. AGN is likely if heavy proteinuria, dysmorphic RBCs in the urine, and RBC casts are observed. Last, fever, rash, and eosinophilia or eosinophiluria, coupled with a history of exposure to specific drugs, strongly suggest AIN. A summary of diagnostic clues to each of these disorders is presented in Table 3-5.

Although a careful, systematic approach will usually lead to the correct detailed in this chapter. Because renal biopsies are not performed in most ARF patients, it must be recognized that presumptive, not definitive, diagnoses are usually made. Thus, during the course of patient follow-up, the

Table 3-5. Laboratory Features in Different Forms of ARF

Disorder	Urine Sediment	U_{Na} (mEq/L)[a]	U_{osm}	U_{prot}	Other
Prerenal azotemia	Normal	<20	>500	0–2+	BUN/Cr >20/1
ATN					
Oliguric	ATN casts	>40	<350	0–2+	—
Nonoliguric	ATN casts	Variable	<350	0–2+	—
AGN	Dysmorphic RBCs, RBC casts	Variable	Variable	2–4+	↓ complements; ANCA, αGBM, ASO, blood cultures, cryoglobulins
AIN					
General	±Pyuria, hematuria	>40	Variable	0–2+	Fever, rash, eosinophilia, eosinophiluria
NSAIDS	±Pyuria, hematuria	<20	Variable	3–4+	Absence of above; ↑ serum K^+
Vasculopathy					
Renal artery, thrombosis/ embolus	Hematuria	>40	<350	0–2+	↑ serum LDH; angiogram
Atheroemboli	Normal	>40	<350	0–2+	↓ C_3, C_4; eosinophilia, ↓ platelets
HUS/TTP	±RBC casts	>40	Variable	Variable	MHA. ↓ platelets
Obstruction	Normal or RBCs	Variable	Variable	0–1+	Ultrasound, CT

Abbreviations: AGN, acute glomerulonephritis; AIN, acute interstitial nephritis; αGBM, antiglomerular basement membrane antibody; ANCA, antineutrophil cytoplasmic antibody; ASO, antistreptolysin O antibody; ARF, acute renal failure; ATN, acute tubular necrosis; BUN/Cr, blood urea nitrogen/creatinine ratio; CT, computed tomography; CT; HUS/TTP, hemolytic uremic syndrome/thrombotic thrombocytopenic purpura; LDH, lactic dehydrogenase; MHA, microangiopathic hemolytic anemia; RBC, red blood cell; U_{osm}, urinary osmolarity; U_{prot}, spot urine protein by dipstick.
[a] U_{Na} of <20 can be equated with a Fe_{Na} of <1%.

possibility of a misdiagnosis needs to be entertained. Unequivocal diagnoses are frequently known only in retrospect, after the disease course and/or its response to therapy have been observed. Thus, a degree of diagnostic skepticism is warranted. If therapy is critically dependent on having a definitive diagnosis, a renal biopsy should be obtained. Unfortunately, this point underscores the fact that important gaps in our diagnostic approach to the ARF patient continue to exist.

REFERENCES

1. Anderson RJ, Schrier RW: Acute tubular necrosis. p. 1413. In Schrier RW, Gottschalk CW (eds): Diseases of the Kidney 4th Ed. Little, Brown, Boston, 1988
2. Kincaid-Smith P, Bennett WM, Dowling JP et al: Acute renal failure and tubular necrosis associated with haematuria due to glomerulonephritis. Clin Nephrol 19:206, 1983
3. Kelleher SP, Berl T: Acute renal failure associated with hypovolemia. p. 233. In Brenner BM, Lazarus JM (eds): Acute Renal Failure. 2nd Ed. Churchill Livingstone, New York, 1988
4. Schlondorff D, Neuwirth R: Platlet activating factor and the kidney. Am J Physiol 251:F1, 1986
5. Brenner BM, Troy JL, Ballerman BJ: Endothelium-dependent vascular responses: mediators and mechanisms. J Clin Invest 84:1373, 1989
6. Bonjour JP, Malvin RL: Renal extraction of PAH, GFR, and $U_{Na}V$ in the rat during infusion of angiotension. Am J Physiol 216:554, 1974
7. Gagnon JA, Keller HL, Kokotis W, Schrier RW: Analysis of role of renin-angiotension system in autoregulation of glomerular filtration. Am J Physiol 219:491, 1970
8. Regoli D, Gauthier R: Site of action of angiotensin and other vasoconstrictors on the kidney. Can J Physiol Pharmacol 49:608, 1971
9. Zimmerman BG, Abboud FM, Eckstein JW: Effects of norepinephrine and angiotensin on total and venous resistance in the kidney. Am J Physiol 206:701, 1964
10. Brenner BM, Troy JL: Postglomerular vascular protein concentration: Evidence for a causal role in governing fluid reabsorption and glomerular tubular balance by the proximal tubule. J Clin Invest 50:336, 1971
11. Burg MB: Renal handling of sodium, chloride, water, amino acids, and glucose. p. 145. In Brenner BM, Rector FC (eds.): The Kidney. 3rd Ed. WB Saunders, Philadelphia, 1986
12. Miller PD, Krebs RA, Neal BJ et al: Polyuric prerenal failure. Arch Intern Med 140:907, 1980
13. Myers BD, Carrie BJ, Yee RR et al: Pathophysiology of hemodynamically mediated acute renal failure in man. Kidney Int 18:495, 1980
14. Myers BD, Hilberman M, Spencer RJ et al: Glomerular and tubular function in non-oliguric acute renal failure. Am J Med 72:642, 1982
15. Myers BD, Moran SM: Hemodynamically mediated acute renal failure. N Engl J Med 314:97, 1986

16. Waugh WH: Functional types of acute renal failure and their early diagnosis. Arch Intern Med 103:686, 1958
17. Welt LG: Clinical Disorders of Hydration and Acid-Base Equilibrium. Little, Brown, Boston, 1955, p 262
18. Espinal CH: The Fe_{Na} test use in the differential diagnosis of acute renal failure. JAMA 236:579, 1976
19. Espinal CH, Gregory AW: Differential diagnosis of acute renal failure. Clin Nephrol 13:73, 1980
20. Handa SP: Diagnostic indices in acute renal failure. Can Med Assoc J 96:78, 1967
21. Miller TR, Anderson RJ, Berns AS et al: Urinary diagnostic indices in acute renal failure. A prospective study. Ann Intern Med 88:47, 1978
22. Anderson RJ, Gross PA, Gabow P: Urinary chloride concentration in acute renal failure. Miner Electrolyte Metab 10:92, 1984
23. Kjellstrand CM, Ebeen J, Davin T: Time of death, recovery of renal function, development of chronic renal failure and need for chronic hemodialysis in patients with acute tubular necrosis. Trans Am Soc Artif Intern Organs 27:45, 1981
24. Levinsky NG, Alexander EA: Acute renal failure, p. 806. In Brenner BM, Rector FC (eds): The Kidney. 1st Ed. WB Saunders, Philadelphia, 1976
25. Rudnick MR, Bastl CP, Elfinbein IB, Narins RG: The differential diagnosis of acute renal failure. p. 177. In (Brenner BM, Lazarus JM (eds): Acute Renal Failure. 2nd Ed. Churchill Livingstone, New York, 1988
26. Zager RA, O'Quigley J, Zager BK et al: Acute renal failure following bone marrow transplantation: a retrospective study of 272 patients. Am J Kidney Dis 13:210, 1989
27. Summerskill WHJ: Hepatic failure and the kidney. Gastroenterology 51:94, 1966
28. Baldus WP, Feichter RN, Summerskill WHJ: The kidney in cirrhosis: I. Clinical and biochemical features of azotemia in hepatic failure. Ann Intern Med 60:353, 1964
29. Baldus WP, Feichter RN, Summerskill WHJ et al: The kidney in cirrhosis. II. Disorders of renal function. Ann Intern Med 60:366, 1964
30. Conn HO: A rational approach to the hepatorenal syndrome. Gastroenterology 65:321, 1973
31. Hecker R, Sherlock S: Electrolyte and circulatory changes in terminal liver failure. Lancet 2:1121, 1956
32. Papper S: The role of the kidney in Laennec's cirrhosis of the liver. Medicine 37:299, 1958
33. Papper S: The hepatorenal syndrome. p. 87. In Epstein M (ed): The Kidney in Liver Disease. 2nd Ed. Elsevier Biomedical, New York, 1983
34. Papper S, Belosky JL, Bleifer KH: Renal failure in Laennec's cirrhosis of the liver: (1) Description of clinical and laboratory features. Ann Intern Med 51:759, 1959
35. Better OS, Chaimovitz C: The hepatorenal syndrome. p. 1489. In Schrier RW, Gottschalk CW (eds.): Diseases of the Kidney. Little, Brown, Boston, 1988
36. Epstein M: The LeVeen shunt for ascites and hepatorenal syndrome. N Engl J Med 302:628, 1980
37. Epstein M: Peritoneovenous shunt in the management of ascites and the hepatorenal syndrome. Gastroenterology 82:790, 1982

38. Iwatsuki S, Popovitzer MM, Corman JL et al: Recovery from "hepatorenal syndrome" after orthotopic liver transplantation. N Engl J Med 289:1155, 1973

39. Dawson JL: Acute postoperative renal failure in obstructive jaundice. Ann R Coll Surg 42:163, 1968

40. Williams RD, Elliot DW, Zolinger RM: The effect of hypotension in obstructive jaundice. Arch Surg 81:182, 1960

41. Levenson DJ, Skorecki KL, Newell GC, Narins RG: Acute renal failure associated with hepatobiliary disease. p. 535 In Brenner BM, Lazarus JM (eds.): Acute Renal Failure. 2nd Ed. Churchill Livingstone, New York, 1988

42. Moore RD, Smith CR, Lipsky TS et al: Risk factors for nephrotoxicity in patients treated with aminoglycosides. Ann Intern Med 100:352, 1984

43. Newell GC: Cirrhotic glomerulonephritis: incidence, morphology, clinical features, and pathogenesis. Am J Kidney Dis 9:183, 1987

44. Fukuda Y: Renal glomerular changes associated with liver cirrhosis. Acta Pathol Jpn 32:361, 1982

45. Manigand G, Taillandier J, Morel-Maroger L et al: La Néphropathie gloméru-laire de cirrhoses du foie. Ann Med Interne (Paris) 132:178, 1981

46. Edmondson HA, Reynolds TB, Jacobson HG: Renal papillary necrosis with special reference to chronic alcoholism: a report of 20 cases. Arch Intern Med 118:255, 1966

47. Patrono C, Dunn MJ: the clinical significance of inhibition of renal prostaglan-din synthesis. Kidney Int 32:1, 1987

48. Clive DM, Stoff JS: Renal syndromes associated with non-steroidal anti-inflammatory drugs. N Engl J Med 310:563, 1984

49. Whelton A, Stout RL, Spilman PS, Klassen DK: Renal effects of ibupro-fin, piroxicam, and sulindac in patients with asymptomatic renal failure: a prospective, randomized, crossover study. Ann Intern Med 112:568, 1990

50. Ciabattoni G, Cinotti GA, Pierucci A et al: Effects of sulindac and ibuprofin in patients with chronic glomerular disease. Evidence for the dependence of renal function on prostacyclin. N Engl J Med 310:279–283, 1984

51. Patrone C, Ciabattoni G, Remuzzi G et al: Functional significance of renal prostacyclin and thromboxane A_2 production in patients with systemic lupus erythematosis. J Clin Invest 76:1011, 1985

52. Galler M, Folkert VW, Schondorff D: Reversible acute renal insufficiency and hyperkalemia following indomethacin therapy. JAMA 264:154, 1981

53. Berheim JL, Rorzets Z: Indomethacin-induced renal failure. Ann Intern Med 91:792, 1979

54. Kimberly RP, Bowden RE, Keiser HR et al: Reduction of renal function by newer nonsteroidal anti-inflammatory drugs. Am J Med 64:804, 1978

55. Abraham RA, Keane WF: Glomerular and interstitial disease induced by non-steroidal anti-inflammatory drugs. Am J Nephrol 4:1, 1984

56. Torres VE: Present and future of the non-steroidal anti-inflammatory drugs in nephrology. Mayo Clin Proc 57:389, 1982

57. Keane WF, Anderson S, Aurell M et al: Angiotensin converting enzyme inhibi-tors and progressive renal insufficiency. Ann Intern Med 111:503, 1989

58. Hricik DE, Browning PJ, Kopelman R et al: Captopril-induced functional renal insufficiency in patients with bilateral renal artery stenosis or renal artery stenosis in a solitary kidney. N Engl J Med 308:373, 1983

59. Jackson B, Matthews PG, McGrath BP, Johnston CI: Angiotensin converting enzyme inhibition in renovascular hypertension: frequency of reversible renal failure, letter. Lancet 1:225, 1984
60. Hollenberg N: Medical therapy of renovascular hypertension: efficacy and safety of captopril in 269 patients. Cardiovasc Rev Rep 4:854, 1983
61. Cahan DH, Ucci AA: Acute renal failure, interstitial nephritis, and nephrotic syndrome with captopril. Kidney Int 25:160, 1984
62. Kahan BD: Drug therapy: cyclosporine. N Engl J Med 321:1725, 1989
63. Perico N, Dadan J, Remuzzi G: Endothelin mediates the renal vasoconstriction induced by cyclosporine in the rat. J Am Soc Nephrol 1:76, 1990
64. Sawaya B, Provenzano R, Kupin WL, Venkat KK: Cyclosporine-induced renal macroangiopathy. Am J Kidney Dis 12:534, 1988
65. Kreisberg JI, Venkatachalam MA: Morphologic factors in acute renal failure. p. 45. In Brenner BM, Lazarus JM (eds): Acute Renal Failure. 2nd Ed. Churchill Livingstone, New York, 1988
66. Hostetter TH, Wilkes BM, Brenner BM: Mechanisms of impaired glomerular filtration in acute renal failure. p. 52. In Brenner BM, Stein JH (eds): Contemporary Issues in Nephrology #6: Acute Renal Failure. Churchill Livingstone, New York, 1979
67. Rasmussen HH, Ibils LS: Acute renal failure. Multivariate analysis of causes and risk factors. Am J Med 96:793, 1982
68. Mustonen J, Pasternack A, Helin H et al: Renal biopsy in acute renal failure. Am J Nephrol 4:27, 1984
69. Bull GM, Joekes AM, Lowe KG: Renal function studies in acute tubular necrosis. Clin Sci 9:379, 1950
70. Sirota JH: Carbon tetrachloride poisoning in man: I. The mechanisms of renal failure and recovery. J Clin Invest 28:1412, 1949
71. Carvallo A, Rukowski TA, Argy WP, Schreiner GE: Acute renal failure following drip infusion pyelography. Am J Med 65:38, 1978
72. D'Elia JA, Kaldeny A, Weinbrauch LA, Buchbinder EM: Inadequacy of fractional excretion of sodium test, letter. Arch Intern Med 141:818, 1981
73. Fang LS, Sirota RA, Ebert TH, Lichenstein NS: Low fractional excretion of sodium with contrast media-induced acute renal failure. Arch Intern Med 140:531, 1980
74. VanZee BE, Hoy WE, Talley TE, Jaenike JR: Renal injury associated with intravenous pyelography in non-diabetic and diabetic patients. Ann Intern Med 89:51, 1978
75. Hou SH, Bushinsky DA, Wish JB, et al: Hospital acquired renal insufficiency: A prospective study. Am J Med 74:243, 1983
76. Luke RG, Briggs JD, Allison MEM, Kennedy AC: Factors determining response to mannitol in acute renal failure. Am J Med Sci 259:168, 1970
77. Eliahou HE, Bata A: The diagnosis of acute renal failure. Nephrology 2:287, 1967
78. Dubrow A, Flamenbaum W: Acute renal failure associated with myoglobinuria and hemoglobinuria. p. 279. In Brenner BM, Lazarus JM (eds): Acute Renal Failure. 2nd Ed. Churchill Livingstone, New York, 1988
79. Gabow P, Kaehny W, Kelleher S: The spectrum of rhabdomyolysis. Medicine 61:141, 1982
80. Better O, Stein J: Early management of shock and prophylaxis of acute renal failure in traumatic rhabdomyolysis. N Engl J Med 322:825, 1990

81. Roth D, Alarcon F, Fernandez J et al: Acute rhabdomyolysis associated with cocaine intoxication. N Engl J Med 319:673, 1988

82. Rubin R, Neugarten J: Cocaine-induced rhabdomyolysis masquerading as myocardial ischemia. Am J Med 86:551, 1989

83. Pogue V, Nurse H: Cocaine-associated acute myoglobinuric renal failure. Am J Med 86:183, 1989

84. Wilke W: Recognition and treatment of cocaine abuse. Cleveland Clin J Med 57:595, 1990

85. Grossman RA, Hamilton RW, Morse BM et al: Non-traumatic rhabdomyolysis and acute renal failure. N Engl J Med 291:807, 1974

86. Koffler A, Friedler RM, Massey SG: Acute renal failure due to non-traumatic rhabdomyolysis. Ann Intern Med 85:23, 1976

87. Chugh KS, Nath IV, Ubroi HS et al: Acute renal failure due to non-traumatic rhabdomyolysis. Postgrad Med J 55:386, 1979

88. Humes HD, O'Connor RP: Aminoglycoside nephrotoxicity. p. 1229. In Schrier RW, Gottschalk CW (eds): Diseases of the Kidney. 4th Ed. Little Brown, Boston, 1988

89. Zager RA, Prior RB: Gentamicin and Gram negative bacteremia. A synergism for the development of experimental nephrotoxic acute renal failure. J Clin Invest 78:196, 1986

90. Zager RA: Gentamicin nephrotoxicity in the setting of acute renal hypoperfusion. Am J Physiol 254:F574, 1988

91. Cronin RE, Bulger RE, Southern P, Henrich WC: Natural history of aminoglycoside nephrotoxicity in the dog. J Lab Clin Med 95:463, 1980

92. Ginsburg DS, Quintanilla AP, Levin M: Renal glycosuria due to gentamicin in rabbits. J Infect Dis 134:119, 1976

93. Beck PR, Thomson RB, Chaudhuri AKR: Aminoglycoside antibiotics and renal function: changes in urinary gamma-glutamyltransferase excretion. J Clin Pathol 30:432, 1977

94. Parfrey PS, Griffiths SM, Barrett BJ et al: Contrast material-induced renal failure in patients with diabetes mellitus, renal insufficiency, or both: a prospective controlled study. N Engl J Med 320:143, 1989

95. Schwab SJ, Hlatky MA, Pieper KS et al: Contrast nephrotoxicity: a randomized controlled trial of a nonionic and an ionic radiographic contrast agent. N Engl J Med 320:149, 1989

96. Martin-Paredero V, Dixon SM, Baker JD et al: Risk of renal failure after major angiography. Arch Surg 118:1417, 1983

97. Harkonen S, Kjellstrand CM: Exacerbation of diabetic renal failure following intravenous pyelography. Am J Med 63:939, 1977

98. Tejler L, Almen T, Holtas S: Proteinuria following nephroangiography. Acta Radiol [Diagn] (Stockh) 18:634, 1977

99. Older RA, Korobkin M, Cleeve DM et al: Contrast-induced acute renal failure; persistent nephrogram as clue to early detection. Am J Roentgenol 134:339, 1980

100. D'Elia JA, Gleason RE, Alday M et al: Nephrotoxicity from angiographic contrast material. A prospective study. Am J Med 72:719, 1982

101. Feldman MA, Goldfarb S, McCurdy DK: Recurrent radiography dye-induced acute renal failure. JAMA 229:72 1974

102. Cohen DJ, Sherman WH, Osserman EF, Appel GB: Acute renal failure in patients with multiple myeloma. Am J Med 76:247, 1989

103. Smolens P: The kidney in dysproteinemic states. Am Kidney Foundation Nephrology Letter 4:27, 1987

104. Schrier RW: Acute renal failure (Nephrology Forum). Kidney Int 15:205, 1979

105. Zager RA: Adenine nucleotide changes in kidney, liver and small intestine during different forms of ischemic injury. Circ Res, 68:185, 1991

106. Zager RA: Ischemic acute renal failure: A multifactorial disease? In Solez K, Racusen L (eds): Acute Renal Failure: Diagnosis, Treatment, and Prevention. Marcel Dekker, New York, 1991

107. Couser WG: Rapidly progressive glomerulonephritis: classification, pathogenetic mechanisms, and therapy. Am J Kidney Dis 11:449, 1988

108. Jennette JC, Falk RS: Diagnosis and management of glomerulonephritis and vasculitis presenting as acute renal failure. Med Clin North Am 73:893, 1990

109. Salant DS, Adler S, Bernard DB, Stilmant M: Acute renal failure associated with renal vascular disease, vasculitis, glomerulonephritis, and nephrotic syndrome. p. 371. In Brenner BM, Lazarus JM (eds): Acute Renal Failure. 2nd Ed. Churchill Livingstone, New York, 1988

110. Nicholson GD, Amin UF, Alleyne GAO: Membranous nephropathy with crescents. Clin Nephrol 5:197, 1975

111. Moorthy A, Zimmerman S, Harrington A, Burkholder P: Progression from membranous glomerulopathy to antiglomerular basement membrane (GBM) antibody mediated crescentic nephritis. Clin Nephrol 6:319, 1976

112. Lyons H, Penn VW, Cortell S et al: Allergic interstitial nephritis causing reversible renal failure in four patients with nephrotic syndrome. N Engl J Med 288:124, 1973

113. Whitworth JA, Morel-Maroger L, Mignon F et al: The significance of extracapillary proliferation: clinical pathological review of 60 patients. Nephron 16:1, 1976

114. Leonard CD, Nagle RB, Striker GE et al: Acute glomerulonephritis with prolonged oliguria. An analysis of 29 cases. Ann Intern Med 73:703, 1970

115. Bacani RA, Velasquez F, Kanter A et al: Rapidly progressive (nonstreptococcal) glomerulonephritis. Ann Intern Med 69:463, 1968

116. Ginsburg JM, Chang BS, Matarese RA, Garella S: Use of single voided urine samples to estimate quantitative proteinuria. N Engl J Med 309:1543, 1983

117. Fairley KF, Birch DF: Hematuria: A simple method for identifying glomerular bleeding. Kidney Int 21:105, 1982

118. Birch DF, Fairley KF, Whitworth JA et al: Urinary erythrocyte morphology in the diagnosis of glomerular hematuria. Clin Nephrol 20:78, 1983

119. Fassett RG, Horgan BA, Mathew TH: Detection of glomerular bleeding by phase contrast microscopy. Lancet 1:1432, 1982

120. Schramek P, Moritsch A, Haschkowitz H et al: In vitro generation of dysmorphic erythrocytes. Kidney Int 36:72, 1987

121. Gibbs DD, Lynn KL: Red cell volume distribution curves in the diagnosis of glomerular and non glomerular hematuria. Clin Nephrol 33:143, 1990

122. Jennette JC, Falk RJ: Antineutrophil cytoplasmic autoantibodies and associated diseases: A review. Am J Kidney Dis 15:517, 1990

123. Falk RJ, Jennette RJ: Anti-neutrophil cytoplasmic autoantibodies with specificity for myeloperoxidase in patients with systemic vasculitis and idiopathic necrotizing and crescentic glomerulonephritis. N Engl J Med 318:1651, 1988

124. ES LA, Wilk A: ANCA: Clinical association and use in disease monitoring. Neth J Med 30:146, 1990

125. Linton AL, Clark WF, Driedgu AA et al: Acute interstitial nephritis due to drugs. Review of the literature with a report of 9 cases. Ann Intern Med 93:735, 1980

126. Richet G, Sraer JD, Kourilsky O, et al: La ponction-biopsie rénale dans l'insuffisance rénale aiguë. Ann Med Interne (Paris) 129:335, 1978

127. Grünfeld JP, Kleinknecht D, Droz D: Acute interstitial nephritis. p. 1461. In Schrier RW, Gottschalk CW (eds): Diseases of the Kidney. 4th Ed. Little, Brown, Boston, 1988

128. Kleinknecht D, Vanhille P, Morel-Maroger L et al: Acute interstitial nephritis due to drug hypersensitivity. An up-to-date review with a report of 19 cases. Adv Nephrol 12:277, 1983

129. Ten RM, Torres VE, Millener DS et al: Acute interstitial nephritis: immunological and clinical aspects. Mayo Clin Proc 63:921, 1988

130. Appel GB, Kunis CL: Acute tubulointerstitial nephritis. Contemp Issues in Nephrol 10:151, 1986

131. Ditlove J, Weidman P, Bernstein M, Massey G: Methicillin nephritis. Medicine 56:483, 1977

132. Galpin JE, Shinaberger JH, Stanley TM et al: Acute interstitial nephritis due to methicillin. Am J Med 65:756, 1978

133. Eknoyan G: Acute renal failure associated with tubulointerstitial nephropathies. p. 491. In Brenner BM, Lazarus JM (eds): Acute Renal Failure. 2nd Ed. Churchill Livingstone, New York, 1988

134. Nolan III, CR, Anger MS, Kelleher SP: Eosinophiluria—a new method of detection and definition of the clinical spectrum. N Engl J Med 315:1516, 1986

135. Wood BC, Sharma JN, Germann DR et al: Gallium citrate Ga[67] imaging in non-infectious interstitial nephritis. Arch Intern Med 138:1665, 1978

136. Brezin JH, Katz SM, Schwartz AB et al: Reversible renal failure and nephrotic syndrome associated with non steroidal anti-inflammatory drugs. N Engl J Med 301:1271, 1979

137. Lee HW: Hemorrhagic fever with renal syndrome (HFRS). Scand J Infect Dis [Suppl] 36:82, 1982

138. Desmyter J, Johnson KM, Deckers C et al: Laboratory rat associated outbreak of haemorrhagic fever with renal syndrome due to Hantaan virus in Belgium. Lancet 2:1445, 1983

139. Stables DP, Fouche RF, DeVillers van Niekerk JP et al: Traumatic renal artery occlusion: 21 cases. J Urol 115:229, 1976

140. Edwards BS, Stanson AW, Holley L et al: Isolated renal artery dissection: Presentation, evaluation, management, and pathology. Mayo Clin Proc 57:564, 1982

141. Hoxie HJ, Coggin CB: Renal infarction: Statistical study of two hundred and five cases and detailed report of an unusual case. Arch Intern Med 65:587, 1940

142. Regan FC, Crabtree EG: Renal infarction: a clinical and possible surgical entity. J Urol 59:981, 1948

143. Lessman RK, Johnson ST, Coburn JW, et al: Renal artery embolism: clinical features and long term follow-up in 17 cases. Ann Intern Med 89:477, 1978

144. Martin DC: Renal artery aneurysm with peripheral embolization of kidney. Urology 15:590, 1980

145. Gault MH, Steiner G: Serum and urinary enzyme activity after renal infarction. Can Med Assoc J 93:1101, 1965

146. Parker MD: Acute segmental renal infarction: difficulty in diagnosis despite multimodality approach. Urology 18:523, 1981

147. Erwin BC, Carroll BA, Walter JF et al: Renal infarction appearing as an echogenic mass. Am J Roentgenol 138:759, 1982

148. Harris RD, Dorros S: Computed tomographic diagnosis of renal infarction. Urology 17:287, 1981

149. Hartenbauer DL, Winston MA, Weiss ER et al: The scintillation camera in embolic acute renal failure. J Urol 104:799, 1970

150. Freeman LM, Meng CH, Richter MW et al: Patency of major renal vascular pathways demonstrated by rapid blood flow scintophotography. J Urol 105:473, 1971

151. Kleinknecht D, Grünfeld JP, Cia Gomez P et al: Diagnostic procedures and long term prognosis in bilateral renal cortical necrosis. Kidney Int 4:390, 1973

152. Grünfeld JP, Ganeval D, Bournérias F: Acute renal failure in pregnancy. Kidney Int 18:179, 1980

153. Donohoe J: Acute bilateral cortical necrosis. p. 252. In Brenner BM, Lazarus JM (eds): Acute Renal Failure. 1st Ed. WB Saunders, Philadelphia, 1983

154. Deutsch V, Frankl O, Drory Y et al: Bilateral renal cortical necrosis with survival through the acute phase with a note on the value of selective nephro-angiography. Am J Med 50:828, 1971

155. Cannon PS, Hassar M, Case DB et al: The relationship of hypertension and renal failure in scleroderma (progressive systemic sclerosis) to structural and functional abnormalities of the renal cortical circulation. Medicine 53:1, 1974

156. Traub YM, Shapiro AP, Rodman GP et al: Hypertension and renal failure in progressive systemic sclerosis. Medicine (Baltimore) 62:335, 1983

157. Levine RJ, Boshell, BR: Renal involvement in progressive systemic sclerosis (scleroderma). Ann Intern Med 52:517, 1960

158. Rodnan GP, Shapiro AP, Krifcher E: The occurrence of malignant hypertension and renal insufficiency in progressive systemic sclerosis (diffuse scleroderma). Ann Intern Med 60:737, 1964

159. LeRoy EC, Fleischmann RM: The management of renal scleroderma: Experience with dialysis, nephrectomy, and transplantation. Am J Med 64:974, 1978

160. Kaplan BS, Drummond KN: The hemolytic uremic syndrome is a syndrome. N Engl J Med 298:964, 1978

161. Ponticelli C, Rivolta E, Imbasciati E et al: Hemolytic uremic syndrome in adults. Arch Intern Med 140:353, 1980

162. Brain MC, Neame PB: Thrombotic thrombocytopenic purpura and the hemolytic uremic syndrome. Semin Thromb Hemost 8:186, 1982

163. Cuttner J: Thrombotic thrombocytopenic purpura: a ten year experience. Blood 56:302, 1980

164. Neill MA, Agosti J, Rosen H: Hemorrhagic colitis with Escherichia coli O157:H7 preceeding adult hemolytic uremic syndrome. Arch Intern Med 145:2215, 1985

165. Kassirer JP: Atheroembolic renal disease. N Engl J Med 280:812, 1969

166. Thurlbeck WM, Castleman B: Atheromatous emboli to the kidneys after aortic surgery. N Engl J Med 257:442, 1957

167. Smith MC, Ghose MK, Henry AR: The clinical spectrum of renal cholestrol embolization. Am J Med 71:174, 1981

168. Gore I, Collins DP: Spontaneous atheromatous embolization: Review of the literature and report of 16 additional cases. Am J Clin Pathol 33:416, 1960

169. Eliot RS, Kanjuh VI, Edwards JE: Atheromatous embolism. Circulation 30:611, 1964
170. Bidani A, Kasinath BS, Corwin HL et al: Eosinophilia in the diagnosis of atheroembolic renal disease. Kidney Int 27:134A, 1985
171. Cosio FG, Zager RA, Sharma HM: Atheroembolic renal disease causes hypocomplementemia. Lancet 2:118, 1985
172. Llach F, Koffler A, Massry SG: Renal vein thrombosis and the nephrotic syndrome. Nephron 19:65, 1977
173. Mukherjee AP, Tog BH, Chan GL: Vascular complications in nephrotic syndrome: relationship to steroid therapy and accelerated thromboplastin generation. Br Med J 4:273, 1970
174. Rosenmann E, Pollak VE, Pirani CL: Renal vein thrombosis in the adult: a clinical and pathologic study based on renal biopsies. Medicine 47:269, 1968
175. McCarthy LJ, Titus JL, Dougherty GW: Bilateral renal vein thrombosis and the nephrotic syndrome in adults. Ann Intern Med 58:837, 1963
176. Harrison CV, Milne MD, Steiner RE: Clinical aspects of renal vein thrombosis. Q J Med 25:285, 1956
177. Clark RA, Wyatt GM, Colley DP: Renal vein thrombosis: an undiagnosed complication of multiple renal abnormalities. Diagn Radiol 132:43, 1979
178. Llach F, Papper S, Massry SG: The clinical spectrum of renal vein thrombosis: acute and chronic. Am J Med 69:819, 1980
179. Verhaeghe R, Vermylen J, Verstraeti M: Thrombosis in particular organ veins. Herz 14:298, 1989
180. Reuther G, Wanjura D, Bauer H: Acute renal vein thrombosis in renal allografts: detection with duplex doppler ultrasound. Radiology 170:557, 1989
181. Llach F: Renal vein thrombosis and the nephrotic syndrome. p. 155. In Llach F (ed): Renal Vein Thrombosis. Futura, New York, 1983
182. Scanlon GT: Radiographic changes in renal vein thrombosis. Radiology 80:208, 1963
183. Llach F: Acute renal vein thrombosis. p. 1447. In Schrier RW, Gottschalk CW (eds): Diseases of the Kidney. 4th Ed. Little, Brown, Boston, 1988
184. Martinez-Maldonado M, Kumjian DA: Acute renal failure due to urinary tract obstruction. Med Clin North Am 74:919, 1990
185. Wilson DR: Urinary tract obstruction. p. 715. In Schrier RW, Gottschalk CW (eds.): Diseases of the Kidney. 4th Ed. Little, Brown, Boston, 1988
186. Hoffman LM, Suki WN: Obstructive uropathy mimicking volume depletion. JAMA 236:2096, 1978
187. Moody TE, Vaughan ED, Gllenwater JY: Relationship between renal blood flow and ureteral pressures during 18 hours of total unilateral ureteral occlusion. Invest Urol 13:246, 1975
188. Batlle DC, Arruda JAL, Kurtzman NA: Hyperkalemic distal renal tubular acidosis associated with obstructive uropathy. N Engl J Med 304:373, 1981
189. Ellenbogen PH, Scheible FW, Talner LB et al: Sensitivity of gray scale ultrasound in detecting urinary tract obstruction. Am J Roentgenol 130:731, 1980
190. Malave SR, Neiman HL, Spies SM et al: Diagnosis of hydronephrosis: Comparison of radionuclide scanning and sonography. Am J Roentgenol 135:1179, 1980
191. Talner LB, Scheible W, Ellenbogen PH et al: How accurate is ultrasonography in detecting hydronephrosis in azotemic patients? Urol Radiol 3:1, 1981

192. Scheible W, Talner LB: Gray scale ultrasound and the genitourinary tract: a review of clinical applications. Radiol Clin North Am 17:281, 1978

193. Stuck KJ, White GM, Granke DS et al: Urinary obstruction in azotemic patients: Detection by sonography. Am J Roentgenol 149:1191, 1987

194. Gottlieb RH, Luhmann K, Oates RP: Duplex ultrasound evaluation of normal native kidneys and native kidneys with urinary tract obstruction. J Ultrasound Med 8:609, 1989

195. Megibow AJ, Mitnick JS, Bosniak MA: The contribution of computed tomography to the evaluation of the obstructed ureter. Urol Radiol 4:95, 1982

196. Powers TA, Grove RB, Bauriedel JK et al: Detection of obstructive uropathy using 99m-technetium diethylenetriaminepentacetic acid. J Urol 124:588, 1980

197. Pitman SW, Frei E, III: Weekly methotrexate-calcium leukovorin rescue. Effect of alkalinization on nephrotoxicity, pharmacokinetics in the CNS, and use in CNS non Hodgkin's lymphoma. Cancer Treat Rep 61:695, 1977

198. Potter JL, Krill CE: Acyclovir crystalluria. Pediatr Infect Dis 5:710, 1986

199. Sawyer MH, Webb DE, Balow JE et al: Acyclovir induced renal failure: Clinical course and histology. Am J Med 84:1067, 1988

200. Reiselbach RE, Bentzel CJ, Cotlove E et al: Uric acid excretion and renal function in the acute hyperuricemia of leukemia. Am J Med 38:872, 1964

201. Kjellstrand CM, Campbell DC III, Hartitzch B, Buselmeier TJ: Hyperuricemic acute renal failure. Arch Intern Med 133:349, 1974

202. Cadman E, Lundberg W, Bertino J: Hyperphosphatemia and hypocalcemia accompanying rapid cell lysis in a patient with Burkitt's lymphoma and Burkitt cell leukemia. Am J Med 62:283, 1977

4

Diabetic Nephropathy

Diagnostic Techniques and Follow-up Evaluation

Rebecca J. Schmidt
Francis Dumler

NATURAL HISTORY

As the single most common cause of end stage renal failure, diabetic nephropathy presents a formidable clinical challenge to internists and nephrologists alike. The devastating renal consequences of diabetes mellitus highlight its potential for significant morbidity and emphasize that better understanding of its pathogenesis is needed to heighten clinical suspicion for early kidney involvement.

The overall prevalence of insulin-dependent diabetes mellitus (IDDM) is 200/100,000 population, while that of non–insulin-dependent diabetes

(NIDDM) is 1,900/100,000 population. Diabetic renal disease etiologically accounts for 30 to 35 percent of diagnoses leading to end stage renal failure.[1] Although both IDDM and NIDDM are associated with nephropathy, end stage renal failure evolves in a greater percentage of IDDM (35 to 45 percent) than NIDDM (3 to 15 percent) patients. That equal numbers of IDDM and NIDDM patients enter end stage renal failure programs nationwide most likely reflects the greater prevalence of NIDDM among the general population. In addition, trend analyses of end stage renal failure program enrollment indicate that the elderly diabetic cohort accounts for most cases of chronic renal failure among whites in the United States.[2]

Similar cumulative frequencies of renal failure in NIDDM and IDDM outlined in recent studies have challenged the accepted notion that end stage renal disease more frequently complicates IDDM.[2,3] The increased cardiovascular mortality seen in NIDDM has been suggested to account for the lesser prevalence of end stage renal failure in these older patients, many of whom are diagnosed with adult-onset diabetes often in the face of silent atherosclerotic disease.[3] Thus, the true risk of developing renal failure in NIDDM patients may be unknown and, indeed, may approach that of IDDM because many adult-onset diabetic patients die cardiac deaths before manifesting renal complications of diabetes.

Only in NIDDM patients has race been found to influence prevalence of renal insufficiency progressing to end stage renal failure. Black diabetic patients more than 50 years old have a reported twofold to fourfold greater risk of developing end stage renal failure when compared to white diabetic cohorts, while Mexican Americans with diabetic nephropathy are six times more likely to progress to end stage renal failure.[4,5] Pima Indians with NIDDM monitored for 20 years were found to have a 41 percent incidence of end stage renal failure, the highest of any group in the United States.[6]

In contrast to NIDDM, the incidence of end stage renal failure in IDDM patients may be decreasing. Studies from Denmark and the Joslin Diabetes Center have reported a 30 to 40 percent decrease in the cumulative frequency of renal failure in IDDM patients whose diabetes began within the last 30 years.[7,8] In the Danish study, the observed decrease in deaths from renal failure paralleled a declining incidence of proteinuria, whereas the death rate in patients with established proteinuria remained unchanged.

In addition to demographic trends, longitudinal observations have also provided insight into the natural history of diabetic nephropathy, facilitating identification of renal involvement in its earliest stages. A most significant advancement has been the recognition that microalbuminuria identifies the diabetic at risk for developing renal insufficiency. The capacity to detect microalbuminuria has become tantamount to the establishment of diabetic renal disease because its presence confers incipient nephropathy and heralds likely progression to end stage renal failure.

The natural history of diabetic nephropathy evolves through five clinical stages, which are most succinctly characterized in IDDM because its onset is distinct and precise in time (Table 4-1).[9] In *stage I,* the earliest phase,

Table 4-1. Stages of Diabetic Nephropathy

Stage	Clinical Term	Histologic Features	Functional Features	Clinical Features
Stage I	Initial stage	Glomerular hypertrophy	Increased GFR	Supranormal ClCr Increased kidney size
Stage II	Early renal involvement	GBM thickening Increased mesangial matrix	Increased GFR Normal UAE rate	Supranormal ClCr
Stage III	Incipient nephropathy	Further GBM thickening and mesangial matrix expansion	Increased UAE rate	Persistently high UAE rates Supranormal to normal ClCr Increase in blood pressure
Stage IV	Clinical nephropathy	Well-defined diffuse and/or nodular diabetic glomerulosclerosis	Proteinuria on routine urinalysis Gradual reduction in GFR	Proteinuria progressing to nephrotic syndrome Established hypertension Gradual increase in SCr
Stage V	End stage renal failure	Significant glomerular closure and obsolescence	GFR < 15 ml/min	Hypertension Anemia Uremic symptoms

Abbreviations: ClCr, creatinine clearance; GFR, glomerular filtration rate; GBM, glomerular basement membrane; SCr, serum creatinine; UAE, urinary albumin excretion.

glomerular hypertrophy predominates. Hyperfunction, as manifested by an increase in mean glomerular filtration rate (GFR) when compared to non-diabetics, occurs in most patients. Unlike stage I, early renal involvement (*stage II*) is characterized by structural lesions, though again, GFR may be increased or normal. In stage II nephropathy, which begins 1 to 2 years after the onset of diabetes, glomerular basement membrane thickening and mesangial expansion are obvious, although urinary albumin excretion rate remains normal.

Histologic changes intensify in *stage III* (incipient nephropathy) and a persistent increase in urinary albumin excretion is measurable by sensitive techniques, while proteinuria remains undetectable by routine urinalysis. The onset of this stage is quite variable, occurring within 5 to 20 years of diagnosis. Blood pressure, although not increased beyond the normal range, frequently increases during this phase. *Stage IV*, clinical nephropathy, is one of overt proteinuria detectable by routine urinalysis. Significant thickening of the glomerular basement membrane and prominent mesangial matrix expansion produce the well-defined histologic lesions of diffuse and/or nodular sclerosis characteristic of diabetic nephropathy. Proteinuria advances to the nephrotic range, while hypertension becomes well established. Glomerular obsolescence intensifies, causing a parallel decline in glomerular filtration and reduction in clinical renal function within 2 to 4 years. End stage renal failure with global glomerular closure defines *stage V* and is reached 2 to 3 years after appearance of nephrotic syndrome. Hypertension is often problematic at this stage, and symptoms related to anemia and uremia compound those that are due to other diabetic sequelae.

The natural course of diabetic nephropathy in NIDDM patients is less clearly characterized because of the difficulty recognizing onset and timing duration of disease. Although the presence of renal hypertrophy and increased GFR is poorly documented, the clinical and histologic evolution of NIDDM probably mirrors that of IDDM. Clinical nephropathy appears to occur earlier in the course of disease, perhaps because time of disease onset is less discrete.[10]

The frequency of progression to end stage renal failure in diabetic nephropathy is listed by sequential stages in Table 4-2. Currently available data suggest that increased GFRs and thickening of the glomerular basement membrane are universal findings in IDDM patients. Similar data are not available for NIDDM. Autopsy studies in NIDDM patients, however, suggest that only 50 percent have histologic lesions suggestive of diabetic nephropathy.[11] The frequency of microalbuminuria and clinical proteinuria or progression to stages III and IV, respectively, is similar in both, averaging 35 to 40 percent of patients.

Two important corollaries derive from demographic data. First, the majority of patients with diabetes mellitus will not develop renal failure; and second, if clinical proteinuria has not developed after 20 to 30 years of diabetes, it is highly unlikely that stage IV (clinical nephropathy) will occur. In sharp contrast, the incidence of diabetic retinopathy, another important

Table 4-2. Frequency of Progression by Stage in Diabetic Nephropathy

Patients Who Reach a Given Stage	IDDM (%)	NIDDM (%)
Stage I: Increased GFR and renal hypertrophy	90–95	?
Stage II: Early histologic changes	90–95	50
Stage III: Microalbuminuria	30–50	30–50
Stage IV: Clinical proteinuria	35–45	20–40
Stage V: End stage renal failure	20–30	5–35

Abbreviations: GFR, glomerular filtration rate; IDDM, insulin-dependent diabetes mellitus; NIDDM, non–insulin-dependent diabetes mellitus.

microangiopathic complication, increases linearly with time. Early detection of the diabetic population at greatest risk for the development of renal failure is of utmost importance. A most significant advancement has been the identification of urinary albumin excretion (microalbuminuria) as a key noninvasive marker of risk for progression to renal failure.

MICROALBUMINURIA

The normal glomerular filtration barrier is highly selective to macromolecules, allowing only minute amounts of protein to pass into the nephron. Total urinary protein excretion varies between 40 and 120 mg/d, of which albumin accounts for 20 percent, with Tamm-Horsfall protein, immunoglobulins, and other plasma proteins comprising the remainder. Normal 24-hour urinary albumin excretion ranges from 2 to 12 μg/min with an upper 95 percent confidence interval at less than 20 μg/min.[12,13]

By international convention, microalbuminuria is defined as a rate of albumin excretion between 20 and 200 μg/min in an overnight or a 24-hour urinary collection demonstrated on at least two of three occasions within a period of 6 months.[14] Values below 20 μg/min are normal, while urinary albumin excretion above 200 μg/min defines clinically overt proteinuria (likely detectable by urinalysis). Reversible (functional) microalbuminuria is not an accurate clinical marker of renal risk. Very poor glycemic control prevailing at the onset of diabetes or during ketosis, urinary tract infections, congestive heart failure, superimposed hypertension, and moderate to strenuous physical exercise may increase urinary albumin excretion to rates usually less than 60 μg/min, which normalize on correction of the triggering event.[15]

Several longitudinal studies have singled out microalbuminuria as a significant risk factor for the development of nephrotic-range proteinuria and end stage renal failure in IDDM.[14] A total of 224 patients were evaluated for microalbuminuria and followed for a mean of 9 years (range: 6 to 14 years). At the time of initial evaluation, 37 patients (17 percent) had microalbuminuria. At the end of the follow-up period, 32 patients with microalbuminuria (86 percent) had progressed to clinical nephropathy (stage IV), compared with only 4 percent of patients initially normoalbuminuric.[12]

Microalbuminuria has emerged as a reliable predictor of ultimate renal demise, but its role in establishing the temporal course of progression has yet to be outlined. Detectable microalbuminuria is speculated to present 5 to 10 years after the initial diagnosis of IDDM. The interval between the appearance of microalbuminuria and nephrotic-range proteinuria is less clear. Interestingly enough, microalbuminuria also portends the development of proliferative diabetic retinopathy and cardiovascular death in diabetic patients.[16]

Lack of microalbuminuria may not ensure the absence of diabetic glomerular pathology, nor does it unequivocally preclude the development of diabetic nephropathy. Significant glomerular structural abnormalities such as thickening of the glomerular basement membrane, expansion of the mesangial matrix, and decreased surface density of the peripheral capillary wall may exist despite normal urinary albumin excretion rates.[17] While cross-sectional studies suggest that microalbuminuria develops in nearly 35 to 40 percent of both IDDM and NIDDM patients, only in 60 to 70 percent will detectable microalbuminuria manifest within the first 10 years of disease.[18,19] Nor does the absence of hypertension exclude the presence of early glomerular pathology since in IDDM, microalbuminuria antedates the onset of diabetes-related hypertension.[20] The temporal relationship between hypertension and the microalbuminuria of NIDDM probably reflects the high prevalence of essential hypertension in these patients.

Mechanisms responsible for the genesis of microalbuminuria include increased intraglomerular pressure, glomerular structural changes, and renal tubular dysfunction. Intraglomerular hypertension and consequent hyperfiltration do not exclusively account for the increase in urinary excretion of albumin because nondiabetic individuals with a solitary kidney exhibit high single kidney filtration rates in the absence of microalbuminuria.[21] Functional clearance studies using negatively charged glycosylated albumin suggest that the loss of glomerular capillary wall barrier charge selectivity is integral to the development of microalbuminuria.[16] Tubular mishandling of albumin is unlikely because normal tubular function is implied by normal urinary excretion of β_2-microglobulin.

For quantitating microalbuminuria, the 24-hour urinary albumin excretion rate is most accurate and reproducible. When 24-hour collections are impractical, a daytime sampling serves as an acceptable alternative.[22] After emptying the bladder, a water load of 300 ml is administered. Urine excreted in the next 30 to 45 minutes is collected, pooled and timed. An albumin excretion rate of 20 μg/min or more constitutes a positive test.

A variety of sensitive immunoassays is available to measure rates of urinary albumin excretion in patients with normal urinalyses. Dye-binding and precipitation methods are inadequate because of their low sensitivity and lack of specificity. An appropriate assay covers a range of 5 to 250 mg/L for undiluted specimens. Samples may be stored at room temperature for a few days or kept refrigerated for up to 2 weeks. The observed coefficient of variation for the analytic assay should be no higher than 12 percent. Radioimmunoassay, accelerated immunoturbidity, and the immunonephelometric methods are most accurate, reproducible, and sensitive. Selection should depend on local expertise and equipment availability.[12]

A simple quantitative office screening procedure for detection of microalbuminuria has been recently introduced (Micro-Bumintest, Miles Inc., Elkhart, IN). Urinary albumin concentrations of 40 to 80 μg/ml or greater produce a bluish-green spot or ring on the reagent tablet. A positive result warrants a repeat test; if positive, microalbuminuria must be confirmed by immunoassay.

Screening for microalbuminuria should begin between three and five years after diagnosis of IDDM. NIDDM patients warrant screening at diagnosis because the duration of their illness cannot be certain. Normoalbuminuric patients should be reassessed at 24-month intervals. Patients undergoing therapeutic interventions aimed at renal salvage (e.g., strict glycemic control, low dietary protein intake, and aggressive blood pressure control) require monitoring at 3- to 4-month intervals to assess the impact of therapy on albuminuria (Table 4-3).

PROTEINURIA

The normal glomerular capillary wall permits the free passage of small solutes but selectively restricts the transfer of macromolecules from the capillary lumen to the urinary space. The capacity for specific permselectivity allows filtration of water and small molecular weight compounds (<6,000 dalton) to occur while impeding the ultrafiltration of albumin (69,000 dalton) and immunoglobulin (IgG) (156,000 dalton).[23]

Three structural components compose the glomerular capillary filter: endothelium, glomerular basement membrane, and epithelium. By virtue of its biochemical and bioelectrical properties, the glomerular basement mem-

Table 4-3. Detection of Microalbuminuria in Patients With Diabetes Mellitus

Definition: Urinary albumin excretion rate of 20–200 μg/min in two of three samples over a 6-month period.

Methodology: • 24-h urine collections are preferred.
 • Methods of choice: Radioimmunoassay
  Accelerated immunoturbidity
  Immunonephelometry

Surveillance: • Within 5 years of diagnosis in IDDM.
 • At diagnosis in NIDDM.
 • Patients with normal results should be tested every 24 mo.
 • Microalbuminuric patients at first testing should be retested twice more within 6–9 mo.
 • Patients undergoing therapeutic interventions should be tested every 3–4 mo to assess the effects of therapy.

Abbreviations: IDDM, insulin-dependent diabetes; NIDDM, non–insulin-dependent diabetes.

brane operates as the primary barrier to the passage of macromolecules. A rich sialoglycoprotein coating confers a strong negative charge on endothelium and epithelium, whereas anionic properties inherent to glomerular basement membrane reflect its high heparan sulfate proteoglycan content. Supplemental barrier activity is provided by the negatively charged endothelial and epithelial cell layers.[24]

Molecular size, shape, and charge together influence glomerular permselectivity. Physiologic studies using neutral dextran clearances have facilitated the construction of a theoretic model of glomerular permselectivity in humans, segregating the glomerular capillary wall into two distinct components: a small-pore ultrafilter and a large-pore filter.[23,25] A majority of the filtration surface functions as a small-pore ultrafilter responsible for the entirety of GFR. The large-pore filter allows passage of neutral dextrans and IgG (Stokes radius 55 Å) but severely restricts negatively charged macromolecules such as serum albumin (Stokes radius 36 Å). This pore model explains why disease processes may clinically present as proteinuria (large-pore permselectivity dysfunction), loss of GFR (small-pore ultrafilter damage), or both. Glomerular lesions that inhibit the making of ultrafiltrate may not be synonymous with those that allow large proteins to leak, thus reflecting damage to different parts of the capillary wall.

Nephrotic-range proteinuria with urinary leakage of large plasma proteins is the hallmark of clinical diabetic nephropathy (stage IV). Mechanisms for proteinuria in IDDM have been attributed to two exclusive glomerular defects: alteration of the electrostatic barrier function and loss of size-selective properties of the glomerular capillary wall.[25,26] A depletion of glomerular glycoproteins rich in negative charges (sialoglycoproteins and heparan sulfate proteoglycans) allows for enhanced transglomerular passage of anionic albumin. Subsequently, large quantities of macromolecules, most notably IgG, are known to accompany leaking albumin consequent to incremental formation of large pores in the glomerular capillary wall. Smaller molecular weight substances are filtered at progressively slower rates because the capillary wall becomes architecturally compromised and surface area available for ultrafiltration becomes diminished.[23] Similar mechanisms likely operate in NIDDM though they have yet to be comprehensively outlined.

Better understanding of the mechanisms underlying proteinuria has heightened interest in the development of interventional strategies aimed at compensating for deranged glomerular permselectivity properties. *Angiotensin-converting enzyme (ACE)* inhibitors were the first class of agents examined for a specific antiproteinuric effect. Without affecting the GFR or renal plasma flow, enalapril improves glomerular permeability by modifying intrinsic membrane properties key to barrier size selectivity.[27] Cessation of enalapril has been linked with a rebound increase in fractional albumin and IgG clearances that had been lowered and nearly normalized by the drug. A reduction in *dietary protein* intake also causes fractional clearances for albumin and IgG to fall.[28] Whether ACE inhibition and low dietary protein intake operate independently or act synergistically to slow glomerular injury is not known. The potential impact of these therapeutic strategies on the natural progression of disease is yet to be determined.

Although important to delineation of pathogenetic mechanisms, dextran permselectivity clearance studies are not clinically applicable to routine care of patients. The effect of treatment regimens on proteinuria should be assessed by serial 24-hour urine collections for measurement of total protein excretion. In the clinical setting, glomerular permselectivity may be monitored by simultaneous measurements of albumin (molecular weight, 69,000 dalton) and IgG (molecular weight, 156,000 dalton) urinary clearance, with the selectivity index expressed as the ratio of Cl_{IgG}/Cl_{alb}.[26] Minimal urinary IgG leakage relative to albumin denotes a preserved capacity for discriminating between smaller (albumin) and larger (IgG) proteins. Conversely, high rates of IgG leakage result from loss of size selectivity within the glomerular capillary wall. Thus, low selectivity index values (less than 0.3) are indicative of better preservation of functional integrity, whereas higher ratios attest to further progression of disease.

GLOMERULAR FILTRATION RATE

Early diabetic nephropathy (stages I to III) is characterized by supranormal GFRs, which normalize as the disease state advances. Along with worsening glomerular protein leak, the damaged glomerular capillary wall loses its capacity for ultrafiltration (stages IV and V), and decline in glomerular filtration rate is unrelenting.

Measurement of glomerular function is imperative to optimal follow-up of patients with renal disease. Assessment of the glomerular filtration rate quantifies the amount of renal function present at a given point in time and, when measured longitudinally, estimates the rate of progression of renal failure. In addition to GFR, sequential measurements of blood pressure, proteinuria, and dietary protein are necessary for comprehensive evaluation and strategic therapeutic planning.

Central to the surveillance of chronic renal failure is identification of the ideal marker for glomerular filtration.[29] Standard research methodology for measurement of GFR has employed inulin, a 5,200-dalton polymer of fructose, because of its complete filtration at the glomerular level without reabsorption or secretion along the course of the renal tubule. Use of this agent is hindered by difficulties obtaining it in adequate supply and lack of commercial methods to perform its assay. A variety of isotopic filtration markers have been used to measure GFR including [131]I- or ^{125}I-labeled iothalamate, ^{99m}Tc-diethylenetriaminepenta-acetic acid (DTPA), [169]Y-DTPA and ^{51}Cr-ethylenediaminetetra-acetic acid (EDTA). While the clearance of such compounds resembles that of inulin, their use is costly, and historically confined to clinical research.

Creatinine clearance and serum creatinine concentration remain the most widely used estimates of renal function. Although a discrepancy between creatinine and inulin clearances is not characteristic of normal kidneys, enhanced tubular secretion of creatinine consequent to renal insufficiency exaggerates creatinine clearance relative to true filtration rates.[30] That creatinine clearance may overstate GFR is compounded by the fact that 24-hour urinary collections are longitudinally imprecise and subject to significant laboratory variability.

Because renal function declines logarithmically, serial serum creatinine concentrations do not accurately portray the rate or degree of renal deterioration. Although a serum creatinine concentration increasing from 1 to 2 mg/dl represents a loss of function approximating 50 percent, the same increase in serum creatinine concentration at poorer levels of renal function (i.e., from 4 to 5 mg/dl) signifies a functional decline of much smaller magnitude (20 percent). Moreover, serum creatinine fails as an acceptable screening test for chronic renal failure because it may remain normal early on when the GFR has already begun to fall. Measurements of glomerular filtration alone accurately establish renal functional status. This concept is best illustrated by IDDM patients with low muscle mass and secondarily reduced creatinine generation who maintain serum creatinine concentrations within the normal range despite a 25 to 30 percent loss of renal function. Among patients with decreased renal function documented by inulin clearance, only 75 percent and 61 percent were correctly identified as such by creatinine clearance and serum creatinine measurements, respectively.[29,31] Serum creatinine concentration becomes more precise as renal failure advances because of diminishing day-to-day variability that accompanies functional deterioration.

Progressing renal failure can be monitored by a variety of methods, the most practical of which employs the reciprocal of serum creatinine concentration. In most patients with glomerular injury, reciprocal serum creatinine concentration values decline linearly with time as renal function worsens.[32,33] This linear relationship suggests that glomerular filtration changes at a constant rate throughout the course of disease. More likely, glomerular filtration changes at a slower rate early on, only to accelerate late in the disease process. To avoid misinterpretation in assessment of renal deterioration rate, the slope of the reciprocal of serum creatinine concentration versus time should be used not as the sole measure but in conjunction with other estimates of glomerular filtration.

Renal function is most comprehensively appraised by quantitating GFR. Even the most precise determination of glomerular filtration, however, may fail to detect subtle changes in function and may inadequately gauge the degree of glomerular damage. The limitations of both creatinine clearance and reciprocal of serum creatinine concentration can be attributed to altered creatinine metabolism consequent to functional deterioration in the kidney. Tubular secretion of creatinine more than doubles during the course of renal failure but exhibits marked variability among patients. Certain therapeutic agents, namely cimetidine, trimethoprim, and probenecid inhibit creatinine secretion, thereby reducing clearance and increasing serum creatinine concentration without truly changing GFR.

Variable tubular capacity for creatinine secretion, coupled with changing extrarenal elimination and total body generation of creatinine, all prejudice measures of creatinine clearance and reciprocal of serum creatinine concentration, confounding interpretation of changing GFRs. An apparent variation in rates of decline in serial creatinine clearance and reciprocal of serum creatinine concentration may follow fluctuations in creatinine metabolism but should not suggest that true GFR has altered its rate of decline.[29,34,35] Frequent sequential determinations of GFR over months to years are imperative to accurate assessment of advancing renal failure.

Key to accurate interpretation of measures of GFR is the recognition that hemodynamic and structural compensatory mechanisms maintain adequate filtration in the face of significant glomerular injury. Individual or single-nephron GFR is a function of net filtration pressure, filtration surface area, and hydraulic permeability of the glomerular capillary wall. Altered interplay of these determinants resulting from glomerular injury can compromise glomerular filtration. Changing arteriolar resistance increases transglomerular filtration pressure, thereby stabilizing filtration rate in the damaged glomerulus. Likewise, hypertrophied glomeruli provide increased capillary surface area for enhanced filtration. Compensatory mechanisms triggered by structural damage are not factored into sequential measurements of GFR. If adaptive responses are indeed operative, then GFR may well underestimate the degree of structural damage and true ultrafiltration capacity.[29]

The progression of renal disease from a functional perspective is best followed by serial clearances, particularly during intensive therapeutic intervention. Techniques using bolus infusion and spontaneous voiding with radioisotopic markers of glomerular filtration are gaining acceptance and becoming commonplace in clinical practice; they will likely become standard in the near future. The convenience and accessibility of serum creatinine concentration and creatinine clearance measurements ensure their continued use. Nevertheless, creatinine-based methods remain limited in their capacity for detecting early renal dysfunction and as exclusive measure of disease progression. In spite of these shortcomings, serum creatinine concentration is still the least expensive and most practical way to estimate renal function.

DIAGNOSIS

The diagnosis of clinical diabetic nephropathy is suspected, founded, and confirmed essentially on clinical grounds. The natural course of most patients with diabetic renal disease proving temporally predictable has rendered histology no longer crucial to diagnosis. Certain clinical settings warrant renal biopsy in that various glomerulonephritides known to occur in concert with diabetic glomerulosclerosis or as solitary renal lesions must be excluded (Table 4-4). The prevalence of nondiabetic renal disease in these patients is not known.

Table 4-4. Clinical Findings Suggestive of Nondiabetic Renal Disease in IDDM and NIDDM

1. Proteinuria in the absence of retinal microangiopathy confirmed by expert ophthalmologic evaluation, particularly in IDDM patients
2. Nephrotic-range proteinuria in IDDM patients with duration of diabetes less than 7–10 yr
3. Nephrotic-range proteinuria in NIDDM with duration of diabetes less than 5 yr
4. Advancing renal failure with monthly declines of GFR greater than 10%
5. Unexplained acute renal failure
6. Renal insufficiency in the absence of significant proteinuria
7. Gross or persistent microscopic hematuria unexplained by urologic pathology; presence of red blood cell casts

Abbreviations: GFR, glomerular filtration rate; IDDM, insulin-dependent diabetes mellitus; NIDDM, non–insulin-dependent mellitus.

Clinical nephropathy (stage IV) presenting before 7 to 10 years of IDDM or 5 years of NIDDM should prompt a search for nondiabetic causes of renal dysfunction. Nephrotic-range proteinuria progressing to advanced renal failure in less than 2 years is not typical of diabetic nephropathy. Rapid monthly declines from normal in GFR exceeding 10 percent are not true to pattern in diabetic glomerulosclerosis and may warrant diagnostic confirmation by biopsy. Massive proteinuria or sudden onset of renal failure should also prompt search for possibly treatable nondiabetic causes. The absence of significant proteinuria in the diabetic patient with renal failure should heighten suspicion for a concomitant or unrelated renal lesion.

Hematuria and red blood cell casts are considered unusual in diabetic patients without urinary tract or isolated glomerular diseases but may be present in up to 20 percent of diabetic patients with renal involvement.[36,37] Because these findings may signify a superimposed nondiabetic process, renal biopsy should be considered to exclude steroid-sensitive glomerulonephritides.

Superimposed idiopathic membranous glomerulopathy is a most frequent diagnosis.[38] A variety of other disease entities—including poststreptococcal, crescentic, and mesangiocapillary glomerulonephritis and less commonly, focal segmental glomerulosclerosis, minimal change disease, granulomatous interstitial nephritis, and IgA nephropathy—have also been described in association with diabetes.[38–41] The prognostic implications of dual renal diseases are formidable because, if effective, treatment of the nondiabetic component may profoundly influence the course of evolving renal failure.

The association of diabetic glomerulosclerosis and superimposed glomerulonephritis has been thought to be more than fortuitous.[41] Functional and biochemical derangements affecting the diabetic glomerulus may predispose to the localization of immunoreactants that hold the potential for perpetuating glomerular injury, though conclusive evidence does not exist for any particular mechanism.

NIDDM patients appear two to three times as likely as their IDDM counterparts to acquire nondiabetic renal disease irrespective of the presence of diabetic glomerulosclerosis.[42] Nondiabetic renal disease is more likely to exist in IDDM patients when disease duration is short, proteinuria is absent, and neuropathy is not evident. NIDDM patients acquiring nondiabetic renal disease are usually whites who developed diabetes at a late age and have no evidence of clinical neuropathy.[43]

Retinal microangiopathy has emerged as a strong clinical correlate of diabetic nephropathy, occurring so predictably in concurrence with renal involvement that diabetics (particularly IDDM patients) without retinal involvement should be considered for renal biopsy. As retinopathy is not easily diagnosed by traditional funduscopic examination,[44] ophthalmologic evaluation and fluorescein angiography are needed to exclude retinal microvasculopathy with certainty before differentiating diabetic and nondiabetic renal disease.

TREATMENT

Effect of Glucose Control on Microvascular Disease

Standard regimens of insulin therapy prevent neither ophthalmologic nor nephrologic microangiopathic complications seen in long-standing diabetes. The concept of strict metabolic control was recently introduced with expectations that near perfect glycemia achieved by continuous subcutaneous insulin infusion would alter the course of diabetic microvascular disease. Initial studies in stage III IDDM patients with supranormal GFRs showed that 6 months of strict metabolic control was associated with improvement in all retinal parameters as well as a fall in the rate of decline of GFR by 9 percent and in urinary albumin excretion by 12 percent.[45] Both retinal and renal parameters worsened in patients maintained on conventional insulin regimens. Similar success in preserving renal function has been reported in IDDM patients receiving multiple subcutaneous insulin injections daily.[46]

A recent 8-year Danish study comparing strict control and standard care regimens associated insulin infusion with a reduction in urinary albumin excretion.[47] In addition, annual loss of GFR was substantially greater (3.7-fold) in patients on conventional therapy. No patient with an initial low range of microalbuminuria (21 to 68 μg/min) maintained with strict control progressed. Moreover, patients with initial urinary albumin excretion between 69 and 200 μg/min given conventional insulin therapy universally developed clinical nephropathy (100 percent) in marked contrast to those strictly controlled (22 percent). Strict metabolic control does not impede progression of renal disease when instituted after proteinuria has become established in stage IV (clinical nephropathy).[48] It seems likely that benefits of stringent glycemic control may be stage dependent and may require implementation before the appearance of high-range microalbuminuria.

Recent observations suggest that poor long-term glycemic control is a significant risk factor for the development of microalbuminuria in IDDM.[49] When glycosylated hemoglobin levels were reviewed in 236 patients, no subjects with levels less than 10 percent above normal had microalbuminuria or retinopathy. Among patients with glycosylated hemoglobin values greater than 1.5 times normal, 29 percent had microalbuminuria and 37 percent had retinopathy. Poor glycemic control, as defined by persistently elevated glycosylated hemoglobin values (equal to or greater than 10 percent) poses significant risk for retinal and glomerular microvasculature, though the mechanisms by which lack of continued normoglycemia hasten microangiopathy in these organs are incompletely understood.[49-51] Likely hemodynamic and metabolic disturbances have integral involvement in the pathogenesis and progression of microangiopathic lesions. Strict metabolic control may reverse the metabolic derangements of renal and glomerular hypertrophy while modulating the evolution of microangiopathy.[52] Altered hemodynamic states will also require attention.

The pathogenetic implications of diabetic-induced glomerular growth on the progression of diabetic nephropathy are of great current interest. Capillary wall tension rises significantly as the radius of the glomerulus increases, making larger glomeruli more susceptible to injury at any given level of intraglomerular pressure.[53] Recent experimental work has demonstrated that renal hypertrophy perpetuates glomerulosclerosis by mechanisms unrelated to hemodynamics,[54,55] lending credence to the concept that reversal of enhanced glomerular growth by insulin replacement therapy may have a beneficial effect on the structural preservation of diabetic glomeruli.

Strict glycemic control may prevent or modify development of microangiopathic complications by inhibiting nonenzymatic glycosylation of structural proteins. Excessively glycosylated proteins undergo inordinate cross-linkage that renders them functionally aberrant while decreasing their turn-over rate.[56,57] Glomerular basement membrane thickening and mesangial matrix expansion characteristic of diabetic nephropathy are in part a result of the accumulation of excessively glycosylated proteins.

Whether strict metabolic control will prevent microangiopathy awaits the conclusion of the Diabetes Control and Complications Trial (DCCT). Clearly, strict glycemic control improves microalbuminuria and possibly retards progression to clinical nephropathy (stage IV). With only 30 percent of the diabetic population at risk for significant renal failure, clinicians need to balance the potential renal advantages of strict metabolic control with its inherent risk for hypoglycemia and sudden death (Table 4-5).[58]

Use of a Low-Protein Diet

Recent studies suggest that dietary protein intake is a key modifier of glomerular response to injury.[59,60] That reduced protein intake conceivably acts counter to the diabetic insult has prompted its move to the therapeutic

Table 4-5. Strict Metabolic Control in the Management of Patients With Diabetes Mellitus

Benefits:	• Reduces rate of loss of glomerular filtration • Reduces urinary albumin excretion rates • Retards progression from microalbuminuria to proteinuria • May minimize risk of developing microalbuminuria
Risks:	• Hypoglycemia and sudden death are more prevalent than with standard glycemic control • Unnecessary morbidity in the 70% of patients who will not progress to end stage renal failure

forefront as a strategy for attenuation of glomerular sclerosis. A high-protein intake unequivocally intensifies morphologic derangement and accelerates renal functional deterioration. Intraglomerular hypertension and hypertrophy, common to diabetes, are exacerbated by a high protein intake.[61-63] In contrast, a low-protein diet opposes the diabetic forces mediating intraglomerular hypertension and hypertrophy, maximizing potential for renal preservation.[61,64]

Until recently, diabetic patients were prescribed dietary regimens providing a relatively high protein content (approximately 20 percent of total caloric intake or 1.2 to 2.4 g/kg/d). When dietary protein intake is not restricted, IDDM patients have GFRs 25 to 45 percent higher than nondiabetic controls.[65-67] A reduction in protein intake lowers glomerular filtration to values only 10 percent higher than those of similarly treated normals.[68] Interestingly, on reduction of dietary protein intake, the largest decreases in GFRs occurred in patients with the highest baseline values.[69] These data demonstrate that a high-protein intake is an important determinant of the supranormal GFR in early diabetes and is potentially deleterious.

Recent therapeutic approaches have focused on dietary protein restriction as a means for retarding the progression of chronic renal failure. Several studies suggest that a low-protein diet (range, 0.4 to 0.8 g/kg/d) slows the rate of glomerular filtration loss in patients with glomerulonephritis, polycystic kidney disease, and pyelonephritis as well as diabetes.[70-77] Preliminary conclusions have prompted the National Institutes of Health to sponsor a multicenter, randomized, controlled trial to assess the impact of low-protein diets on preservation of renal function in progressive renal disease. The Modification of Diet in Renal Disease (MDRD) study is now underway.[35]

The effect of protein intake on proteinuria has been most extensively studied in IDDM. In patients with clinical nephropathy (stage IV), a reduction in protein intake from 1.44 g/kg/d to 0.7 g/kg/d was causally related to a 50 percent decrease in protein excretion without changes in glomerular filtration or blood pressure.[78,79] Stage IV patients maintained on regular-protein diets had a 90 percent increase in urinary protein excretion during concurrent observation. In patients with incipient nephropathy (stage III), a reduction in protein intake was also associated with a comparable decrease in microalbuminuria.[80]

The mechanisms by which low dietary protein intake promote reduced proteinuria are poorly understood but likely mediated by metabolic and hemodynamic effects unrelated to changes in systemic blood pressure, glycemic control, or serum protein concentration. The simultaneous decline in albumin and IgG urinary excretion rates suggests that low-protein diet restores glomerular permselectivity. Of particular clinical impact is that alleviation of nephrotic syndrome occurs as a direct consequence of this antiproteinuric effect.

A judicious dietary protein intake has been recommended by the American Diabetes Association (0.8 g/kg/d) for all diabetics.[81] Patients at risk (stage III or greater) should be offered specific therapeutic intervention in the form of further protein restriction (0.6 to 0.8 g/kg/d). Though nutritional assessments have not linked stringent protein restriction (0.6 g/kg/d) and protein malnutrition,[82] close surveillance by clinician and dietitian is essential. Dietary protein intake should be monitored by history and by periodically assessing the 24-hour urinary urea nitrogen (UUN) excretion. In practice, these measurements are made every 3 to 4 months after initiating a protein-restricted diet.

Assuming a subject is in steady-state nitrogen balance, excreted nitrogen will equal its intake. The two measurable sources of nitrogen excretion are UUN and a smaller extrarenal component. The latter value, derived from meticulous balance studies,[83,84] indicates that on average, nonrenal nitrogen losses are equivalent to 11 g/d of catabolized protein. Daily balance studies in stable subjects have identified a linear correlation between a defined protein intake and the amount of UUN excretion. The factor 9.35 is derived from plotting a known protein ingestion (grams per day) against the measured urea nitrogen excreted (milligrams per day); indeed, the product of 9.35 and the milligrams per minute of UUN equals the grams per day of protein ingestion in the steady state. Thus dietary protein ingestion (DPI) is derived from the following formula:

$$DPI\ (g/d) = \left[\frac{UUN\ (mg/d)}{1,440\ min/d} \right] \times 9.35 + [11]$$

Urinary yield of DPI   Average extrarenal
                              yield of DPI

Other formulae for DPI incorporate body weight or total body water to individualize nonrenal urea nitrogen losses[84] but are cumbersome and no more practical in a clinical setting than the method described previously (Table 4-6).

Management of Hypertension

A most exciting discovery has been the demonstration that control of arterial hypertension effectively retards progressing renal injury in diabetic nephropathy.[85,86] The recognition that sustained lowering of blood pressure

Table 4-6. Calculation of Dietary Protein Intake From Urinary Urea Nitrogen Measurements

Patient data
    Sex: male
    Age: 45 yr
    Weight: 70.4 kg
    Urinary urea nitrogen: 11,628 mg/24 h

Calculations

$$\text{DPI (g/d)} = \frac{\text{UUN (mg/d)}}{1{,}440 \text{ min/d}} \times 9.35 + 11$$

$$\text{DPI (g/d)} = \frac{11{,}628 \text{ (mg/d)}}{1{,}440 \text{ min/d}} \times 9.35 + 11$$

DPI (g/d) = 8.075 × 9.35 + 11
DPI (g/d) = 75.50 + 11 = 86.5
DPI (g/kg/d) = 86.5 g/d/70.4 kg = 1.23 g/kg/d

Abbreviation: DPI, dietary protein intake.

is integral to preserving renal function has sparked hopes that glomerular injury could be virtually arrested.

Advancing diagnostic capabilities have facilitated earlier identification of (microalbuminuric) patients with the propensity for developing renal micro-angiopathy. Concomitant hypertension in proteinuric patients is highly prevalent (greater than 50 percent) and as renal failure develops is essentially universal.[87] The temporal importance of early intervention is underscored by observations that stage IV diabetic nephropathy has not regressed consequent to antihypertensive therapeutic strategy.

Given the pathogenetic evolution of glomerulosclerosis with its accompaniment of deranged renal hemodynamics, the phenomenon of glomerular hypertension has commanded much attention but has not proven an exclusive force in diabetic nephropathy. Although systemic hypertension clearly warrants intervention, attenuation of intraglomerular hypertension may offer additional advantage in renal diabetes. Most antihypertensive agents do not specifically address intraglomerular pressure, though glomerular capillary hemodynamic benefit is possibly obtained by indirect systemic effects. The emphasis on intraglomerular physiology has brought ACE inhibitors and calcium channel blockers to the forefront for their purported effects on systemic and renal hemodynamics and a narrowed spectrum of side effects. Therapeutic success remains difficult to predict but appears to depend on an interplay of multiple factors including type of diabetes, presence of hypertension, and most importantly, the stage of nephropathy.

A dramatic reduction in urinary albumin excretion (40 percent) was observed in normotensive IDDM patients with stage III nephropathy given an ACE inhibitor (captopril or enalapril).[88,89] In normotensive patients with early stage IV nephropathy given captopril, the antiproteinuric effect was of lesser magnitude.[90] In hypertensive NIDDM patients with more advanced stage IV nephropathy, the mitigating effect of ACE inhibition on proteinuria was also favorable (40 percent), though most likely magnified by the improvement in blood pressure control.[91,92] This response may be highly dependent on near-normal levels of glomerular function because, in patients with mild to moderate renal insufficiency, captopril's effect on proteinuria has been inconsistent at best.[93] The reduction of proteinuria in diabetic patients with normal renal function by ACE inhibitors likely depends on vasodilatation of the efferent arteriole. In advanced stages of diabetic nephropathy where extreme sclerosis compromises glomerular function, efferent vasodilatation may be pharmacologically unachievable, prohibiting the antiproteinuric activity.

Renal hemodynamics in hypertensive NIDDM patients with stage IV nephropathy have been favorably influenced by two calcium channel blockers, nicardipine and diltiazem.[91,92] Nicardipine, used singly and in combination with captopril, significantly lowered blood pressure and urinary albumin excretion, though filtration fraction fell only when ACE inhibition was used alone. Filtration fraction was not altered by calcium channel blockade in the face of equivalent reductions in urinary albumin excretion, which suggests that additional mechanisms for lowering proteinuria other than efferent vasodilation must be at play. In contrast, a third calcium channel blocker, nifedipine, has been shown to worsen urinary protein leakage except at the lowest rates of urinary albumin excretion.[89,94,95] Indeed, in normotensive IDDM patients with stage III (incipient) nephropathy given a 6-week course of nifedipine, urinary albumin excretion climbed nearly 40 percent. The divergent intrarenal actions of calcium channel blockers on proteinuria have yet to be elucidated but appear to be independent of intraglomerular capillary hydraulic pressure changes.

Historically, blood pressure control achieved with furosemide, β-blockers, and hydralazine in various combinations dramatically slowed the rate of glomerular filtration loss (50 to 60 percent) and diminished proteinuria (40 to 50 percent) without impacting intraglomerular hemodynamics. ACE inhibitors and calcium channel blockers are now clearly established as agents of choice for treating systemic hypertension in the diabetic patient. In addition to their antihypertensive potential, these newer agents are well tolerated, have few side effects, and are not deleterious to carbohydrate metabolism. Hyperkalemia may occur with the use of ACE inhibitors, making calcium channel blockers a better choice for patients who have preexisting potassium imbalance. ACE inhibitors may precipitate acute renal failure in patients receiving nonsteroidal antiinflammatory drugs or with underlying renovascular disease or volume depletion, in whom efferent arteriolar vasoconstriction is essential to maintain a glomerular hydraulic pressure gradient necessary for filtration. Calcium channel blockers known to favor regression of proteinuria have side effects not directly related to renal hemodynamics. Like ACE inhibitors, these agents hold promise for their effects on systemic hypertension and urinary protein excretion. The contribution of preferential efferent arteriolar vasodilatation by ACE inhibitors remains to be validated.

Table 4-7. Antihypertensive Agents Used in the Management of Patients With Diabetes Mellitus

Preference	Therapeutic Agent	Renal-Related Side Effects
First choice	Angiotensin-converting enzyme inhibitors, calcium channel blockers	Loss of GFR; hyperkalemia Some may increase proteinuria
Second choice	Prazosin, β_1-blockers, clonidine	
Third choice	Minoxidil	Sodium retention; edema
Diuretics	Thiazides, metolazone, loop diuretics	Prerenal azotemia

Abbreviation: GFR, glomerular filtration rate.

Therapeutically, most important to minimizing loss of glomerular filtration is control of systemic blood pressure. Because IDDM patients may initially have normal blood pressure, serial measures are needed to detect the earliest signs of increase. A rise in systolic blood pressure by 20 mmHg is a definite indication for antihypertensive treatment even if peak blood pressure levels are contained within normal ranges. In any event, antihypertensive therapy is warranted in IDDM patients once blood pressure reaches 130/80 mmHg, the comparable threshold value being 140/90 mmHg in NIDDM (Table 4-7).

Early diagnosis of renal involvement is critical to optimal management of diabetic patients. Microalbuminuria is now a recognized risk factor for progression of early stage nephropathy to end stage renal failure (Fig. 4-1). In IDDM patients, microalbuminuria precedes hypertension; the latter constitutes a late manifestation of renal damage. Normotensive diabetic patients with microalbuminuria may benefit from treatment with ACE inhibitors and calcium channel blockers with antiproteinuric effect in hopes of arresting progression to end stage renal failure. NIDDM patients in whom hypertension often antedates nephropathy may also derive advantage from early intervention, depending on level of blood pressure and renal function. Optimal control of blood pressure has far reaching consequences, because hypertension may perpetuate progression of macrovascular and microvascular disease. Effective antihypertensive treatment in diabetic nephropathy has been associated with a threefold reduction in cumulative mortality at 10 years.[86] Short of the introduction of insulin, control of hypertension has become second in importance to promoting survival and enhancing quality of life in diabetic patients. Good glycemic control and dietary protein restriction are also of paramount importance. Despite a myriad of technologic and pharmacologic advances, management of the diabetic patient continues to challenge the clinician. Ultimate clinical success requires insightful orchestration of multiple diagnostic and therapeutic modalities (Fig. 4-2).

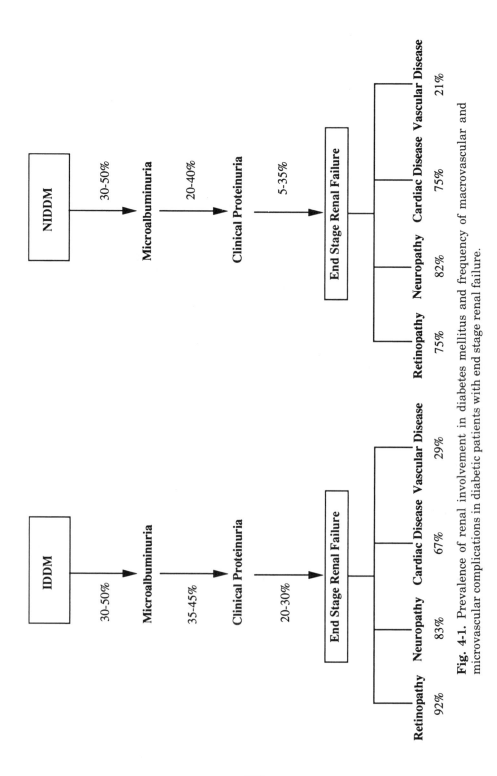

Fig. 4-1. Prevalence of renal involvement in diabetes mellitus and frequency of macrovascular and microvascular complications in diabetic patients with end stage renal failure.

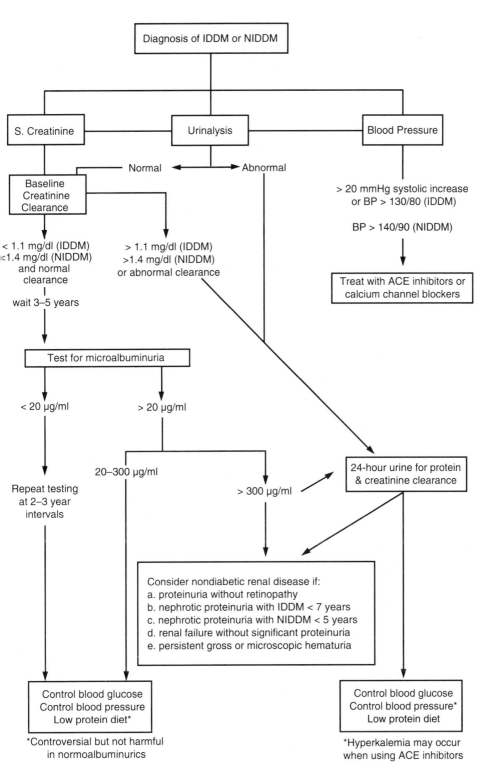

Fig. 4-2. Renal surveillance of diabetic patients. BP, blood pressure; IDDM, insulin-dependent diabetes mellitus; NIDDM, non–insulin-dependent diabetes mellitus; ACE, angiotensin-converting enzyme.

REFERENCES

1. Eggers PW: Effect of transplantation on the Medicare end-stage renal disease program. N Engl J Med 318:223, 1988
2. Humphrey LL, Ballard DJ, Frohnert PP et al: Chronic renal failure in non-insulin-dependent diabetes mellitus. A population-based study in Rochester, Minnesota. Ann Intern Med 111:788, 1989
3. Hasslacher CH, Ritz E, Wahl P, Michael C: Similar risks of nephropathy in patients with type I or II diabetes mellitus. Nephrol Dial Transplant 4:859, 1989
4. Kappel DF, Van Tuinen M: Trends in the incidence of treated end-stage renal disease secondary to diabetic nephropathy: 1975–1984. Am J Kidney Dis 8:234, 1986
5. Pugh JA, Stern MP, Haffner SM et al: Excess incidence of treatment of end-stage renal disease in Mexican Americans. Am J Epidemiol 127:135, 1988
6. Nelson RG, Neuman JM, Knowler WC et al: Incidence of end-stage renal disease in type 2 (non-insulin-dependent) diabetes mellitus in Pima Indians. Diabetologia 31:730, 1988
7. Krolewski AS, Warram JH, Christlieb AR et al: The changing natural history of nephropathy in type I diabetes. Am J Med 78:785, 1985
8. Kofoed-Enevoldsen A, Borch-Johnsen K, Kreiner S et al: Declining incidence of persistent proteinuria in type I (insulin-dependent) diabetic patients in Denmark. Diabetes 36:205, 1987
9. Mogensen CE: Prevention and treatment of renal disease in insulin-dependent diabetes mellitus. Semin Nephrol 10:260, 1990
10. Tung P, Levin SR: Nephropathy in non-insulin-dependent diabetes mellitus. Am J Med 85(suppl 5A):131, 1988
11. Dumler F, Kumar V, Romanski RN et al: Renal involvement in type 2 diabetes mellitus: a clinicopathologic study of the Henry Ford Hospital experience. Henry Ford Hosp Med J 35:221, 1987
12. Rowe DJF, Dawnay A, Watts GF: Microalbuminuria in diabetes mellitus: review and recommendations for the measurement of albumin in urine. Ann Clin Biochem 27:297, 1990
13. Feldt-Rasmussen B: Microalbuminuria and clinical nephropathy in type 1 (insulin-dependent) diabetes mellitus: pathophysiologic mechanisms and intervention studies. Danish Med Bull 36:405, 1989
14. Mogensen CE: Prediction of clinical diabetic nephropathy in IDDM patients: alternatives to microalbuminuria? Diabetes 39:761, 1990
15. Mogensen CE: Microalbuminuria as a predictor of clinical diabetic nephropathy. Kidney Int 31:673, 1987
16. Deckert T, Feldt-Rasmussen B, Borch-Johnsen K et al: Albuminuria reflects widespread vascular damage: the Steno hypothesis. Diabetologia 32:219, 1989
17. Chavers BM, Bilous RW, Ellis EN et al: Glomerular lesions and urinary albumin excretion in type I diabetes without overt proteinuria. N Engl J Med 320:966, 1989
18. Marshall SM, Alberti KGMM: Comparison of the prevalence and associated features of abnormal albumin excretion in insulin-dependent and non-insulin-dependent diabetes. Q J Med 261:61, 1989

19. Nelson RG, Kunzelman CL, Pettitt DJ et al: Albuminuria in type 2 (non-insulin-dependent) diabetes mellitus and impaired glucose tolerance in Pima Indians. Diabetologia 32:870, 1989

20. Mathiesen ER, Rønn B, Jensen T et al: Relationship between blood pressure and urinary albumin excretion in development of microalbuminuria. Diabetes 39:245, 1990

21. Schmits A, Christensen CK, Christensen T, Sølling K: No microalbuminuria or other adverse effects of long-standing hyperfiltration in humans with one kidney. Am J Kidney Dis 13:131, 1989

22. Wiegmann TB, Chonko AM, Barnard MJ et al: Comparison of albumin excretion rate obtained with different times of collection. Diabetes Care 13:864, 1990

23. Tomlanovich S, Deen WM, Jones III HW et al: Functional nature of glomerular injury in progressive diabetic glomerulopathy. Diabetes 36:556, 1987

24. Kanwar YS: Biology of disease. Biophysiology of glomerular filtration and proteinuria. Lab Invest 51:7, 1984

25. Myers BD, Winetz JA, Chui F, Michaels AS: Mechanisms of proteinuria in diabetic nephropathy: a study of glomerular barrier function. Kidney Int 21:633, 1982

26. Deckert T, Feldt-Rasmussen B, Djurup R, Deckert M: Glomerular size and charge selectivity in insulin-dependent diabetes mellitus. Kidney Int 33:100, 1988

27. Morelli E, Loon N, Meyer T et al: Effects of converting-enzyme inhibition on barrier function in diabetic glomerulopathy. Diabetes 39:76, 1990

28. Rosenberg ME, Swanson JE, Thomas BL, Hostetter TH: Glomerular and hormonal responses to dietary protein intake in human renal disease. Am J Physiol 253:F1083, 1987

29. Levey AS: Measurement of renal function in chronic renal failure. Kidney Int 38:167, 1990

30. Rosenbaum RW, Hruska KA, Anderson C et al: Inulin: an inadequate marker of glomerular filtration rate in kidney donors and transplant recipients? Kidney Int 16:179, 1979

31. Shemesh O, Golbetz H, Kriss JP, Myers BD: Limitations of creatinine as a filtration marker in glomerulopathic patients. Kidney Int 28:830, 1985

32. Mitch WE, Walser M, Buffington GA, Lemann Jr J: A simple method of estimating progression of chronic renal failure. Lancet 2:1326, 1976

33. Rowe PA, Richardson RE, Burton PR et al: Analysis of reciprocal creatinine plots by two-phase linear regression. Am J Nephrol 9:38, 1989

34. Walser M, Drew HH, LaFrance ND: Creatinine measurements often yield false estimates of progression in chronic renal failure. Kidney Int 34:412, 1988

35. Modification of Diet in Renal Disease (MDRD) study group: Assessing the progression of renal disease in clinical studies: effects of duration of follow-up and regression to the mean. J Am Soc Nephrol 1:1087, 1991

36. O'Neill WM, Wallin JD, Walker PD: Hematuria and red cell casts in typical diabetic nephropathy. Am J Med 74:389, 1983

37. Hommel E, Carstensen H, Skøtt P et al: Prevalence and causes of microscopic hematuria in type 1 (insulin-dependent) diabetic patients with persistent proteinuria. Diabetologia 30:627, 1987

38. Kasinath BS, Mujais SK, Spargo BH, Katz AI: Nondiabetic renal disease in patients with diabetes mellitus. Am J Med 75:613, 1983

39. Carstens SA, Hebert LA, Garancis JC et al: Rapidly progressive glomerulonephritis superimposed on diabetic glomerulosclerosis: recognition and treatment. JAMA 247:1453, 1982
40. Rao KV, Crosson JT: Idiopathic membranous glomerulonephritis in diabetic patients. Report of three cases and review of the literature. Arch Intern Med 140:624, 1980
41. Cavallo T, Pinto JA, Rajaraman S: Immune complex disease complicating diabetic glomerulosclerosis. Am J Nephrol 4:347, 1984
42. Grenfell A, Watkins PJ: Clinical diabetic nephropathy: natural history and complications. Clin Endocrinol Metab 15:783, 1986
43. Amoah E, Glickman JL, Malchoff CD et al: Clinical identification of nondiabetic renal disease in diabetic patients with type I and type II disease presenting with renal dysfunction. Am J Nephrol 8:204, 1988
44. Frank RN, Hoffman WH, Podgor MJ et al: Retinopathy in juvenile-onset type I diabetes of short duration. Diabetes 31:874, 1982
45. Steno Study Group: Effect of 6 months of strict metabolic control on eye and kidney function in insulin-dependent diabetics with background retinopathy. Lancet 1:121, 1982
46. Holman RR, Dornan TL, Mayon-White V et al: Prevention of deterioration of renal function and sensory-nerve function by more intensive management of insulin-dependent diabetic patients. A two-year randomized prospective study. Lancet 1:204, 1983
47. Feldt-Rasmussen B, Mathiesen ER, Jensen T et al: Effect of improved metabolic control on loss of kidney function in type 1 (insulin-dependent) diabetic patients: an update of the Steno studies. Diabetologia 34:164, 1991
48. Reichard P, Rosenqvist U: Nephropathy is delayed by intensified insulin treatment in patients with insulin-dependent diabetes mellitus and retinopathy. J Intern Med 226:81, 1989
49. Chase HP, Jackson WE, Hoops SL et al: Glucose control and the renal and retinal complications of insulin-dependent diabetes. JAMA 261:1155, 1989
50. Kalk WJ, Osler C, Taylor D, Panz VR: Prior long term glycaemic control and insulin therapy in insulin-dependent diabetic adolescents with microalbuminuria. Diabetes Res Clin Practice 9:83, 1990
51. Howard-Williams J, Hillson RM, Bron A et al: Retinopathy is associated with higher glycaemia in maturity-onset type diabetes. Diabetologia 27:198, 1984
52. Feldt-Rasmussen B, Mathiesen ER, Hegedüs L, Deckert T: Kidney function during 12 months of strict metabolic control in insulin-dependent diabetic patients with incipient nephropathy. N Engl J Med 314:665, 1986
53. Daniels BS, Hostetter TH: Adverse effects of growth in the glomerular microcirculation. Am J Physiol 258:F1409, 1990
54. Yoshida Y, Fogo A, Ichikawa I: Glomerular hemodynamic changes vs. hypertrophy in experimental glomerular sclerosis. Kidney Int 35:654, 1989
55. O'Donnell MP, Kasiske BL, Schmitz PG, Keane WF: High protein intake accelerates glomerulosclerosis independent of effects on glomerular hemodynamics. Kidney Int 37:1263, 1990
56. Garlick RL, Bunn HF, Spiro RG: Nonenzymatic glycation of basement membranes from human glomeruli and bovine sources. Diabetes 37:1144, 1988
57. Brownlee M, Cerami A, Vlassara H: Advanced glycosylation end products in tissue and the biochemical basis of diabetic complications. N Engl J Med 318:1315, 1988

58. The DCCT Research Group: Epidemiology of severe hypoglycemia in the diabetes control and complications trial. Am J Med 90:450, 1991
59. Klahr S, Buerkert J, Purkerson ML: Role of dietary factors in the progression of chronic renal disease. Kidney Int 24:579, 1983
60. Zeller KR: Review: effects of dietary protein and phosphorus restriction on the progression of chronic renal failure. Am J Med Sci 294:328, 1987
61. Zatz R, Meyer TW, Rennke HG, Brenner BM: Predominance of hemodynamic rather than metabolic factors in the pathogenesis of diabetic glomerulopathy. Proc Natl Acad Sci USA 82:5963, 1985
62. Mauer SM, Steffes MW, Azar S, Brown DM: Effects of dietary protein content in streptozotocin-diabetic rats. Kidney Int 35:48, 1989
63. Collins DM, Coffman TM, Ruiz P, Klotman PE: High-protein feeding stimulates renal thromboxane production in rats with streptozotocin-induced diabetes. J Lab Clin Med 114:545, 1989
64. Wen S-F, Huang T-P, Moorthy AV: Effects of low-protein diet on experimental diabetic nephropathy in the rat. J Lab Clin Med 106:589, 1985
65. Carr S, Mbanya J-C, Thomas T et al: Increase in glomerular filtration rate in patients with insulin-dependent diabetes and elevated erythrocyte sodium-lithium countertransport. N Engl J Med 322:500, 1990
66. Mogensen CE: Early glomerular hyperfiltration in insulin-dependent diabetics and late nephropathy. Scand J Clin Lab Invest 46:201, 1986
67. Sandahl Christiansen J, Gammelgaard J, Frandsen M, Parving H-H: Increased kidney size, glomerular filtration rate and renal plasma flow in short-term insulin-dependent diabetics. Diabetologia 20:451, 1981
68. Kupin WL, Cortes P, Dumler F et al: Effect on renal function of change from high to moderate protein intake in type I diabetic patients. Diabetes 36:73, 1987
69. Rudberg S, Dahlquist G, Aperia A, Persson B: Reduction of protein intake decreases glomerular filtration rate in young type 1 (insulin-dependent) diabetic patients mainly in hyperfiltering patients. Diabetologia 31:878, 1988
70. Ihle BU, Becker GJ, Whitworth JA et al: The effect of protein restriction on the progression of renal insufficiency. N Engl J Med 321:1773, 1989
71. Hannedouche T, Chaveau P, Fehrat A et al: Effect of moderate protein restriction on the rate of progression of chronic renal failure. Kidney Int 36(suppl 27):S-91, 1989
72. Rosman JB, Langer K, Brandl M et al: Protein-restricted diets in chronic renal failure: a four year follow-up shows limited indications. Kidney Int 36(suppl 27):S-96, 1989
73. Oldrizzi L, Rugiu C, Maschio G: The Verona experience on the effect of diet on progression of renal failure. Kidney Int 36(suppl 27):S-103, 1989
74. Evanoff GV, Thompson CS, Brown J, Weinman EJ: The effect of dietary protein restriction on the progression of diabetic nephropathy. Arch Intern Med 147:492, 1987
75. Barsotti G, Ciardella F, Morelli E et al: Nutritional treatment of renal failure in type 1 diabetic nephropathy. Clin Nephrol 29:280, 1988
76. Walker JD, Bending JJ, Dodds RA et al: Restriction of dietary protein and progression of renal failure in diabetic nephropathy. Lancet 2:1411, 1989
77. Zeller K, Whittaker E, Sullivan L et al: Effect of restricting dietary protein on the progression of renal failure in patients with insulin-dependent diabetes mellitus. N Engl J Med 324:78, 1991

78. Ciavarella A, Di Mizio G, Stefoni S et al: Reduced albuminuria after dietary protein restriction in insulin-dependent diabetic patients with clinical nephropathy. Diabetes Care 10:407, 1987
79. Bending JJ, Dodds RA, Keen H, Vibert GC: Renal response to restricted protein intake in diabetic nephropathy. Diabetes 37:1641, 1988
80. Wiseman MJ, Bognetti E, Dodds R et al: Changes in renal function in response to protein restricted diet in type 1 (insulin-dependent) diabetic patients. Diabetologia 30:154, 1987
81. American Diabetes Association: Nutritional recommendations and principles for individuals with diabetes mellitus: 1986. Diabetes Care 10:126, 1987
82. Levine SE, D'Elia JA, Bistrian B et al: Protein-restricted diets in diabetic nephropathy. Nephron 52:55, 1989
83. Maroni BJ, Steinman TI, Mitch WE: A method for estimating nitrogen intake of patients with chronic renal failure. Kidney Int 27:58, 1985
84. Kosanovich JM, Dumler F, Horst M et al: Use of urea kinetics in the nutritional care of the acutely ill patient. JPEN 9:165, 1985
85. Sawacki PT, Mühlhauser I, Baba T, Berger M: Do angiotensin converting enzyme inhibitors represent a progress in hypertension care in diabetes mellitus? Diabetologia 33:121, 1990
86. Parving H-H: Impact of blood pressure and antihypertensive treatment on incipient and overt nephropathy, retinopathy, and endothelial permeability in diabetes mellitus. Diabetes Care 14:260, 1991
87. Hamilton BPM: Diabetes mellitus and hypertension. Am J Kidney Dis 16(suppl 1):20, 1990
88. Marre M, Chatellier G, Leblanc H et al: Prevention of diabetic nephropathy with enalapril in normotensive diabetics with microalbuminuria. Br Med J 294:1448, 1987
89. Mimran A, Insua A, Ribstein J et al: Comparative effect of captopril and nifedipine in normotensive patients with incipient diabetic nephropathy. Diabetes Care 11:850, 1988
90. Parving H-H, Hommel E, Nielsen MD, Giese J: Effect of captopril on blood pressure and kidney function in normotensive insulin-dependent diabetics with nephropathy. Br Med J 299:533, 1989
91. Stornello M, Valvo EV, Scapellato L: Hemodynamic, renal, and humoral effects of the calcium entry blocker nicardipine and converting enzyme inhibitor captopril in hypertensive type II diabetic patients with nephropathy. J Cardiovasc Pharm 14:851, 1989
92. Bakris GL: Effects of diltiazem or lisinopril on massive proteinuria associated with diabetes mellitus. Ann Intern Med 112:707, 1990
93. Valvo E, Bedogna V, Casagrande P et al: Captopril in patients with type II diabetes and renal insufficiency: systemic and renal hemodynamic alterations. Am J Med 85:344, 1988
94. Demarie BK, Bakris GL: Effects of different calcium antagonists on proteinuria associated with diabetes mellitus. Ann Intern Med 113:987, 1990
95. Melbourne Diabetic Nephropathy Study Group: Comparison between perindopril and nifedipine in hypertensive and normotensive diabetic patients with microalbuminuria. Br Med J 302:210, 1991

5

Serologic Diagnostic Techniques in Renal Disease

J. Charles Jennette
Ronald J. Falk

145

Cryoglobulin Assay
IgA-Fibronectin Aggregate Assays

COMPLEMENT ANALYSIS

Complement Abnormalities in Patients With the Nephrotic Syndrome
Complement Abnormalities in Patients With Glomerulonephritis

AMYLOID AND IMMUNOGLOBULIN PARAPROTEIN ANALYSIS

DIAGNOSTIC APPLICATION OF SEROLOGIC TESTS IN RENAL DISEASE

Nephritic Syndrome
Concurrent Renal and Extrarenal Disease
Nephrotic Syndrome

CONCLUSIONS

INTRODUCTION

Diagnostic serologic tests are of greatest value when their capabilities and limitations are thoroughly understood. This requires a knowledge of the technical quality of a given analytic procedure, as well as a knowledge of the diagnostic utility of positive and negative results generated by the procedure. Diagnostic utility is determined from data reported in the literature that allow calculation of the specificity, sensitivity, and predictive value of tests.[1] One of the most challenging aspects of using serologic data for patient care is developing the capacity to critically analyze the sometimes conflicting data in the literature to discern the diagnostic and prognostic capabilities and limitations of a particular test.

The following chapter discusses the general principles of serologic test interpretation, followed by a series of descriptions of serolgic tests that have utility for diagnosing renal disease, and concludes with a commentary on the use of serologic tests in resolving differential diagnoses in patients with various clinical and pathologic expressions of renal disease.

PRINCIPLES OF SEROLOGIC
TEST INTERPRETATION

Quality

The *quality* of the analytic procedure depends on the technical limitations of the procedure itself, and the capabilities of the laboratory performing the test. Accuracy and precision data should be available to inform the clinician about the analytic quality of a test being performed by a given laboratory.

Precision is the agreement between replicate assays on the same sample. Knowledge of the precision of a test is required to decide whether changes in test results over time are within the expected range of analytic variation or are real changes in the patient's status.

Accuracy is the agreement between a test result and the "true value." Poor accuracy can result in an unacceptably greater number of false-positive or false-negative results, and therefore will adversely affect the specificity, sensitivity, and predictive value of the test.

Serologic methodologic pitfalls and ways to avoid them are reviewed in two reports of the World Health Organization (WHO) Working Group.[2,3]

Sensitivity and Specificity

The *sensitivity* of a test for a disease is the percentage of patients with the disease who have a positive test result (i.e., positivity in disease). The *specificity* of a test for a disease is the percentage of individuals without the disease who have a negative test result (i.e., negativity in the absence of the disease). These parameters are not always easy to determine for a given serologic test, in part because the definition of "true-positives," i.e., patients with the disease, may differ among investigators.

With many analytic tests, including serologic tests, the specificity and sensitivity of a positive test result are oppositely affected by raising or lowering the positive threshold (i.e., sensitivity and specificity vary with the strength of the signal). For example, if 1:40 is considered the positive threshold for an antinuclear antibody assay, the test has a higher sensitivity but lower specificity for systemic lupus erythematosus (SLE) than when the positive threshold is 1:80. Realization of this relationship allows more circumspect use of serologic data, for example, using negative results at low titer to help exclude a diagnosis, and positive results at high titer to help confirm a diagnosis, while being more cautious about the significance of intermediate titer positives. In other words, even though two values are both positive, a stronger positive should be considered to have greater specificity than a weaker positive.

Positive and Negative Predictive Value

The most important, and least understood, concept of diagnostic laboratory medicine is predictive value. The *positive predictive value* is the probability that the disease is present in a patient who has a positive test result, i.e., the percentage of patients with a positive test result who in fact have the disease.[1] The *negative predictive value* is the probability that the disease is absent in a patient who has a negative test result, i.e., the percentage of patients with negative test results who in fact do not have the disease.[1]

The most important concept about predictive value that must be understood is the profound influence of disease prevalence on the calculation of both positive and negative predictive values. The positive predictive value of a test is directly proportional to the prevalence of the disease in the population studied (i.e., the higher the disease prevalence in the population being tested, the better the positive predictive value) (Fig. 5-1); whereas the negative predictive value is inversely proportional to the disease prevalence.

A disease's prevalence is different in asymptomatic normal individuals compared to patients with signs of symptoms characteristic of the disease. For example, the prevalence of systemic lupus erythematosus in asymptomatic individuals is markedly less than in patients with malar rash, arthralgias, and hematuria; therefore, the positive predictive value of an antinuclear antibody assay is much greater in the latter than the former. Likewise, the positive predictive value of an elevated antistreptolysin O (ASO) titer for the poststreptococcal glomerulonephritis is much greater in a patient with nephritis than in the general population. Thus, physicians improve the positive predictive value of serologic assays by ordering tests for diseases that are of relatively high prevalence in patients with the signs and symptoms manifested by the patient being tested. In this setting, in which the positive predictive value is high, serologic tests are useful for confirming

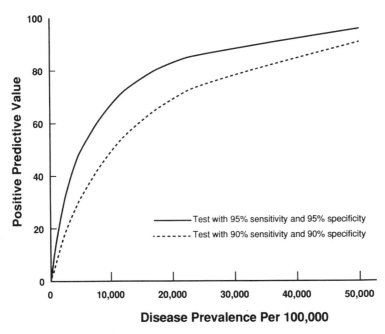

Fig. 5-1. Relationship between the positive predictive value of a test and disease prevalence. Even for tests with very good sensitivity and specificity, the positive predictive value of a test is good only when the signs and symptoms of disease in the patient being tested indicate a high prevalence of the disease being tested for.

specific diagnoses. For a laboratory test to provide optimum diagnostic information, data from the history and physical examination should predict that the patient has a probability of the disease being tested for in the range of 40 to 60 percent.[4]

However, in a setting where the disease prevalence is too low, or where the test is too insensitive or nonspecific to provide definitive predictive value, a serologic test can still be of value by influencing the likelihood that a disease is present.[5] For example, a serologic test with a positive predictive value of only 20 percent, if positive, can increase the likelihood that a disease is present by 50 times (i.e., the post-test probability of the disease is substantially higher than the pretest probability).[5] This serves to adjust the differential diagnosis and suggests what additional tests might be most appropriate.

Combining Multiple Tests

In clinical practice, diagnoses are rarely based on individual laboratory tests but rather on the predictive value of combined tests. Once the likelihood of a disease is increased by one serologic test, this in effect increases the predicted prevalence of that disease in the patient, thus affording a higher positive predictive value to an additional (confirmatory) serologic test. For example, in a patient with nephritis, a positive test for hypocomplementemia adjusts the differential diagnosis (i.e., increases the likelihood or prevalence of certain diagnoses) but is not definitive for a specific diagnosis. However, this increased likelihood or prevalence of particular diseases afforded by the demonstration of hypocomplementemia sets the stage for using an additional serologic assay as a confirmatory test, e.g., ASO for poststreptococcal glomerulonephritis, C3 nephritic factor for membranoproliferative glomerulonephritis, and anti-DNA antibody for lupus nephritis.

Combinations of serologic tests with different qualities can be useful. For example, a test with high sensitivity but low specificity (e.g., an indirect immunofluorescence antinuclear antibody assay) can be combined with a test with high specificity but low sensitivity (e.g., an anti-Smith antibody assay). Using antinuclear antibody and anti-Sm to diagnose SLE, good negative predictive value is imparted by the antinuclear antibody assay and good positive predictive value by the anti-Sm assay.

Combinations of tests also can be used to monitor disease activity. For example, Swaak et al. have observed that combined complement and anti-DNA assays are better predictors of development of renal impairment than any one test alone.[6]

Resolving Differential Diagnoses

To use serologic tests for facilitating diagnosis of a patient with renal disease, the first step is to formulate a differential diagnosis that includes diseases that are likely given the available clinical and laboratory data (i.e., diseases that have a high prevalence in patients with the clinical and laboratory features of the patient being tested). As noted, for a serologic test to have good positive predictive value, the signs and symptoms in the patient should indicate that the patient has a predicted pretest prevalence of 40 to 60 percent for the disease for which the serologic test is a marker. Under this circumstance, a test with good sensitivity and specificity would provide greater than 90 percent positive predictive value (Fig. 5-1); i.e., it would confirm the diagnosis with acceptable confidence. A negative result from a test with high sensitivity would help exclude a diagnosis. Under conditions that would not allow confident confirmation or exclusion of a diagnosis, test results would at least adjust the hierarchy within the differential diagnosis.

Therefore, a knowledge of not only the performance characteristics of specific serologic tests but also the signs and symptoms of specific renal diseases is required for proficient use of serology to diagnose renal diseases. In the following sections, the characteristics of serologic tests that are used to diagnose renal diseases are described, followed at the end of the chapter by a discussion of the use of these assays in patients with particular renal disease syndromes (e.g., nephritis, systemic vasculitis, pulmonary-renal syndrome, nephrotic syndrome, and thrombotic microangiopathy).

SEROLOGIC ANALYSIS OF ANTIBODIES TO HETEROLOGOUS ANTIGENS

Antistreptococcal Antibodies

Antistreptococcal antibodies are useful for demonstrating that a patient has had a streptococcal infection but are of no value in predicting the development of poststreptococcal glomerulonephritis or its severity.

Assays for ASO and anti-DNase B are the most widely used serologic tests for group A β-hemolytic streptococcal infection. Different serologic tests for antistreptococcal antibodies have different sensitivities and specificities for streptococcal infections.[7] ASO is elevated in approximately 75 percent of patients with acute poststreptococcal glomerulonephritis caused by pharyngitis, and additional patients are positive for anti-DNase B. ASO titer is elevated in approximately 60 percent of patients with acute poststreptococcal glomerulonephritis caused by pyoderma, whereas anti-DNase B is elevated in 90 percent of these patients.[8] Antihyaluronidase antibodies are also more sensitive for streptococcal pyoderma than are ASO antibodies. For greatest sensitivity, combined ASO and anti-DNase B testing is recommended.

The sensitivity of antistreptococcal antibody assays for antecedent streptococcal infections is reduced by antibiotic treatment; therefore, a negative result in a patient who has received antibiotics is not as useful in reducing the likelihood of poststreptococcal glomerulonephritis. Especially in children, who have a high frequency of streptococcal infections, a positive serologic test does not prove that concurrent nephritis is of poststreptococcal pathogenesis. If hematuria, proteinuria, or hypocomplementemia persist past 2 months, alternative diagnoses should be considered, particularly IgA nephropathy if hematuria is the major persistent feature, and membranoproliferative glomerulonephritis if proteinuria and hypocomplementemia persist.

Antihepatitis B Antibodies

A small minority of patients with symptomatic or asymptomatic hepatitis B infection develop glomerulonephritis and/or systemic vasculitis with immunohistologic evidence for vessel wall localization of immune complexes containing hepatitis B antigens (e.g., HB_sAg, HB_cAg, and especially HB_eAg). The systemic vasculitis usually manifests as microscopic polyarteritis nodosa. The glomerulonephritis can have a variety of structural manifestations, including proliferative glomerulonephritis, type I membranoproliferative glomerulonephritis, and most often, membranous glomerulopathy. The possibility of hepatitis B-induced glomerulonephritis should be suspected in young patients with membranous glomerulopathy, especially young black males,[9] and in patients with immune complex-mediated glomerulonephritis accompanied by systemic arteritis.

Antitreponemal Antibodies

Syphilis is a rare cause of immune complex-mediated glomerulonephritis.[10,11] Less than 1 percent of patients with secondary syphilis and approximately 5 percent of patients with congenital syphilis develop syphilitic glomerulopathy. As is true with other immune complex-mediated glomerulopathies that are caused by persistent infections, the glomerular lesions are variable and span a continuum from membranous glomerulopathy to proliferative glomerulonephritis to type-I membranoproliferative glomerulonephritis. The clinical manifestations vary according to the underlying glomerular lesion. The most frequent presentation is membranous glomerulopathy with nephrotic syndrome.

The most widely used serologic tests for syphilis are the Venereal Disease Research Laboratory (VDRL) test and the fluorescent *Treponema pallidum* antibody-adsorption (FTA-ABS) test; but there are additional enzyme-linked immunosorbent assay (ELISA) and hemagglutination assays for antitreponemal antibodies. The FTA-ABS assay is more sensitive and more specific for syphilis than the VDRL assay. False-positive VDRL results occur in patients with a variety of infections, systemic lupus erythematosus, antiphospholipid antibody syndrome, and age in the eighth decade or older.

Although glomerular disease caused by syphilis is uncommon, its recognition is important because it is a potentially curable disease.[10]

Antihuman Immunodeficiency Virus (HIV) Antibodies

A form of focal glomerular sclerosis occurs in HIV-infected patients and causes nephrotic syndrome and progressive renal failure.[12,13] This HIV-associated nephropathy can be the initial clinical manifestation of HIV infection or can be associated with acquired immunodeficiency syndrome (AIDS) or AIDS-related complex (ARC). Especially in patients with risk factors for HIV infection, serologic evaluation of patients with the nephrotic syndrome should include assay for anti-HIV antibodies by ELISA or Western blot analysis. Anti-HIV antibodies also should be measured in a patient who has renal biopsy findings suggestive of HIV-associated nephropathy, e.g., focal glomerular sclerosis with focal dilation of tubules and endothelial tubuloreticular inclusions.[12,13]

Although HIV-associated nephropathy is most common, other renal lesions are sometimes observed in renal biopsies from patients with anti-HIV antibodies, e.g., renal infection (especially cytomegalovirus and fungus), and immune complex-mediated infection-associated glomerulopathies.

Antitoxigenic Bacteria Antibodies

Hemolytic uremic syndrome associated with enteropathogenic *Escherichia coli* infection may be the most common cause for acute renal failure in children.[14] The enteric pathogens produce toxins that putatively injure endothelial cells. Serologic demonstration of infection by toxin-producing strains of pathogens or serologic demonstration of the toxins are useful in the diagnosis of hemolytic uremic syndrome.[15-18] The most common pathogen responsible for hemolytic uremic syndrome in the United States and the United Kingdom is verotoxin-producing *E. coli* (VTEC) serotype O157:H7.[15,16] Once VTEC is identified as the cause, administration of immune globulin-containing toxin-neutralizing antibodies is a novel treatment option.[19]

SEROLOGIC ANALYSIS OF AUTOANTIBODIES

Antiglomerular Basement Membrane Antibodies

Antiglomerular basement membrane (anti-GBM) antibodies, attached to basement membranes and in the serum, are found in patients with Goodpasture's syndrome and patients with anti-GBM antibody-mediated glomerulonephritis. Anti-GBM glomerulonephritis also occurs as recurrent or de novo glomerulonephritis in renal transplants.[20]

Goodpasture's syndrome was initially defined as the clinical coexistence of pulmonary hemorrhage and glomerulonephritis.[21] Subsequent studies demonstrated that some cases of pulmonary-renal syndrome are associated with tissue and serum anti-basement membrane antibodies.[22,23] Because of this association, and as proposed by Martinez and Kohler,[24] Goodpasture's syndrome currently is usually defined as coexistent pulmonary hemorrhage and glomerulonephritis that are both mediated by anti-GBM antibodies. Anti-GBM glomerulonephritis can occur alone, or as a component of Goodpasture's syndrome. Goodpasture's syndrome is only one of several immunohistopathologic variants of pulmonary-renal syndrome, and anti-GBM glomerulonephritis is only one of many variants of aggressive glomerulonephritis. Therefore, as discussed in more detail later, serologic analysis is very useful in the diagnostic evaluation of patients with pulmonary-renal syndrome and in patients with rapidly progressive glomerulonephritis. Recurrence of clinically significant anti-GBM glomerulonephritis in an allograft is unlikely if transplantation is delayed until after serum anti-GBM antibodies are no longer detectable.[20]

Direct immunofluorescence microscopy of renal biopsy specimens from patients with anti-GBM glomerulonephritis demonstrates characteristic linear immunostaining of the GBM, and sometimes tubular basement membranes, with anti-IgG antisera. Because nonspecific linear GBM IgG localization can be misinterpreted as anti-GBM binding, serologic identification of anti-GBM antibodies is a useful confirmatory test for anti-GBM glomerulonephritis. ELISA or radioimmunoassay (RIA) assays are preferable to indirect immunofluorescence microscopy assays because they have much better sensitivity and specificity. A number of rapid immunoassays are available for the serologic detection of anti-GBM antibodies.[25,26] Particular attention should be given to the selection of the collagen substrate for anti-

GBM detection (preferably a substrate containing type IV collagen NC1 domain) because anticollagen antibodies with specificity for non-NC1 domain determinants may be present in a variety of glomerulonephritides.[27]

The major antigen with which anti-GBM autoantibodies react is in the noncollagenous NC1 domain of type IV collagen; however, some patients also have low-titer antibodies reactive with the 7S domain of type IV collagen, laminin, and entactin.[28] Saxena et al. have recently reported the presence of anti-entactin antibodies in patients with a pathologically heterogenous group of glomerulonephritides.[29]

Tubulointerstital nephritis caused by antitubular basement membrane (anti-TBM) antibodies has been reported, but is rare.[30] Anti-TBM antibodies have been observed in the serum and allograft tissue of renal transplant patients but do not correlate with graft injury.[31] Anti-TBM antibodies are usually detected by indirect immunofluorescence microscopy assay.

Antinuclear Antibodies

The disease states with renal involvement in which antinuclear antibodies are found in high frequency are SLE, systemic sclerosis, and overlap syndromes with mixed features of lupus and systemic sclerosis.

Approximately 95 percent of patients with active, untreated lupus nephritis have a positive antinuclear antibody result in an indirect immunofluorescence (IIF) assay; however, this test is not highly specific, unless only high-titer results are considered. IIF assays using rodent tissue as substrate are more sensitive than assays using human cell lines.[32] IIF assays for antinuclear antibodies have very poor specificity for SLE; e.g., when the IIF assay is used as a screening test on unselected patients, only 35 percent of individuals with positive results using rodent tissue and 15 percent of positives with human cell lines have lupus.[32]

Once a positive IIF antinuclear antibody result is obtained, more specific immunoassays should be performed using purified nuclear antigens as substrate. A serologic marker with good specificity for SLE is anti-Smith (anti-Sm), which reacts with small nuclear rebonucleoproteins. Anti-Sm antibodies have a positive predictive value of 90 percent for SLE[32] but have a sensitivity of only 25 to 30 percent. Antibodies to proliferating cell nuclear antigen (PCNA), which react with an auxiliary protein of DNA polymerase,[33] have virtually 100 percent specificity and positive predictive value but have extremely low sensitivity (i.e., 5 percent).[32]

Depending on the immunoassays, anti-dsDNA antibodies are detected in 40 to 75 percent of lupus patients, and anti-ssDNA in 70 to 95 percent of patients, with the former being more specific. Different serologic tests for anti-DNA antibodies have different causes for false-negative and false-positive results.[34] In patients with rheumatologic symptoms, anti-dsDNA antibodies have a positive predictive value of greater than 90 percent for SLE.[32]

For assessing disease activity on the basis of anti-DNA titer, ELISA or Farr assays are better than the *Crithedia luciliae* assay.[35] In patients with SLE, serial anti-dsDNA titers are a better predictor of disease exacerbations, including nephritis, than C3 and/or C4 levels.[35] Swaak et al. have observed that combined complement and anti-DNA assays are better predictors of development of nephritis than one test alone.[6]

Antinuclear antibodies with specificity for histones are detected in only 25 percent of patients with SLE, but are much more sensitive for drug-induced lupus erythematosus,[36] although these patients usually do not have significant renal disease. Antihistone antibodies are present in over 95 percent of patients with procainamide-induced lupus and in approximately 75 percent of those with hydralazine-induced lupus.[32] Some patients with drug-induced lupus also have antimyeloperoxidase autoantibodies.

Antinuclear antibodies are observed in patients with systemic sclerosis, who can have renal disease as a manifestation. The sensitivity of antinuclear antibodies for systemic sclerosis has been variably reported from 40 to 98 percent, with some of this variability caused by the use of different substrates for indirect immunofluorescence microscopy assay.[36] Using indirect immunofluorescence microscopy, a speckled pattern is most often observed in patients with systemic sclerosis. More specific immunoassays can identify the molecular nuclear specificity of autoantibodies that are associated with systemic sclerosis, e.g., anti-Scl-70 antibodies specific for DNA topoisomerase I,[37] and anti-centromere antibodies specific for kinetochore.[38] Antinucleolar and anticentriole autoantibodies also have been reported in patients with systemic sclerosis.[39] Anti-Scl-70 and anticentromere antibodies are greater than 98 percent specific for systemic sclerosis, although their sensitivity is only 25 to 35 percent. Therefore, they have much better positive predictive value than negative predictive value.

There is a correlation between autoantibody specificity and disease expression of systemic sclerosis. Most anticentromere antibodies (96 percent) are found in patients with limited cutaneous scleroderma (including CREST syndrome), who do not have renal disease; but this antibody has only 43 percent sensitivity for cutaneous scleroderma.[36] Two thirds of patients with anti-Scl-70 have diffuse systemic sclerosis; although this antibody has only 33 percent sensitivity for diffuse systemic sclerosis.[36] Therefore, in patients with renal disease that is suspected of being induced by systemic sclerosis, assay for anti-Scl-70 antibodies are a specific test with high (greater than 90 percent) positive predictive value for systemic sclerosis, but it is insensitive and therefore is not good for excluding systemic sclerosis. In patients with systemic sclerosis, the presence or absence of anti-Scl-70 antibodies us not a predictor of the likelihood of renal involvement or patient survival[36]; however, the presence of anticentromere antibodies reduces the likelihood of developing renal complications.

Antineutrophil Cytoplasmic Autoantibodies

The most common type of rapidly progressive (i.e., crescentic) glomerulonephritis has no evidence by direct immunofluorescence microscopy or serology for mediation by immune complexes or anti-GBM antibodies and therefore is designated idiopathic or pauciimmune crescentic glomerulonephritis.[40,41] Approximately 80 percent of these patients with pauciimmune crescentic glomerulonephritis have a serologic marker of disease, i.e., antineutrophil cytoplasmic autoantibodies (ANCAs).[42–44] Patients with ANCA-associated glomerulonephritis can have either renal-limited disease (i.e., idiopathic crescentic glomerulonephritis) or systemic vasculitis (e.g., Wegener's granulomatosis, polyarteritis nodosa, leukocytoclastic angiitis, or Churg-Strauss syndrome).

ANCAs were first reported by Davies et al. in 1982 in patients with crescentic and necrotizing glomerulonephritis who had no glomerular immune deposits and varying degrees of clinical evidence for systemic vasculitis.[45] ANCAs have specificity for constituents of neutrophil granules (usually primary granules) and monocyte lysosomes.[43] In an analogous fashion to antinuclear antibodies, ANCAs have multiple specificities that can be differentiated by ELISA and, to a lesser extent, by indirect immunofluorescence microscopy assay.

The most widely used serologic assay for ANCA detection uses alcohol-fixed neutrophils as substrate for indirect immunofluorescence microscopy. ANCAs in serum samples that bind to antigens in the substrate neutrophils are detected using fluorochrome-labeled anti-Ig antibodies. As with antinuclear antibodies, ANCA of different specificities produce different staining patterns. The two major staining patterns are cytoplasmic (C-ANCA) and perinuclear (P-ANCA) (Fig. 5-2). The perinuclear staining distribution is the result of in vitro translocation of certain soluble, nucleophilic cytoplasmic antigens (e.g., myeloperoxidase and elastase) to the nucleus during substrate preparation.[46] When the standard indirect immunofluorescence assay is used, nuclear staining caused by P-ANCA cannot be confidently distinguished from nuclear staining caused by antinuclear antibodies. This problem is resolved by using immunoassays with purified antigens as substrate. Figure 5-3 demonstrates the frequency of P-ANCA and C-ANCA detected by indirect immunofluorescence microscopy in patients with various types of renal disease. ANCAs are greater than 80 percent sensitve for pauciimmune crescentic glomerulonephritis whether or not it occurs as a renal-limited disease (i.e., "idopathic" crescentic glomerulonephritis) or as a component of systemic vasculitis (e.g., Wegener's granulomatosis or polyarteritis nodosa). Note that a minority of patients with anti-GBM and immune complex-mediated glomerulonephritis also have ANCA.

ELISA and RIA assays can also be used to detect and quantify ANCA. Currently, the greatest problem with this technology is the use of different nonstandardized substrates in different laboratories. Immunoassays can use complex substrates to screen for multiple ANCA specificities (Fig. 5-4) or

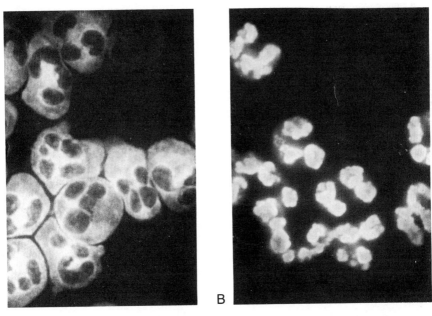

Fig. 5-2. Indirect immunofluorescence microscopy assay for antineutrophil cytoplasmic autoantibodies (ANCA) using alcohol-fixed normal human neutrophils as substrate. **(A)** cytoplasmic staining (C-ANCA) produced by PR3-ANCA. **(B)** Perinuclear staining (P-ANCA) produced by myeloperoxidase-ANCA (MPO-ANCA). (From Jennette and Falk,[43] with permission.)

purified proteins to detect ANCAs of a particular antigen specificity (Fig. 5-5). In patients with glomerulonephritis or systemic vasculitis, the major C-ANCA antigen specificity is for an elastinolytic serine proteinase usually designated proteinase 3 (PR3-ANCA), and the major P-ANCA specificity is for myeloperoxidase (MPO-ANCA).[43]

There is controversy over the disease sensitivity, specificity, and predictive value of ANCA.[43,47] There are investigators who conclude that C-ANCA/PR3-ANCAs are extremely sensitive and specific for Wegener's granulomatosis.[48] There is no doubt that C-ANCAs are a sensitive serologic markers of Wegener's granulomatosis (probably greater than 95 percent sensitive for active untreated disease); however, most investigators who have studied large numbers of patients have identified C-ANCA/PR3-ANCA in patients without Wegener's granulomatosis, as well as P-ANCA/MPO-ANCA in a few patients with typical Wegener's granulomatosis. Therefore, the absence of C-ANCA has good negative predictive value for Wegener's granulomatosis, but a positive C-ANCA must be interpreted in the context of the patient's disease manifestations to determine whether the appropriate diagnosis is Wegener's granulomatosis, microscopic polyarteritis nodosa, or idiopathic crescentic glomerulonephritis.[43,47] The indirect immunofluorescence micros-

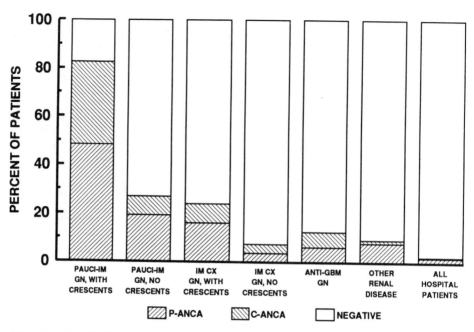

Fig. 5-3. Results from indirect immunofluorescence microscopy assay for antineutrophil cytoplasmic autoantibodies (ANCA) in 397 patients (without lupus) who underwent renal biopsy and 1,029 consecutive unselected hospital patients. (From Jennette,[47] with permission.)

copy ANCA assay is more than 95 percent specific for ANCA-associated glomerulonephritis and vasculitis, with the C-ANCA pattern even more specific than the P-ANCA pattern.[47]

As discussed in more detail later, in a patient with ANCA-associated glomerulonephritis, the presence, organ distribution, and histologic character of systemic vasculitis must be determined for proper diagnostic categorization. Dahlberg et al. have evaluated the sensitivity, specificity, and predictive value of what they consider to be "safe" procedures (i.e., skin, muscle, and rectal biopsies) and "invasive" procedures (i.e., arteriography, lung biopsy, and kidney biopsy) for detecting systemic vasculitis.[49] None of these procedures alone had high predictive value. Combined procedures and procedures directed at involved tissues (e.g., lung biopsy when pulmonary disease is prominent) were most likely to be diagnostic. Albert et al. have also concluded that multiple diagnostic procedures are usually required to confirm the presence of systemic vasculities.[50,51]

Changes in ANCA titers over time correlate to a degree with disease activity, although, as is true for most serologic markers, there are exceptions to this general trend. Most patients have a fall in titer with institution of immunosuppressive therapy and improvement of disease manifestations, and in many patients, the titer will remain low or negative during post-

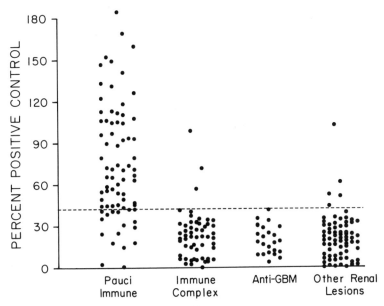

Fig. 5-4. Results of a screening enzyme-linked immunosorbent assay (ELISA) for antineutrophilic cytoplasmic antibody (ANCA) using a substrate isolated from neutrophil cytoplasm that reacts with both cytoplasmic ANCA (C-ANCA) and perinuclear ANCA (P-ANCA). Note that the majority of 76 patients with crescentic pauci-immune glomerulonephritis are positive, compared with only a few of the 55 patients with nonlupus immune complex-mediated glomerulonephritis, and none of the 24 patients with anti-GBM glomerulonephritis are positive. The dashed line is the positive threshold and is the normal control mean plus two standard deviations. (From Jennette et al.,[42] with permission.)

treatment quiescence. Subsequent exacerbations of disease activity are accompanied by rises in ANCA titer. The most frequent exceptions to these patterns are occasional patients who continue to have high titers in spite of treatment and clinical improvement and occasional patients with post-treatment quiescent disease who have a precipitous rise in titer without clinical evidence for disease exacerbation. This occasional disjunction of ANCA titer and disease activity may be the result of a multifactorial pathogenesis in which ANCAs are required, but not sufficient, for mediating tissue injury.[52]

Antiendothelial Antibodies

Antiendothelial antibodies have been detected in the serum of patients with renal disease caused by glomerulonephritis and thrombotic microangiopathies; but assays for antiendothelial antibodies have not been widely used as diagnostic tools, in part because of their technical difficulty. A variety of serologic assays have been used, e.g., complement-mediated endothelial ly-

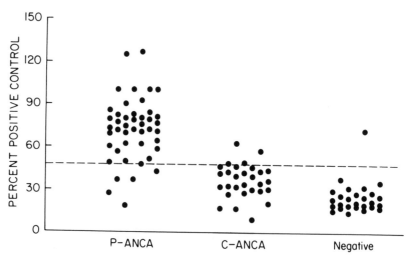

Fig. 5-5. Results of an enzyme-linked immunosorbent assay (ELISA) using purified myeloperoxidase (MPO) as antigen to detect anti-MPO autoantibodies in 101 patients with glomerulonephritis who by indirect immunofluorescence antineutrophilic cytoplasmic antibody (ANCA) assay were either perinuclear ANCA (P-ANCA) positive (45 patients), cytoplasmic ANCA (C-ANCA) positive (29 patients), or ANCA negative (27 patients). Note the strong correlation between anti-MPO activity in this ELISA and a positive P-ANCA result in the indirect immunofluorescence assay. The dashed line is the positive threshold and is the negative mean plus two standard deviations. (From Jennette et al.,[42] with permission.)

sis,[53] antibody-dependent endothelial cell cytotoxicity,[54] and endothelial cell surface ELISA.[55]

Antiendothelial antibodies are in the serum of some patients with thrombotic microangiopathies and may be involved in the pathogenesis of these diseases by injuring endothelial cells. Leung et al. have detected antiendothelial cell antibodies in the serum of patients with hemolytic uremic syndrome and thrombotic thrombocytopenic purpura.[53] Using an endothelial lysis assay, they detected complement-fixing IgG and IgM antiendothelial antibodies in 13 of 14 children with hemolytic uremic syndrome, and in 3 of 5 adults with thrombotic thrombocytopenic purpura. Using an antibody-dependent cell cytotoxicity assay, Marks et al. detected antiendothelial antibodies in 19 percent of patients with systemic sclerosis.[54]

Antiendothelial antibodies have been reported in the serum of patients with nephritis caused by SLE, systemic vasculitis, and IgA nephropathy; but their pathogenic importance in these settings is unknown. Ferraro et al. detected antiendothelial antibodies in 2 of 5 Wegener's granulomatosis patients and in 9 of 10 microscopic polyarteritis nodosa patients using a cell-surface RIA.[56] Yap et al. reported the presence of antiendothelial antibodies in 32 percent of IgA nephropathy patients.[55] Antiendothelial antibodies also have been demonstrated in patients with Kawasaki disease,[57] but these patients usually do not develop renal disease.

Antiphospholipid Antibodies

Antiphospholipid antibodies (e.g., anticardiolipin antibodies) were first identified in patients with SLE, in which setting they are sometimes called "lupus anticoagulant," because they inhibit in vitro coagulation assays, although in vivo they paradoxically enhance coagulation. Because the phospholipid antigens recognized by these autoantibodies are similar to the antigen used in the VDRL assay for syphilis, patients with antiphospholipid antibodies tend to have false-positive VDRL assay results.[32] In patients with SLE, Kalunian et al. observed that the presence of anticardiolipin antibodies was associated with thrombosis, fetal loss, and thrombocytopenia; but not with overall severity of disease or with nephritis.[58]

Recently, D'Agati et al. have reported an association between serum anticardiolipin antibodies and renal injury that has a thrombotic microangiopathy pattern.[59] Of the three patients reported, one had primary antiphospholipid syndrome with thrombotic complications, one a mild lupus-like syndrome, and one mild SLE.

Anti-C3 Convertase Antibodies (C3 and C4 Nephritic Factors)

There are autoantibodies that react with neoantigens expressed by the C3 convertase complexes of the alternative complement activation pathway (C3 nephritic factors) and classical pathway (C4 nephritic factors). As discussed later in the section on complement analysis, patients with diseases associated with nephritic factors often have hypocomplementemia. This may be induced, at least in part, by stabilization of C3 convertase and enhanced consumption of complement.

C3 nephritic factor is an autoantibody that binds to a neoantigen on the alternative complement activation pathway C3 convertase, i.e., the C3bBb complex.[60] C3 nephritic factor is more frequent in type II membranoproliferative glomerulonephritis (43 percent) than in type I membranoproliferative glomerulonephritis (20 percent).[61] Different sensitivities of C3 nephritic factor for membranoproliferative glomerulonephritis that are reported in the literature are most likely the result of different assay methods.[60] C3 nephritic factor is also present in a minority of patients with glomerulonephritis secondary to lupus, cryoglobulinemia, and infected ventriculoatrial shunt. Therefore, C3 nephritic factor is not a very sensitive or specific serologic marker for membranoproliferative glomerulonephritis. The presence of C3 nephritic factor is associated with more rapid deterioration of renal function; but serial quantitation of C3 nephritic factor in a given patient is not a good method for monitoring disease activity.[61]

An interesting observation is that C3 nephritic factors from different individuals have a shared idiotype.[62] If this is true, it may be possible to design a highly specific serologic test for C3 nephritic factor based on the detection of antibodies with this common idiotype in patient serum.

C4 nephritic factor is an autoantibody that binds to a neoantigen on the classical complement activation pathway C3 convertase, i.e., the C4b2a complex.[63] C4 nephritic factor has been detected in patients with postinfectious glomerulonephritis, lupus glomerulonephritis, and type I membranoproliferative glomerulonephritis.[63,65] Seino et al. have suggested that C4 nephritic factor is a useful serologic marker of type I membranoproliferative glomerulonephritis in the same way that C3 nephritic factor is a marker for type II membranoproliferative glomerulonephritis.[63] However, C4 nephritic factor is not a very sensitive marker for type I membranoproliferative glomerulonephritis, and its diagnostic utility is not yet well established.

A nephritic factor in patients with membranoproliferative glomerulonephritis that stabilizes conversion of not only C3, but also C5 and C9 has been reported.[66] This properdin-dependent nephritic factor may enhance terminal complement component activation.

Anti-C1q Antibodies

Antibodies directed against the collagen-like portion of C1q have been identified in the serum of patients with SLE[67–69] and in patients with hypocomplementemic urticarial vasculitis syndrome.[70] Both of these diseases often have nephritis with hypocomplementemia as a conspicuous clinical feature.

Anti-C1q antibodies have been detected in the serum of approximately 50 percent of SLE patients.[68,69] These autoantibodies are most frequent in patients with decreased CH50 and C1q.[67] Anti-C1q antibodies can cause false-positive results in C1q binding assays for circulating immune complexes, and this may explain the high positive rate for these assays in lupus patients.[67]

Anti-C1q antibodies also have been observed in patients with hypocomplementemic urticarial vasculitis syndrome.[70] These patients typically have urticaria and/or angioedema, glomerulonephritis, arthralgias with or without arthritis, and uveitis; but are negative for antinuclear antibodies. The glomeruli and cutaneous vessels have immunohistologic evidence for immune complex deposition with prominent complement activation.

SEROLOGIC ANALYSIS OF CIRCULATING IMMUNE COMPLEXES

Serologic Methods for Immune Complex Detection

Dozens of serologic tests have been devised to detect immune complexes in the circulation.[71,72] None of these tests have proven to be of great diagnostic or even prognostic value. In addition to insensitivity, a major problem with almost all of these tests is that they detect immune complexes without determining the constituent antigen and antibody. Most immune complex assays discriminate between immunoglobulin in immune complexes and free immunoglobulin on the basis of physiochemical characteristics (especially size and precipitability); reactivity with receptors (e.g., complement receptors and Fc receptors); or activation of or binding to complement components (e.g., C1q binding). Table 5-1 lists the most widely used circulating immune complex assays.

A major problem with almost all of the assays in Table 5-1 is that they do not discriminate between immunoglobulin in immune complexes and nonspecifically aggregated immunoglobulin. If a single assay system is to be used, the WHO Working Group recommends a C1q binding assay or a conglutinin binding assay.[3] Because of different specificities, sensitivities, and adverse analytic influences, use of multiple immune complex assays is preferred if the presence or absence of circulating immune complexes is to be determined with reasonable accuracy.

Utility of Serologic Immune Complex Assays

The diagnostic utility of current assays for circulating immune complexes is marginal at best.[3,71,72] Immune complex-mediated diseases (e.g., immune complex-mediated glomerulonephritis) can be present without detectable circulating immune complexes, and assays for circulating immune complexes are often positive in patients with no evidence for immune complex-mediated tissue inflammation.[2] In a patient with documented immune complex-mediated disease (e.g., glomerulonephritis with immune complex localization demonstrated by direct immunofluorescence microscopy) who has a positive assay for circulating immune complexes, serial immune complex levels may be of value in monitoring disease activity and treatment response; but this assertion is based mainly on anecdotal reports.

The capacity of assays for circulating immune complexes to detect immune complexes has been demonstrated in patients with serum sickness. For example, Nielsen et al. followed the time course of circulating immune complex generation in a patient who received 100 ml of horse antivenom globulin after a rattlesnake bite and observed that a C1q binding assay and a complement consumption assay detected circulating immune complexes at the predicted time during the course of the serum sickness.[73] Therefore, in this archetypical form of immune complex-mediated disease, immune complex assays did document the circulating pathogenic factors.

Table 5-1. Circulating Immune Complex Assays

C1q binding assay	Staphylococcal protein A binding assay
Raji cell assay	Rheumatoid factor binding assay
Conglutinin binding assay	Cryoprecipitation assay
Complement activation assay	Fibronectin aggregate assay
Platelet aggregation assay	Density gradient centrifugation assay
Ultracentrifugation assay	Polyethylene glycol precipitation assay

Circulating immune complex assays have been studied most extensively in patients with systemic autoimmune diseases of presumed immune complex pathogenesis. McDougal et al.[71] have compared the performance of five commonly used immune complex assays in patients with SLE, rheumatoid arthritis, vasculitis, and miscellaneous other rheumatic diseases. The assays they studied were the bovine conglutinin assay, C1q binding assay, staphylococci binding assay, Raji cell assay, and monoclonal rheumatoid factor assay. The specificity of these assays (determined by analysis of normal sera) ranged from 94 to 98 percent. Rheumatoid factor was a source of false-positive results in all assays. Compared to specificity, sensitivity was much more variable among tests and among the disease groups. For example, the sensitivity for SLE of the various assays ranged from 20 to 67 percent.

Cryoglobulin Assay

Virtually by definition, serologic demonstration of cryoglobulins is required for diagnosing renal disease secondary to cryoglobulinemia. More than half of the patients with disease caused by mixed cryoglobulinemia have renal involvement, although an even higher proportion have cutaneous angiitis and polyarthralgias. Mixed cryoglobulins are immune complexes composed of antiimmunoglobulin antibodies (i.e., rheumatoid factors, usually IgM) complexed with immunoglobulins (usually IgG). In addition to cryoglobulins, patients with mixed cryoglobulinemia often have hypocomplementemia, polyclonal hyper-γ-globulinemia, and positive rheumatoid factor assays.[74]

The serologic demonstration of cryoglobulins is not specific for the syndrome of mixed cryoglobulinemia with nephritis. For example, positive cryoglobulin assay results also occur with lupus nephritis and postinfectious glomerulonephritis. False-negative results can result from improper handling of the blood sample before assay. The sample must be kept at 37°C until it is clotted and the serum removed for cryoprecipitation.

IgA-Fibronectin Aggregate Assays

A variety of serologic abnormalities has been observed in patients with IgA nephropathy. Approximately half of the patients have elevated serum IgA levels, especially polymeric IgA.[75,76] Circulating immune complexes, especially those containing IgA, have been detected in IgA nephropathy patients,[75–77] but most assay systems have not had good enough sensitivity or specificity to be of diagnostic value. A recent methodologic innovation that may overcome this insensitivity and nonspecificity is the use of IgA-fibronectin aggregate assay.[78–81]

The relationship of the fibronectin to the IgA in the aggregates is not conclusively determined. These likely are IgA immune complexes in which the fibronectin could be the antigen attached to the IgA Fab region, or could be attached to the IgA Fc region, or to the antigen.[81]

Serum IgA-fibronectin aggregates can be detected and quantified using ELISA with collagen or heparin as substrate to bind to the collagen-binding or heparin-binding domains of fibronectin. ELISA with immobilized antifibronectin to capture the IgA-fibronectin aggregates in serum also can be used. Using an ELISA system with collagen as substrate, Jennette et al. demonstrated IgA-fibronectin aggregates in 93 percent of 30 patients with IgA nephropathy, compared to 12 percent of 103 patients with other forms of glomerular disease and 7 percent of normal controls[81] (Fig. 5-6). IgA-fibronectin aggregates were identified in patients with primary IgA nephropathy, IgA nephropathy with Henoch-Schönlein purpura, and recurrent IgA nephropathy in transplants. The diagnostic utility of IgA-fibronectin aggregate assays has not been definitively determined, but this serologic test may prove to be a useful noninvasive means of supporting a diagnosis of IgA nephropathy.

COMPLEMENT ANALYSIS

There are patterns of complement-component and complement-control protein alterations that are typical for certain types of renal disease,[82–84] but

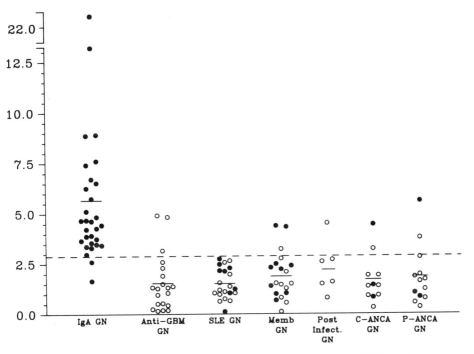

Fig. 5-6. Results of an enzyme-linked immunosorbent assay (ELISA) for serum IgA-fibronectin aggregates showing good sensitivity and specificity for IgA nephropathy. The dashed line is the positive threshold and is the normal control mean plus two standard deviations. (From Jennette et al.,[81] with permission.)

these are too variable and nonspecific to have strong positive predictive value alone, although they can be helpful in combination with other serologic tests for confirming a diagnosis. Complement-component assays also may be useful for evaluating disease activity. Because of the broad reference range for normal complement-component levels, changes over time in an individual patient are sometimes as useful as values outside the normal range.

The two major mechanisms of complement-component depletion in patients with renal disease are (1) urinary loss and tubular epithelial catabolism caused by the nephrotic syndrome and (2) consumption caused by the inflammatory events of glomerulonephritis (especially activation by immune complexes). Rare patients with glomerulonephritis and decreased CH50 activity will be found to have a primary complement-component deficiency that has secondarily predisposed to the development of immune complex-mediated glomerulonephritis. Such patients usually have deficiency of C1 or C2, which probably impairs opsonization and clearance of nephritogenic immune complexes from the circulation.[32]

Complement Abnormalities in Patients With the Nephrotic Syndrome

In patients with the nephrotic syndrome, some complement components and control proteins are often decreased while other are increased. Although substantial variability occurs among diseases and patients, in general, C1q, C2, C8, C9, factor B, and factor I are decreased by nephrosis, whereas C1s, C4, C3, C5, C6, properdin, C1INH and factor H are elevated.[83,85,86] The greatest degree of decrease is in C1q, C2, C8, and factor B.[83] Therefore, because low levels of C1q and C2 can be caused by renal excretion and catabolism, low levels of C4 are the only reliable marker of classic pathway complement activation in a patient with the nephrotic syndrome.

Patients with the nephrotic syndrome and decreased C3 levels should be suspected of having some form of glomerular diseases that is associated with hypocomplementemia, e.g., membranoproliferative glomerulonephritis,[60] or membranous glomerulopathy secondary to SLE.[87]

A recent approach to analyzing glomerular complement activation in patients with the nephrotic syndrome is to measure levels of membrane attack complexes in the urine. Hebert et al. have reported that 8 of 12 patients with membranous glomerulopathy had elevated urine SC5b-9, as well as 4 of 12 patients with other causes for the nephrotic syndrome.[88]

Complement Abnormalities in Patients With Glomerulonephritis

Some forms of immune complex-mediated glomerulonephritis are frequently associated with depletion of plasma complement components, presumably caused by consumption during formation of immune complexes either in the circulation or in situ in vessel walls. Glomerulonephritides associated with hypocomplementemia include acute postinfectious glomerulonephritis, lupus glomerulonephritis, membranoproliferative glomerulonephritis, cryoglobulinemic glomerulonephritis, and endocarditic glomerulonephritis (including shunt nephritis). Glomerulonephritides not associated with hypocomplementemia include anti-GBM disease, ANCA-associated disease (e.g., idiopathic crescentic glomerulonephritis, Wegener's granulomatosis, and most cases of polyarteritis nodosa), and IgA nephropathy (including Henoch-Schölein purpura).

Approximately 90 percent of patients with acute poststreptococcal glomerulonephritis have hypocomplementemia during the acute phase of the illness; but a small proportion never have hypocomplementemia.[89] Total hemolytic complement (CH50), C3 and C5 are decreased. Only 5 percent of patients have decreased C4.[83] With respect to terminal pathway components, C6, C7, and C9 are normal, but C8 may be low.[83] Decreased complement components usually return to normal within 1 to 8 weeks. Prolongation of hypocomplementemia past 2 months casts doubt on a diagnosis of acute poststreptococcal glomerulonephritis and raises the possibility of more persistent forms of immune complex-mediated glomerulonephritis, such as membranoproliferative glomerulonephritis, including membranoproliferative glomerulonephritis caused by persistent infections such as indolent endocarditis or osteomyelitis.

As discussed earlier, most patients with membranoproliferative glomerulonephritis have hypocomplementemia and serum autoantibodies specific for C3 convertase complexes (i.e., C3 nephritic factor and C4 nephritic factor).[60-66] Approximately 70 percent of patients with membranoproliferative glomerulonephritis have hypocomplementemia at the time of diagnosis, and approximately 80 percent have hypocomplementemia at some time during follow-up; with type II having more frequent, more severe, and more persistent hypocomplementemia than type I membranoproliferative glomerulonephritis. C3 is low in all membranoproliferative glomerulonephritis patients with hypocomplementemia. Classic pathway components (e.g., C4) are normal in type II membranoproliferative glomerulonephritis.[83]

Approximately 75 percent of patients with active lupus nephritis have hypocomplementemia. Most patients with hypocomplementemia show evidence for consumption of both classic and alternative pathway components, with decreased levels of C1q, C2, C3, and C4.[83] C5 is decreased in only around 10 percent of patients. The terminal components C6, C7, and C9 are never decreased, but many patients with active disease will have decreased C8.[84] Changes in C4 provide a more sensitive indicator of disease activity than changes in C3.[90] With disease exacerbations, C4 is decreased more often than C3 and decreases before C3.

Demonstration of complement-component consumption is an indirect means of detecting complement activation in lupus patients, but a more direct method is to measure activation fragments or complement component complexes. Falk et al. used a monoclonal antibody specific for a neoantigen on poly C9 in an RIA to measure the complement attack complex (i.e.,

SC5b-9) in serum.[91] They detected elevated levels of SC5b-9 in 13 of 14 SLE patients with active disease. The SC5b-9 level was a more sensitive measure of disease activity than C3, C4, or CH50.

Patients with hypocomplementemic urticarial vasculitis syndrome may have antibody-mediated activation of C1 by anti-C1q antibodies.[70] The hypocomplementemia is characterized by reduced C1, C2, C3, and C5.[83,92]

Mixed cryoglobulinemic glomerulonephritis is often accompanied by hypocomplementemia.[74] Typically, C1q, C3, and C4 are decreased.

Two diseases that can be clinically misdiagnosed as immune complex-mediated glomerulonephritis or systemic vasculitis are atherembolic disease and thrombotic microangiopathy, both of which can cause hypocomplementemia,[93,94] acute renal failure, hematuria, and evidence for systemic vascular injury. The presence of eosinophilia supports the possibility of atheroembolism, and the presence of a microangiopathic hemolytic anemia and thrombocytopenia supports thrombotic microangiopathy.

AMYLOID AND IMMUNOGLOBULIN PARAPROTEIN ANALYSIS

Light chain deposition disease and amyloidosis injure renal glomeruli and other renal vessels, as well as the tubulointerstitial compartment. Serologic detection of quantitatively and qualitatively abnormal serum immunoglobulins is useful in diagnosing some, but not all, cases of light chain deposition disease and amyloidosis composed of immunoglobulin light chains (AL amyloidosis).

Definitive diagnosis of amyloidosis still requires demonstration of amyloid in tissue specimens; however, certain serum assays can suggest or support the possibility of amyloidosis in a given patient with renal disease, especially nephrosis and renal insufficiency in an older adult. Different types of amyloid are composed of different amyloidogenic proteins that have serum precursors that are sometimes elevated in patients with the derivative form of amyloidosis. Protein constituents of different types of amyloid include immunoglobulin light chains (AL amyloid); amyloid A protein (AA amyloid, familial Mediterranean fever); transthyretin (prealbumin) (senile cardiac amyloid, autosomal dominant familial amyloid); β-protein (Alzheimer's and cerebral amyloid); and β_2-microglobulin (hemodialysis associated amyloid). Elevated serum levels of the precursor proteins may be present in patients with amyloid, but this is not a sensitive or specific diagnostic marker. For example, serum β_2-microglobin levels can be 40 to 50 times higher than normal in chronic hemodialysis patients, but the presence or degree of elevation does not correlate well with the development of β_2-microglobulin amyloidosis.[95]

Detection of monoclonal immunoglobulin in serum or urine is useful in diagnosing AL amyloidosis.[95,96] Of patients with AL amyloidosis, approximately 60 percent have serum monoclonal immunoglobulin, 75 percent urine monoclonal immunoglobulin, 85 percent urine or serum monoclonal immunoglobulin, 75 percent bone marrow plasmacytosis, and 20 percent overt multiple myeloma. AL amyloid is usually derived from λ-light chains. Very rarely, amyloid can be composed of abnormal heavy chains.[97]

Light chain deposition disease has extensive nonfibrillar deposits of light chains in glomeruli, vessels, and tubular basement membranes, often resulting in a nodular glomerulosclerosis that may resemble diabetic glomerulosclerosis by light microscopy.[96,98] This is much more often caused by monoclonal κ-light chain deposition than by λ-light chain deposition; and therefore has been called κ-light chain nephropathy. Of patients with light chain deposition disease, approximately 60 percent have serum monoclonal immunoglobulin, 75 percent urine monoclonal immunoglobulin, 80 percent urine or serum monoclonal immunoglobulin, 70 percent bone marrow plasmacytosis, and 45 percent overt multiple myeloma.

Thus, it appears that the renal pathogenicity of excess λ- and κ-light chains is different, possibly because λ-light chains are more amyloidogenic. This difference in disease associations between serum and urine monoclonal κ- and λ-light chains should influence the differential diagnosis in a patient with proteinuria, and Bence Jones proteinuria and paraproteinemia. AL amyloidosis is most likely if monoclonal λ-light chains are identified, whereas nonamyloidotic light chain deposition disease is most likely if monoclonal κ-light chains are present.

AA amyloid is an insoluble fibrillar tissue derivative of serum amyloid A (SAA) protein that has been altered by proteolytic cleavage of the carboxy end of the molecule. This raises the possibility that quantitation of serum SAA might be of diagnostic value. A variety of assay procedures quantify SAA, most of which use ELISA techniques.[99] Although SAA is elevated in patients with amyloidosis, this does not correlate well with the type of amyloidosis; and increased SAA occurs in many diseases other than amyloidosis, including neoplastic diseases (e.g., lung cancer) and inflammatory diseases (e.g., rheumatoid arthritis).[100] Therefore, SAA analysis is too nonspecific to be of diagnostic value for AA amyloidosis.

DIAGNOSTIC APPLICATION OF SEROLOGIC TESTS IN RENAL DISEASE

Nephritic Syndrome

The differential diagnosis of a patient with nephritis can be substantially refined by serologic analysis. As shown in Table 5-2, the most frequent forms of glomerulonephritis have serologic markers that facilitate diagnosis.

A useful first step in the serologic categorization of patients with nephritis is to consider the complement status.[101] Hypocomplementemia is a sensitive marker for postinfectious glomerulonephritis and lupus glomerulonephritis and is a less sensitive marker for membranoproliferative glomerulonephritis and cryoglobulinemic glomerulonephritis. Hypocomplementemia is not observed with IgA nephropathy, idiopathic (pauciimmune) glomerulonephritis, or anti-GBM glomerulonephritis.

Table 5-2. Serologic Findings in the Nephritic Syndrome

Serologic demonstration of	*Increases likelihood of*
Hypocomplementemia and	
Antistreptococcal antibodies	Poststreptococcal glomerulonephritis
Antinuclear antibodies	Lupus proliferative glomerulonephritis
C3 nephritic factor	Membranoproliferative glomerulonephritis
Mixed cryoglobulins	Cryoglobulinemic glomerulonephritis
Normocomplementemia and	
IgA fibronectin aggregates	IgA nephropathy
Antineutrophil cytoplasmic antibodies	Idiopathic crescentic glomerulonephritis
Anti-GBM antibodies	Anti-GBM glomerulonephritis

Abbreviations: GBM, glomerular basement membrane.

Serologic tests for the antibodies listed in Table 5-2 are more specific than hypocomplementemia for particular forms of glomerulonephritis, but as discussed, they are not totally specific. For example, although it is most frequent in membranoproliferative glomerulonephritis, C3 nephritic factor also occurs in a minority of patients with lupus, cryoglobulinemic, and postinfectious glomerulonephritis. Therefore, combined positive and negative test results are required for the most confident serologic conclusions; e.g., a good diagnostic profile for membranoproliferative glomerulonephritis would be positive results for hypocomplementemia and C3 nephritic factor, combined with negative results for elevated antistrep antibodies, antinuclear antibodies, and cryoglobulins.

The most common form of indolent, normocomplementemic glomerulonephritis is IgA nephropathy. Serologic assay for IgA-fibronectin aggregates may prove useful in the diagnosis of this disease (Fig. 5-6).

Timely diagnosis is particularly important in the evaluation of patients with rapidly progressive glomerulonephritis. As diagramed in Figure 5-7, serologic analysis combined with clinical distribution of disease is required to classify patients with rapidly progressive glomerulonephritis. Although the patient's initial manifestations of disease may be exclusively renal, especially among patients referred to nephrologists, the presence of rapidly progressive glomerulonephritis raises the possibility of unrecognized or nascent systemic disease.

Concurrent Renal and Extrarenal Disease

As shown in Table 5-3, there are serologic markers that help diagnose the cause of renal disease that is secondary to systemic disease.

Glomerulonephritis is a form of vascular inflammation; therefore, it is not surprising that some patients have glomerulonephritis as one component of vasculitis affecting other organ systems, e.g., lungs, skin, and gut. On the basis of immunopathology, glomerulonephritis and vasculitis that affects the kidney can be divided into immune complex-mediated, anti-GBM an-

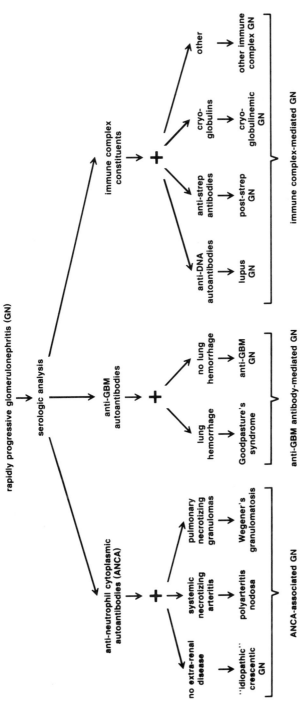

Fig. 5-7. Algorithmic diagram of the categorization of rapidly progressive glomerulonephritis based on a combination of serologic and clinicopathologic data. (From Jennette and Falk,[41] with permission.)

Table 5-3. Serologic Findings in Combined Renal and Extrarenal Disease

Serologic demonstration of	*Increases likelihood of*
Anti-GBM antibodies	Goodpasture's syndrome
ANCA (especially C-ANCA)	Wegener's granulomatosis
ANCA (C-ANCA or P-ANCA)	Polyarteritis nodosa
IgA fibronectin aggregates	Henoch-Schönlein purpura
Antihepatitis B antibodies	Polyarteritis nodosa
Antinuclear antibodies	Systemic lupus erythematosus
Mixed cryoglobulins	Cryoglobulinemic vasculitis
Anti-C1q antibodies	Hypocomplementemic urticarial vasculitis
Anticardiolipin antibodies	Thrombotic microangiopathy
Antiverotoxin antibodies	Hemolytic uremic syndrome
Anti-Scl 70	Systemic sclerosis
Monoclonal immunoglobulin	AL amyloidosis

Abbreviations: AL, amyloid of light chain origin; ANCA, antineutrophil cytoplasmic autoantibodies; C-ANCA, cytoplasmic ANCA; GBM, glomerular basement membrane; P-ANCA, perinuclear ANCA.

tibody-mediated, and ANCA-associated disease (Figs. 5-7 and 5-8).[41,47] Figure 5-8 depicts the relative frequency and degree of overlap of these immunopathogenic categories and also depicts the relationship of these categories to various clinicopathologic categories of glomerulonephritis and systemic vasculitis. C-ANCA is depicted as a very sensitive marker for Wegener's granulomatosis (i.e., almost all Wegener's granulomatosis patients fall within the C-ANCA sphere), but it is not completely specific (i.e., some patients within the C-ANCA sphere have glomerulonephritis alone, microscopic polyarteritis nodosa, or pulmonary-renal syndrome without granulomas).

Serologic evaluation is particularly useful in the evaluation of pulmonary-renal syndrome. As diagrammed in Figure 5-8, pulmonary renal syndrome can be caused by anti-GBM antibodies (e.g., Goodpasture's syndrome), immune complexes (e.g., cryoglobulinemia), or can be associated with ANCA. ANCA-associated pulmonary-renal syndrome is most frequent.[41] The lung injury of C-ANCA pulmonary-renal syndrome frequently has granulomatous inflammation (i.e., is Wegener's granulomatosis), whereas that of P-ANCA pulmonary-renal syndrome is usually characterized by hemorrhagic capillaritis without granulomatous inflammation.[42,43,47]

Systemic vasculitis that usually does not have pulmonary involvement also has different immunopathologic variants that have different serologic markers. Henoch-Schönlein purpura has IgA-fibronectin aggregates, cryoglobulinemic vasculitis has mixed cryoglobulins, hypocomplementemic urticarial vasculitis syndrome has anti-C1q antibodies, and pauciimmune microscopic polyarteritis nodosa has ANCA.

Renal disease associated with systemic organ dysfunction also can be caused by the thrombotic microangiopathies. The renal injury in the thrombotic microangiopathies is characterized pathologically by edematous intimal expansion in arteries, fibrinoid necrosis of arterioles, and expansion of

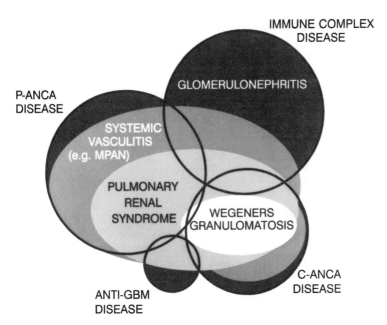

Fig. 5-8. Diagram depicting the major immunopathologic categories of glomeru-lonephritis and systemic necrotizing vasculitis (circles) and the relationship of these to various clinicopathologic syndromes (shaded areas). A patient often can be po-sitioned in the appropriate circles by serologic analysis, but additional data are required to determine the appropriate specific diagnosis. (From Jennette,[47] with permission.)

the subendothelial zone in glomerular capillaries, sometimes with superim-posed platelet-rich thrombosis. All of these changes are most likely caused by endothelial injury with resultant insudation of plasma constituents into vessel walls. Clinically, the thrombotic microangiopathies are characterized by a microangiopathic hemolytic anemia and thrombocytopenia caused by destruction of erythrocytes and platelets as they pass through the injured vessels. Differences in cause and organ system distribution allow further clinicopathologic categorization of the thrombotic microangiopathies: e.g., hemolytic uremic syndrome, thrombotic thrombocytopenic purpura, acute postpartum renal failure, and systemic sclerosis renal crisis. Patients with a thrombotic microangiopathy often present with renal failure that may be difficult to distinguish from the renal failure of glomerulonephritis because these patients often exhibit hematuria and proteinuria and sometimes hypo-complementemia.[94] Serologic analysis can help by reducing the likelihood of other systemic diseases (e.g., negative antinuclear antibody assay, negative ANCA assay, negative cryoglobulin assay) and by identifying serologic markers for the thrombotic microangiopathies.

Serologic tests that can identify various etiologic agents of the thrombotic microangiopathies can be useful; e.g., tests demonstrating the presence of a toxin-producing pathogen (e.g., serotype O157:H7 *E. coli*), or a pathogenic autoantibody. Etiologic agents include bacterial toxins (especially verotoxin and Shiga toxin),[14–17] drugs (especially cyclosporin A, mitomycin C, and cisplatin),[102–105] and autoantibodies (e.g., antiendothelial antibodies and antiphospholipid antibodies).[53,54,59]

Nephrotic Syndrome

As shown in Table 5-4, there are serologic markers that can assist with the diagnosis, or elucidation of the pathogenesis of a number of causes of the nephrotic syndrome. Also bear in mind that the glomerulonephritides listed in Table 5-2 also can cause nephrotic range proteinuria.

Serologic analysis is sometimes useful even after a diagnosis of the pathologic cause for nephrotic syndrome has been determined by renal biopsy. This is because most glomerular lesions occur as both primary (idiopathic) and secondary forms, and causes for the latter may be identifiable by serology.

Especially in children or young adults, the possibility of secondary rather than primary membranous glomerulopathy should be considered. Pathologically, the presence of mesangial deposits, in addition to the prerequisite subepithelial deposits, raises the possibility of secondary rather than primary membranous glomerulopathy. Serologic analysis helps identify causes for secondary membranous glomerulopathy, e.g., SLE,[87] hepatitis B,[106,107] syphilis,[10,11] thyroiditis,[108] and carcinoma (e.g., assay for serum carcinoembryonic antigen). Especially when the renal biopsy demonstrates intense glomerular immunostaining for C1q, or endothelial tubuloreticular inclusions by electron microscopy, serologic analysis for lupus should be pursued.[87]

Experimental studies of Heyman nephritis suggest that idiopathic membranous glomerulopathy may be caused by autoantibodies directed against glomerular visceral epithelial cell antigens.[109,110] If this is true in humans, in the future a serologic assay for this nephritogenic autoantibody may be developed and could be used to diagnose idiopathic membranous glomerulopathy.

Table 5-4. Serologic Findings in the Nephrotic Syndrome

Serologic demonstration of	*Increases likelihood of*
Antinuclear antibodies	Lupus membranous glomerulopathy
Antihepatitis B antibodies	Membranous glomerulopathy
Antitreponemal antibodies	Membranous glomerulopathy
Carcinoembryonic antigen	Membranous glomerulopathy
Antithyroid antibodies	Membranous glomerulopathy
C 3 nephritic factor	Membranoproliferative glomerulonephritis
Anti-HIV antibodies	Focal glomerulosclerosis
λ-monoclonal immunoglobulin	AL amyloidosis
κ-monoclonal immunoglobulin	Light chain deposition disease

Abbreviations: AL, amyloid of light chain origin; HIV, human immunodeficiency virus.

As discussed earlier, in patients with focal glomerulosclerosis who have risk factors for HIV infection, or who have renal biopsy findings suggesting HIV nephropathy, serologic analysis for HIV is warranted.

In nephrotic patients in their seventh decade or older, analysis of serum for monoclonal immunoglobulins, which would support a diagnosis of AL amyloidosis, and carcinoembryonic antigen, which would support a diagnosis of carcinoma-induced membranous glomerulopathy, are reasonable components of the laboratory evaluation.

CONCLUSIONS

No serologic test is 100 percent specific or sensitive for a given disease, and no serologic test has 100 percent positive or negative predictive value, although some tests come closer to these ideals than others. Therefore, serologic tests cannot be used as the sole means of making or excluding a diagnosis. Nevertheless, when used appropriately, serologic tests are a powerful diagnostic adjunct.

To draw conclusions from serologic test data, the approximate specificity, sensitivity, and predictive value of the test must be known. The predictive value is dramatically affected by disease prevalence. The best positive predictive value is obtained when a serologic test is applied in a patient who has clinical signs and symptoms that already predict a pretest prevalence of the suspected disease of 40 percent or better. Even when sensitivity, specificity, or predictive value are too low for a serologic test to have definitive diagnostic value, positive or negative results can substantially alter the likelihood of a disease in the patient being tested and thus can refine the differential diagnosis and point the way for additional tests. Knowledgeably selected combinations or sequences of serologic tests have more diagnostic power than individual tests.

REFERENCES

1. Galan SG, Gambino SR: Beyond Normality: The Predictive Value and Efficacy of Medical Diagnosis. John Wiley & Sons, New York, 1975
2. Bentwich Z, Biancon N, Jager L et al: Use and abuse of laboratory tests in clinical immunology: critical considerations of eight widely used diagnostic procedures. Clin Immunol Immunopathol 24:122, 1982
3. Bentwich Z, Beverley PCL, Hammarstrom L et al: Laboratory investigations in clinical immunology; methods, pitfalls, and clinical indications. Clin Immunol Immunopathol 49:478, 1988
4. Lichtenstein MJ, Pincus T: How useful are combinations of blood tests in "rheumatic panels" in diagnosis of rheumatic diseases? J Gen Intern Med 3:435, 1988
5. Gambino SR: The misuse of predictive value—or why you must consider the odds. Lab Report 11:65, 1989

6. Swaak AJG, Groenwold J, Bronsveld W: Predictive value of complement profiles and anti-dsDNA in systemic lupus erythematosus. Ann Rheum Dis 45:359, 1986

7. Bisno AL, Ofek I: Serologic diagnosis of streptococcal infection. Comparison of a rapid hemagglutination technique with conventional antibody tests. Am J Dis Child 127:676, 1974

8. Dillon HC: Post-streptococcal glomerulonephritis following pyoderma. Rev Infect Dis 1:935, 1979

9. Southwest Pediatric Nephrology Study Group: Hepatitis B surface antigenemia in North American children with membranous glomerulonephropathy. J Pediatr 106:571, 1985

10. Yuceoglu AM, Sagel, Treser G et al: The glomerulopathy of congenital syphilis. A curable immune-deposit disease. J Am Med Assoc 229:1085, 1974

11. Gamble CN, Reardon JB: Immunopathogenesis of syphilitic glomerulonephritis: elution of antitreponemal antibody from glomerular immune complex deposits. N Engl J Med 292:449, 1975

12. D'Agati V, Suh J-I, Carbone L et al: Pathology of HIV-associated nephropathy: a detailed morphologic and comparative study. Kidney Int 35:1358, 1989

13. Glassock RJ, Cohen AH, Danovitch G, Parsa KP: Human immunodeficiency virus (HIV) infection and the kidney. Ann Intern Med 112:35, 1990

14. Rose PE, Clark AJ: Haematology of the haemolytic uraemic syndrome. Blood Rev 3:136, 1989

15. Whittam TS, Wachsmuth IK, Wilson RA: Genetic evidence of clonal descent of Escherichia coli O157:H7 associated with hemorrhagic colitis and hemolytic uremic syndrome. J Infect Dis 157:1124, 1988

16. Scotland SM, Rowe B, Smith HR et al: Vero cytotoxin-producing strains of *Escherichia coli* from children with haemolytic uraemic syndrome and their detection by specific DNA probes. J Med Microbiol 25:237, 1988

17. Chart H, Scotland SM, Smith HR et al: Antibodies to Escherichia coli O157 in patients with haemorrhagic colitis and haemolytic uraemic syndrome. J Clin Pathol 42:973, 1989

18. Chart H, Scotland SM, Rowe B: Serum antibodies to Escherichia coli serotype O157:H7 in patients with hemolytic uremic syndrome. J Clin Microbiol 27:285, 1989

19. Ashkenazi S, Cleary TG, Lopez E et al: Anticytotoxin-neutralizing antibodies in immune globulin preparations: potential use in hemolytic-uremic syndrome. J Pediatr 113:1008, 1988

20. Mathew TH: Recurrence of disease following renal transplantation. Am J Kidney Dis 12:85, 1988

21. Stanton MC, Tange JD: Goodpasture's syndrome (pulmonary haemorrhage associated with glomerulonephritis). Austr Ann Med 7:132, 1958

22. Scheer RL, Grossman MA: Immune aspects of the glomerulonephritis associated with pulmonary hemorrhage. Ann Intern Med 60:1009, 1964

23. Lerner R, Glassock RJ, Dixon FL: The role of anti-glomerular basement membrane antibody in the pathogenesis of human glomerulonephritis. J Exp Med 126:989, 1967

24. Martinez JS, Kohler PF: Variant "Goodpasture's syndrome"? The need for immunologic criteria in rapidly progressive glomerulonephritis and hemorrhagic pneumonitis. Ann Intern Med 75:67, 1971

25. Wheeler J, Simpson J, Morley AR: Routine and rapid enzyme linked immuno-sorbent assays for circulating anti-glomerular basement membrane antibodies. J Clin Pathol 41:163, 1988

26. Saxena R, Isaksson B, Bygren P, Wieslander J: A rapid assay for circulating anti-glomerular basement membrane antibodies in Goodpasture syndrome. J Immunol Methods 118:73, 1989

27. Bygren P, Cederholm B, Heinegard D, Wieslander J: Non-Goodpasture anti-GBM antibodies in patients with glomerulonephritis. Nephrol Dial Transplant 4:254, 1989

28. Hudson BG, Wieslander J, Wisdom BJ, Noelkey ME: Goodpasture syndrome: molecular architecture and function of basement membrane antigen. Lab Invest 61:256, 1989

29. Saxena R, Bygren P, Cederholm B, Wieslander J: Circulating anti-entactin antibodies in patients with glomerulonephritis. Kidney Int 39:996, 1991

30. Brentjens JR, Matsuo S, Fakatsu A et al: Immunologic studies in two patients with antitubular basement membrane nephritis. Am J Med 86:603, 1989

31. Rotellar C, Noel LH, Droz D et al: Role of antibodies directed against tubular basement membranes in human renal transplantation. Am J Kidney Dis 7:157, 1986

32. Schur PH: Serologic tests in the evaluation of rheumatic diseases. Immunol Allergy Pract 13:138, 1991

33. Bravo R, Frank R, Blundell PA et al: Cyclin/PCNA is the auxiliary protein of DNA polymerase-delta. Nature 316:515, 1987

34. Monier JC, Sault C, Veysseyre C, Bringuier JP: Discrepancies between two procedures for ds-DNA antibody detection: Farr test and indirect immuno-fluorescence on Crithidia luciliae. J Clin Lab Immunol 25:149, 1988

35. ter Borg EJ, Horst G, Hummel EJ et al: Measurement of increases in anti-double-stranded DNA antibody levels as a predictor of disease exacerbation in systemic lupus erythematosus. A long-term, prospective study. Arthritis Rheum 33:634, 1990

36. Fritzler MJ, Tan EM: Antibodies to histones in drug induced and idiopathic lupus erythematosus. J Clin Invest 62:560, 1978

37. Guldner HH, Szostecki S, Vosberg HP et al: Scl 70 autoantibodies from sclero-derma patients recognize a 95 KDa protein identified as DNA topoisomerase I. Chromosoma 94:132, 1986

38. Moroi Y, Peebles C, Fritzler MJ et al: Autoantibody to centromere (kineto-chrore) in scleroderma sera. Proc Natl Acad Sci USA 77:1627, 1980

39. Pinnas JL, Northway JD, Tan EM: Antinucleolar antibodies in human sera. J Immunol 111:996, 1973

40. Couser WG: Rapidly progressive glomerulonephritis: classification, pathogenetic mechanisms, and therapy. Am J Kidney Dis 11:449, 1988

41. Jennette JC, Falk RJ: Diagnosis and management of glomerulonephritis and vasculitis presenting as acute renal failure. In Mandal AK, Hebert LA (ed): Medical Clinics of North America: Renal Failure and Transplantation. WB Saunders, Philadelphia, 74:893, 1990

42. Jennette JC, Wilkman AS, Falk RJ: Anti-neutrophil cytoplasmic autoantibody-associated glomerulonephritis and vasculitis. Am J Pathol 135:921, 1989

43. Jennette JC, Falk RJ: Anti-neutrophil cytoplasmic autoantibodies and associated diseases: a review. Am J Kidney Dis 15:517, 1990

44. Cohen Tervaert JW, Goldschmeding R, Elema JD et al: Autoantibodies against myeloid lysosomal enzymes in crescentic glomerulonephritis. Kidney Int 37:799, 1990

45. Davies DJ, Moran JE, Niall JF et al: Segmental necrotizing glomerulonephritis with antineutrophil antibody: possible arbovirus aetiology? Br Med J 285:606, 1982

46. Charles LA, Falk RJ, Jennette JC: Reactivity of anti-neutrophil cytoplasmic autoantibodies with HL-60 cells. Clin Immunol Immunopathol 53:243, 1989

47. Jennette JC: Anti-neutrophil cytoplasmic autoantibody-associated diseases: a pathologist's perspective. Am J Kidney Dis 18:164, 1991

48. Nolle B, Specks U, Lüdemann J et al: Anticytoplasmic autoantibodies: their immunodiagnostic value in Wegener's granulomatosis. Ann Intern Med 111:28, 1989

49. Dahlberg PJ, Lockhart JM, Overholt EL: Diagnostic studies for systemic necrotizing vasculitis. Sensitivity, specificity, and predictive value in patients with multisystem disease. Arch Intern Med 149:161, 1989

50. Albert DA, Rimon D, Silverstein JD: The diagnosis of polyarteritis nodosa: I. A literature-based decision analysis approach. Arthritis Rheum 31:1117, 1988

51. Albert DA, Silverstein MD, Paunicka K et al: The diagnosis of polyarteritis nodosa: II. Empirical verification of a decision analysis model. Arthritis Rheum 31:1128, 1988

52. Falk RJ, Terrell RS, Charles LA, Jennette JC: Anti-neutrophil cytoplasmic autoantibodies induce neutrophils to degranulate and produce oxygen radicals in vitro. Proc Natl Acad Sci USA 87:4115, 1990

53. Leung DYM, Moake JL, Havens PL et al: Lytic antiendothelial cell antibodies in haemolytic-uraemic syndrome. Lancet 2:183, 1988

54. Marks RM, Czerniecki M, Andrews BS, Penny R: The effects of scleroderma serum on human microvascular endothelial cells. Arthritis Rheum 31:1524, 1988

55. Yap HK, Sakai RS, Bahn L et al: Antivascular endothelial cell antibodies in patients with IgA nephropathy: frequency and clinical significance. Clin Immunol Immunopathol 49:450, 1988

56. Ferraro G, Meroni PL, Tincani A et al: Anti-endothelial cell antibodies in patients with Wegener's granulomatosis and micropolyarteritis. Clin Exp Immunol 79:47, 1990

57. Leung DYM, Geha RS, Newburger JW, et al: Two monokines, interleukin 1 and tumor necrosis factor, render cultured vascular endothelial cells susceptible to lysis by antibodies circulating during Kawasaki syndrome. J Exp Med 164:1958, 1986

58. Kalunian KC, Peter JB, Middlekauff HR et al: Clinical significance of a single test for anti-cardiolipin antibodies in patients with systemic lupus erythematosus. Am J Med 85:602, 1988

59. D'Agati V, Kunis C, Williams G, Appel GB: Anti-cardiolipin antibody and renal disease: a report of three cases. J Am Soc Nephrol 1:777, 1990

60. Ohi H, Watanabe S, Fujita T et al: Detection of C3bBb-stablizing activity (C3 nephritic factor) in the serum from patients with membranoproliferative glomerulonephritis. J Immunol Methods 131:71, 1990

61. Schena FP, Pertosa G, Stanziale P et al: Biological significance of the C3 nephritic factor in membranoproliferative glomerulonephritis. Clin Nephrol 18:240, 1982

62. Tsokos GC, Stitzel AE, Patel AD et al: Human polyclonal and monoclonal IgG and IgM complement 3 nephritic factors: evidence for idiotypic commonality. Clin Immunol Immunopathol 53:113, 1989

63. Seino J, Kinoshita Y, Sudo K et al: Quantitation of C4 nephritic factor by an enzyme-linked immunosorbent assay. J Immunol Methods 128:101, 1990

64. Halbwachs L, Leveille M, Lesavre P et al: Nephritic factor of the classical pathway of complement. Immunoglobulin G autoantibody directed against the classical pathway C3 convertase enzyme. J Clin Invest 65:1249, 1980

65. Daha MR, Hazevoet JM, Van Es LA, Cats A: Stabilization of the classical C3 convertase, C42, by a factor, F-42, isolated from serum of patients with systemic lupus erythematosus. Immunology 40:417, 1980

66. Clardy CW, Forristal J, Strife CF, West CD: A properdin dependent nephritic factor slowly activating C3, C5, and C9 in membranoproliferative glomerulonephritis, types I and III. Clin Immunol Immunopathol 50:333, 1989

67. Antes U, Heinz H-P, Loos M: Evidence for the presence of autoantibodies to the collagen-like portion of C1q in systemic lupus erythematosus. Arthritis Rheum 31:457, 1988

68. Uwatoko S, Mannik M: Low-molecular weight C1q-binding immunoglobulin G in patients with systemic lupus erythematosus consists of autoantibodies to the collagen-like region of C1q. J Clin Invest 82:816, 1988

69. Wener MH, Uwatoko S, Mannik M: Antibodies to the collagen-like region of C1q in sera of patients with autoimmune rheumatic diseases. Arthritis Rheum 32:544, 1989

70. Wisnieski JJ, Naff GB: Serum IgG antibodies to C1q in hypocomplementemic urticarial vasculitis syndrome. Arthritis Rheum 32:1119, 1989

71. McDougal JS, Hubbard M, Strobel PL, McDuffie FC: Comparison of five assays for immune complexes in the rheumatic diseases; performance characteristics of the assays. J Lab Clin Med 100:705, 1982

72. Ritzmann SE, Daniels JC: Immune complexes: characteristics, clinical correlations, and interpretive approaches in the clinical laboratory. Clin Chem 28:1259, 1982

73. Neilsen H, Sorensen H, Faber V, Svehag SE: Circulating immune complexes, complement activation kinetics and serum sickness following treatment with heterologous anti-snake venom globulin. Scand J Immunol 7:25, 1978

74. Gorevic PD, Kassab HJ, Levo Y et al: Mixed cryoglobulinemia: clinical aspects and long-term follow-up of 40 patients. Am J Med 60:287, 1980

75. Emancipator SN, Lamm ME: IgA nephropathy: pathogenesis of the most common form of glomerulonephritis. Lab Invest 60:168, 1989

76. Hernando P, Egido J, de Nicolas R, Sancho J: Clinical significance of polymeric and monomeric IgA complexes in patients with IgA nephropathy. Am J Kidney Dis 8:410, 1986

77. Jackson S: Immunoglobulin-antiimmunoglobulin interactions and immune complexes in IgA nephropathy. Am J Kidney Dis 12:425, 1988

78. Cederholm B, Wieslander J, Bygren P, Heinegard D: Circulating complexes containing IgA and fibronectin in patients with primary IgA nephropathy. Proc Natl Acad Sci USA 85:4865, 1988

79. Peter JB, Hollingsworth PN, Dawkins RL et al: Serologic diagnosis of IgA nephropathy: clinical utility of assay for IgA-fibronectin aggregates, abstracted. J Am Soc Nephrol 1:565, 1990

80. Jennette JC, Wieslander J, Tuttle R, Falk RJ: Diagnostic utility and pathogenetic implications of serum IgA-fibronectin aggregates in IgA nephropathy, abstracted. Lab Invest 64:98A, 1991

81. Jennette JC, Wieslander J, Tuttle R et al: Serum IgA-fibronectin aggregates in patients with IgA nephropathy and Henoch-Schönlein purpura: diagnostic value and pathogenic implications. Am J Kidney Dis 18:466, 1991

82. Dalmasso AP: Complement in the pathophysiology and diagnosis of human diseases. CRC Crit Review Clin Lab Sci 24:123, 1986

83. West CD: The complement profile in clinical medicine. Inherited and acquired conditions lowering the serum concentrations of complement components and control proteins. Complement Inflamm 6:49, 1989

84. Hebert LA, Cosio FG, Neff JC: Diagnostic significance of hypocomplementemia. Kidney Int 39:811, 1991

85. Lewis EJ, Carpenter CB, Schur PH: Serum complement component levels in human glomerulonephritis. Ann Intern Med 75:555, 1971

86. Strife CF, Jackson EC, Forristal J, West CD: Effect of the nephrotic syndrome on the concentration of serum complement components. Am J Kidney Dis 8:37, 1986

87. Jennette JC, Iskandar SS, Dalldorf FG: The diagnostic accuracy of pathologic differentiation between nonlupus and lupus membranous glomerulopathy. Kidney Int 14:377, 1983

88. Hebert LA, Ogrodowski JL, Ricker DM et al: Membrane attack complex (SC5b-9, MAC) in urine of patients with nephrotic syndrome, abstracted. J Am Soc Nephrol 1:560, 1990

89. Strife CF, McAdams AJ, McEnery PT et al: Hypocomplementemic and normocomplementemic acute nephritis in children. A comparison with respect to etiology, clinical manifestations, and glomerular morphology. J Pediatr 84:29, 1974

90. Lloyd W, Schur P: Immune complexes, complement, and anti-DNA in exacerbations of systemic lupus erythematosus (SLE). Medicine, Baltimore 60:208, 1981

91. Falk RJ, Dalmasso AP, Kim Y et al: Radioimmunoassay of the attack complex of complement in serum from patients with systemic lupus erythematosus. N Engl J Med 312:1594, 1985.

92. Waldo FB, Leist PA, Strife CF et al: Atypical hypocomplementemic vasculitis syndrome in a child. J Pediatr 106:745, 1985

93. Cosio FG, Zager RA, Sharma HM: Atheroembolic renal disease causes hypocomplementemia. Lancet 2:118, 1985

94. Monnens L, Molenaar J, Lambert PH et al: The complement system in hemolytic-uremic syndrome in children. Clin Nephrol 13:168, 1980

95. Stone MJ: Amyloidosis: a final common pathway for protein deposition in tissues. Blood 75:531, 1990

96. Buxbaum JN, Chuba JV, Hellman GC et al: Monoclonal immunoglobulin deposition disease: light chain and light and heavy chain deposition diseases and their relation to light chain amyloidosis. Clinical features, immunopathology, and molecular analysis. Ann Intern Med 112:455, 1990

97. Eulitz M, Weiss DT, Solomon A: Immunoglobulin heavy-chain-associated amyloidosis. Proc Natl Acad Sci USA 87:6542, 1990

98. Gallo G, Picken M, Buxbaum J, Frangione B: The spectrum of monoclonal immunoglobulin deposition disease associated with immunocyte dyscrasias. Sci Hematol 26:234, 1989

99. Sipe JD, Gonnerman WA, Loose LD et al: Direct binding enzyme-linked immunosorbent assay (ELISA) for serum amyloid A (SAA). J Immunol Methods 125:125, 1989

100. Benson MD, Cohen AS: Serum amyloid A protein in amyloidosis, rheumatic, and neoplastic diseases. Arthritis Rheum 22:36, 1979

101. Madio MP, Harrington JT: The diagnosis of acute glomerulonephritis. N Engl J Med 309:1299, 1983.

102. Merganthaler HG, Binsack T, Wilmanns W: Carcinoma-associated hemolytic-uremic syndrome in a patient receiving 5-fluorouracil-adriamycin-mitomycin C combination chemotherapy. Oncology 45:11, 1988

103. Lesesne JB, Rothschild N, Erickson B et al: Cancer-associated hemolytic-uremic syndrome: analysis of 85 cases from a national registry. J Clin Oncol 7:781, 1989

104. Nizze H, Mihatsch MJ, Zollinger HU et al: Cyclosporine-associated nephropathy in patients with heart and bone marrow transplants. Clin Nephrol 30:248, 1988

105. Remuzzi G, Bertani T: Renal vascular and thrombotic effects of cyclosporine. Am J Kidney Dis 13:261, 1989

106. Hattori S, Furuse A, Matsuda I: Presence of HBe antibody in glomerular deposits in membranous glomerulonephritis is associated with hepatitis B virus infection. Am J Nephrol 8:384, 1988

107. Lee HS, Koh HI: Hepatitis Be antigen-associated membranous nephropathy. Nephron 52:356, 1989

108. Sato Y, Sasaki M, Kan R et al: Thyroid antigen-mediated glomerulonephritis in Graves' disease. Clin Nephrol 31:49, 1989

109. Ronco P, Allegri L, Brianti E et al: Antigenic targets in epimembranous glomerulonephritis. Experimental data and potential application in human pathology. Appl Pathol 7:85, 1989

110. Fukatsu A, Yuzawa Y, Brentjens J et al: Renal immune deposits induced by antibodies reactive with cell-surface antigens in laboratory animals and in man. Am J Nephrol 9 suppl. 1:27, 1989

6

Renal Transplantation Rejection

Approach to Diagnosis and Follow-up Evaluation

Bedri Yousif
Joao Chequer Bou-Habib
Marvin R. Garovoy

INTRODUCTION

Since the first successful renal transplantation over 30 years ago, the practice of this branch of medicine has seen tremendous advances. It is a tribute to the many men and women who have been involved in transplantation that patient survival at 1 year exceeds 93 percent and that allograft survival in the majority of transplant centers ranges from 77 to 89 percent.[1] However, even today renal transplantation is beset by the same problem that was present in its infancy, i.e., allograft rejection. Indeed, rejection continues to be the Achilles heel of transplantation.

The purpose of this chapter is to explore the various techniques that are now clinically employed to establish a diagnosis of rejection and also discuss some of the techniques that are of theoretic interest. Even though great strides have been made in the overall management of the renal transplant patient, the search for a diagnostic test for rejection that is sensitive and specific remains a long-term goal.

PERCUTANEOUS RENAL BIOPSY

The transplant biopsy remains the benchmark by which other techniques are measured. It is the most precise and definitive means of diagnosing cellular or humoral rejection.

The histopathologic pattern, pathogenesis, and timing allow renal allograft rejection to be classified into four types.

Hyperacute Rejection

Hyperacute rejection can be mediated by ABO antibodies or, more commonly, by preformed human leukocyte antigen (HLA) antibodies induced by a previous transplant, multiple pregnancies, or previous blood transfusions. The existing antibodies may be deposited on the endothelium and cause damage by triggering the complement cascade and coagulation. The reaction takes place *within minutes to hours of transplantation*. The allograft, which was firm and pink initially, turns soft and cyanotic and ceases to produce urine.

Histopathologically, it is characterized by engorgement of small blood vessels and polymorphonuclear leukocyte infiltrates within the glomeruli and peritubular capillaries. There are also small lakes of hemorrhage at the corticomedullary junction and platelet aggregation in blood vessels.

With increased awareness of ABO compatibility and more sensitive lymphocytotoxic crossmatching techniques between donor and recipient, the incidence of this complication has now been reduced to less than 2 percent. However, as an increasing number of sensitized patients accumulates on transplant waiting lists, a continuous vigil is needed to further reduce the incidence and to prevent hyperacute rejection from assuming any larger proportion.

Acute Rejection

Acute rejection can occur anywhere from as few as *7 days to a few months post-transplantation.*[2] It may also be superimposed on chronic rejection.[3] It is mediated by cellular and/or humoral mechanisms producing fairly distinct cellular or vascular pathologic patterns.

The gross appearance of the kidney depends on the time course of the rejection. With rejection episodes occurring within days of transplantation, the kidney becomes swollen, appears darker and congested. In late acute rejection episodes, the kidney looks large and pale.

Microscopically, acute cellular rejection is characterized by interstitial edema and cellular infiltrates consisting of small and large lymphocytes, immunoblasts, plasma cells, monocytes/macrophages, eosinophils, and polymorphonuclear leukocytes.[4, 5] Interstitial hemorrhage may also be a feature. Tubulitis characterized by lymphocytes interspersed between tubules is a sign of rejection.[6, 7] There is no correlation between the degree of cellular infiltration and the functional severity of acute rejection. Glomerular involvement is limited to an increase in mesangium without immunoglobulin deposition.

The vascular changes of acute rejection are varied. In mild to moderate cases there may be only subendothelial mononuclear infiltrates, or fibrin deposition. Fibrinoid necrosis with loss of the arterial structural integrity is a hallmark of severe acute vascular rejection. Vascular rejection is usually difficult to reverse by current immunosuppressive agents and may occur alone or may accompany cellular rejection.

Accelerated Rejection

Clinically, this form of rejection can present as either prolonged *delayed graft function* or rapid deterioration *within 4 to 5 days of transplantation* after an initial period of short-lived function. Histologically, the lesions are similar to severe forms of acute rejection with tubulitis and vasculitis.

Chronic Rejection

This last type of rejection is often insidious in onset, usually appearing *6 or more months post-transplantation.*[8] It is characterized by hypertension, gradual deterioration of renal function, and proteinuria. Chronic rejection is probably the most common cause of post-transplant nephrotic syndrome.[9] The kidney may be small or normal in size. Histopathologically, it is characterized by a fibroobliterative endarteritis or arteriolopathy. With attending ischemic changes, we see tubular atrophy, thickened basement membrane, glomerular basement membrane, collapse and interstitial fibrosis.

The transplant biopsy has also been extremely helpful in cases of primary nonfunction where acute rejection can coexist with acute tubular necrosis

(ATN). Another important clinical situation where biopsy is indicated is in steroid-resistant rejection. Demonstration of cellular rejection is an indication for changing therapy, or alternatively, the presence of significant vascular rejection could signal discontinuation of aggressive immunosuppressive therapy.

CLINICAL DIAGNOSIS OF ACUTE REJECTION

For the sake of brevity and meaningful analysis, we will restrict ourselves to the discussion of acute rejection. Clinically, acute rejection can manifest itself as fever, allograft tenderness, hypertension, and oliguria accompanied by an increase in serum creatinine. This is indeed a classic presentation and one that was observed in patients on conventional immunosuppressive therapy, i.e., azathioprine and prednisone. It is not commonly seen in the majority of cyclosporine (CSA)-treated patients. In the cyclosporine era, the first and perhaps the only sign of acute rejection may be a rise in serum creatinine accompanied by oliguria. Therefore, the diagnosis of acute rejection is a diagnosis of exclusion as there is no single pathognomonic finding with any of the noninvasive modalities that are currently used. The approach to the diagnosis of rejection in the transplant recipient is similar to the approach to renal dysfunction in the nontransplanted patient. The diagnosis of rejection and the complications that are unique to the post-transplant period are merely added to considerations of prerenal, renal, and post-renal causes of renal dysfunction.

DIFFERENTIAL DIAGNOSIS OF REJECTION

Surgical Causes of Acute Rejection

Classification of the causes of early graft dysfunction into surgical and medical causes is very helpful (Table 6-1). The surgical causes appearing early in the post-transplantation period require immediate intervention. Impairment of allograft function due to *arterial stenosis* immediately following transplatation is rare. However, hypertension and renal ischemia resulting from this condition can potentially lead to the eventual deterioration of renal function. The true incidence of late renal artery stenosis is not known because sequential arteriography or duplex sonography is not routinely performed. This diagnosis has been made in up to 30 percent of patients whose blood pressure was difficult to control. Angiotensin-converting enzyme (ACE) inhibitors can be used as a diagnostic probe in those patients suspected of having transplant arterial stenosis. In patients with hemodynamically significant renal artery stenosis and who are also volume depleted, ACE inhibitors, by preferentially decreasing the efferent arteriolar resistance can decrease the glomerular filtration rate (GFR). Transplant arterial stenosis could be secondary to immunologic rejection or to flow

Table 6-1. Differential Diagnosis of Acute Rejection

Surgical
    Arterial complication
        Stenosis
        Thrombosis
        Rupture with hemorrhage
        Perigraft hematoma with ureteral obstruction
    Lymphatic complication
        Lymphocele with obstruction
    Urologic complication
        Urine extravasation
        Ureteral stenosis
        Bladder leak
    Perirenal abscess
Medical
    Acute tubular necrosis
    Urinary tract infection
    Drug-induced nephrotoxicity
    Acute cytomegalovirus infection
    Recurrent glomerulopathy
    De novo glomerulonephritis
    Hypovolemia

turbulence at the anastamotic site. In cadaveric transplantation, this complication has become less frequent because aortic cuffs are now used for the anastomosis.

Anuria can develop following *acute thrombosis of allograft vessels*.[12] Arterial thrombosis with complete or segmental infarction of the kidney, though rare, can occur in kidneys with multiple renal arteries, which more commonly cause technical difficulties with the anastomosis, or if recipient or donor vessels are very sclerotic.[13] Venous thrombosis is believed by some to be more common since the advent of CSA.[14] Placement of a kidney in a tight or scarred retroperitoneal space may also lead to venous thrombosis.[13] Salvage of the kidney, which involves thrombectomy or revascularization, depends on rapid diagnosis by arteriography, renal scan, or duplex sonography.

Perinephric fluid leading to compression of the ureter and subsequent oliguria and increase in serum creatinine could result from a lymphocele, urinary leakage, or from a hematoma. The clinical setting can favor one diagnosis over the other. A hematoma should be considered, e.g., in a hypotensive patient or dialysis and receiving heparin. After the diagnosis, an immediate exploration is warranted. Urinary leakage, on the other hand, manifests itself in an escalating fashion. The patient may present with ascites, and swelling of the labia or scrotum, while urine output decreases and serum creatinine increases gradually. A lymph collection can mimic a urinary leakage. These could be easily differentiated by performing simultaneous determinations of creatinine from the leaking fluid, serum, and urine. The creatinine concentration of lymph and serum are identical whereas that in urine is substantially higher.

Medical Causes of Graft Dysfunction

Acute tubular necrosis is a common cause of oligoanuria. Donor problems that are often associated with ATN in the recipient are hemodynamic instability requiring vasoactive agents and prolonged cold and warm ischemia times. Recipient causes such as hypovolemia with a decreased mean pulmonary arterial pressure, are also sensitive to this condition.[15] Because CSA has been shown to prolong the anuric state, many institutions[16] have adopted a sequential immunosuppressive regimen that involves the initial use of antilymphocyteglobulin (ALG) or OKT3, azathioprine, and prednisone. CSA is added, and the ALG is discontinued after the serum creatinine has fallen to a near normal value (2.5 mg/dl) and when diuresis is well established.

The presentation of *urinary tract infection* (UTI) with fever, allograft tenderness, and oliguria can mimic acute rejection. UTI is the most common infection during the first year following transplantation.[17] Its incidence has been reported to be 35 to 79 percent.[18–20] It may also account for 60 percent of the bacteremias in these patients.[20–22] There are a number of predisposing factors for UTI. Urinary reflux through the short and denervated ureter, and in-dwelling catheter, and a noncompliant and contracted bladder after several years on dialysis conspire to make patients susceptible to such infections. Other predisposing factors to infection include ischemia, rejection, and trauma to the allograft.[23, 24] Before embarking on antirejection therapy, one is well advised to undertake simple urinalysis and blood cultures to eliminate the possibility of a UTI or to initiate the appropriate antibiotic therapy. With increased attention to urologic complications and the use of antibiotic prophylaxis, the incidence of UTI has decreased significantly. In a controlled study using oral trimethoprim-sulphamethoxazole during the first 4 months after renal transplantation, the incidence of UTI and septicemia decreased from approximately 40 percent to 5 percent or less.[25]

Drug-induced renal impairment is an ever present threat. Cyclosporine-induced renal impairment, always a consideration, has been classified into (1) functional toxicity without significant morphologic lesions, and (2) morphologic forms of toxicity with tubular and/or vascular interstitial lesions.[26] CSA-induced functional toxicity appears to be reversible and is believed to be due to the vasconstrictive action of CSA on the afferent glomerular arterioles. There is also evidence that CSA decreases the ultrafiltration coefficient of the glomerulus. Stimulation of the renin–angiotensin system[27,28] and the sympathetic nervous system and its effect on prostanoids may contribute to the vasoconstrictive effect of CSA. It has been shown that CSA increases the synthesis of the vasoconstrictive eicosanoid, thromboxane.[29,30] The functional toxicity that is due to CSA may augment the oligoanuria that is due to ischemic injury to the allograft.

Different morphologic changes have been attributed to CSA nephrotoxicity. Within the tubules, there may be vacuolization, giant mitochondria, and microcalcification. Although the tubular toxicity may be reversible, the appearance of vascular-interstitial changes may be more ominous. Clinically, this may lead to slowly progressive deterioration of renal function.[31] The most frequent lesions and hallmarks of vascular-interstitial toxity are arteriolopathy and interstitial fibrosis, with tubular atrophy.[32-35]

Although cyclosporine levels of 400 ng/ml (whole blood) or 300 ng/ml (plasma) are associated with a greater incidence of toxicity, individual sensitivities vary quite widely. In some patients, levels as low as 200ng/ml (whole blood) can be associated with toxicity. Observing the response to lowered CSA doses and/or the absence of signs of immune system activation (see section on interleukin-2 receptor) and renal biopsy are the few approaches available to diagnose CSA nephrotoxicity.

Coadministration of certain drugs with CSA may affect the renal allograft by either increasing CSA levels (e.g., erythromycin, ketoconazole, diltiazem), and thus leading to nephrotoxicity, or decreasing CSA levels, and thereby making the kidney susceptible to allograft rejection.[36, 37] Most anticonvulsants lead to a decrease in CSA blood levels, e.g., phenobarbital, phenytoin, and carbamazepine. Valproate does not appear to have this effect and may be the medication of choice in patients with seizure disorders.[38] Antituberculous medication such a rifampin and isoniazid also decrease CSA blood levels.[36]

Cimetidine and trimethoprine, by inhibiting the tubular secretion of creatinine, can lead to a functional elevation of serum creatinine.[39] Other potentially nephrotoxic medications such as aminoglycosides and amphotericin can exacerbate the nephrotoxicity of CSA. One must also consider antibiotics or other drugs that can lead by themsleves to interstitial nephritis and renal failure.

The risk of *cytomegalovirus (CMV) infection* is a function of the immunosuppressive therapy. CMV infection may influence the graft in several ways: the fever accompanying the viremia may nonspecifically impair renal function. The level of immunosuppressive agents, which are usually decreased as a result of the developing CMV-induced leukopenia , can spawn a rejection. Acute renal colonization by CMV may be associated with interstitial nephritis.[40] Some investigators have suggested that the appearance of HLA class II antigen on the vascular endothelium induced by CMV infection may correlate with increased risk of allograft rejection.[41] Others have suggested an immune complex-mediated mechanism.[42]

Until recently, clinicians depended on the detection of CMV antibody for diagnosis. In primary and often secondary infection, CMV-specific IgM antibody determined by a fluorescent antibody technique is diagnostic for CMV infection. In the absence of CMV-specific IgM, the appearance of CMV-specific IgG in primary infection and a fourfold increase in secondary infection are sufficient for diagnosis. Because the rise of antibody levels to a significant degree may require a few days to a few weeks, other techniques provide greater clinical utility. CMV can be isolated in human fibroblast cell cultures from urine, saliva, throat, and cervix. CMV can also be cultivated from peripheral blood lymphocytes. Because demonstration of a cytopathic effect takes 5 to 28 days, the viral culture has been modified to enable detection within 16 to 18 hours.[43] The technique involves centrifugation on to fibroblast-coated shell vials. After an incubation period of 16 to 18 hours, monoclonal antibodies are used to detect immediate early CMV antigen. This technique has a sensitivity of more than 90 percent.

Recurrent disease after renal transplantation is assuming a greater relative importance, as graft survival increases.[44] Postoperative recurrence of such primary glomerular diseases, as antiglomerular basement membrane disease,[45,46] focal segmental sclerosis,[47,48] type I[48,49] and type II mesangioproliferative glomerulonephritis and IgA nephropathy[48,52] have been amply documented. Clinically, recurrence is characterized by proteinuria, hematuria, and in some cases, impaired renal function. Systemic diseases that secondarily affect the glomeruli are also know to recur and may subsequently destroy the kidney. Such diseases include progressive systemic sclerosis[53, 54] and primary oxalosis.[55] Other secondar glomerular diseases, such as type I diabetes[56] and systemic lupus erythematosus (SLE)[57] are characterized by recurrence, but rarely are associated with graft loss.

Post-transplantation de novo membranous glomerulonephritis and focal glomerulosclerosis have been described. The incidence of de novo membranous glomerulonephritis was 0.83 percent,[58] and its clinical course is generally as benign as that of idiopathic membranous glomerulonephritis. The incidence of de novo focal glomerulosclerosis, however, was higher, in the range of 8.7 percent.[59] The authors suggested that microvascular rejection and obliterative arteriolopathy could be etiologic mechanisms. The use of heterologous antilymphocyte preparations has been implicated by some investigators in the development of de novo glomerulonephritis.[60] The antilymphocyte globulin is believed to crossreact with the glomerular basement membrane leading to membranoproliferative glomerulonephritis.[60]

The *postoperative fluid management* of the transplant recipient is crucial to the outcome of both patient and graft survival. The majority of living donor recipients exhibit a brisk diuresis shortly after transplantation. However, 20 percent of cadaveric renal recipients develop (ATN) and therefore show a variable urine output. Any substantial abrupt decrease in the hourly urine output in the living donor recipient and significant oliguria in the cadaveric recipient is a cause for initiating a workup for oliguria (Fig. 6-1). Sterile irrigation of the bladder with saline is initiated once oliguria is established. The patient's volume status is evaluated if irrigation does not reestablish the diuresis. Early correction of extracellular fluid (ECF) volume contraction can result in the resumption of diuresis. Fluid resuscitation should be attempted on the "apparently" euvolemic patient before administering a loop diuretic. Failure to respond to the loop diuretic is declared only after a second larger dose. At this point a renal scan is performed. A positive uptake scan without excretion points toward ATN, obstruction, or possibly, urinary leakage. In the latter case, there will be extravasation of the radionuclide. A negative uptake and excretion of the radionuclide may be due to the hyperacute rejection or renal artery thrombosis. The latter requires immediate surgical intervention.

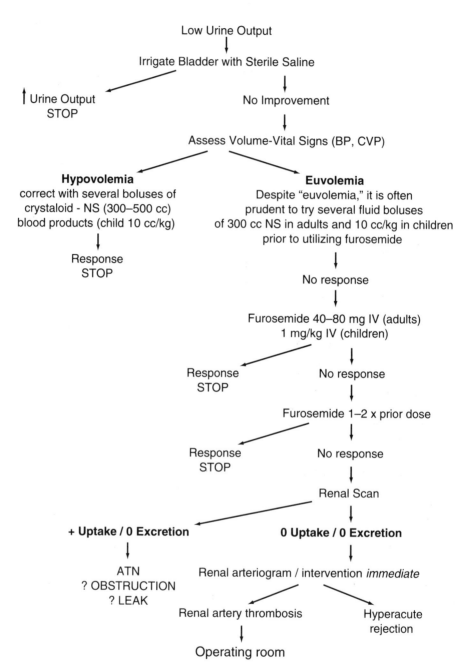

Fig. 6-1. Recommended management of oliguria after an initial diuresis.

NONINVASIVE TESTS: RENAL IMAGING

Renal Scan

The ancillary radiologic procedures that are commonly employed in the differential diagnostic workup for rejection will now be considered. For renal scans either ^{131}I OIH (orthoiodohippurate) or [99m]Tc (DTPA) diethylinetria-minepenta-acetic acid (DTPA) commonly are used. Approximately 88 percent of intravenously injected ^{131}I OIH is excreted from the body by renal tubular secretion, and the remaining 12 percent is excreted by passive glomerular filtration.[61] In contrast, ^{99m}Tc DTPA is excreted only by glomerular filtration.[61] Either one could be used to evaluate the real complications arising in the post-transplant period.

A typical imaging protocol using ^{131}I-hippurate aims the scintillation camera at the transplant recipients lower abdomen. The hippurate is injected intravenously, and six time-lapse 4-minute images are obtained. At the same time, the image data are computer acquired at four frames per minute. At the end of the study, the computer data are summed into one composite image, and regions of interest over the graft, the bladder, and background are chosen. The computer is then instructed to generate background corrected time-activity histograms from the kidney and bladder. Several parameters can be mathematically extracted from these curves and used for objective serial comparison.

In normal patients, renal activity peaks within 4 to 6 minutes of that in the the aorta. Intensity of renal activity matches or exceeds that of the aorta.[61] The presentation of normal blood flow is confirmed by the rapidly rising and falling activity on serial images. The radiopharmaceutical material appears in the bladder within 0 to 4-minute image (Fig. 6-2).

In a patient with urinary extravasation, one will see increasing concentration of the radiopharmaceutical material outside the confines of the ureter and the bladder. The most common site is the ureteral–vesical anastomotic junction, where rupture can be due to either mechanical failure or rejection (Fig. 6-3).

In parenchymal failure that is due to ATN or transplant rejection, there is impaired concentration and a prolonged transit of the radiopharmaceutical. The collecting system is not visualized, and in the presence of anuria the bladder is not demonstrable (Fig. 6-4).

Ultrasonography

Renal ultrasonograph suffers from a low sensitivity and specificity in distinguishing between three causes of acute graft dysfunction: ATN, acute rejection, and CSA nephrotoxicity. The sonographic findings that are often used to diagnose rejection are renal sinus fat and size, corticomedullary ratio, sharpness and conspicuity, focal parenchymal abnormalities and pelvic wall thickness. In *acute rejection*, the size and echogenicity of the renal

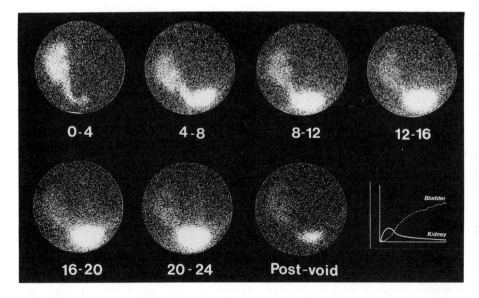

Fig. 6-2. An excellently functioning kidney several days after transplantation. Note the prompt uptake of hippurate, and the short transit time demonstrated by the exit of renal activity by the 20- to 24-minute image. Bladder activity is seen in the 0- to 4-minute image and is abundant in the 20- to 24-minute image. Voiding efficiency is determined by comparing the pre- and postvoid images. The computer-generated renogram and excreted activity curves are shown in the lower right. (From Hattner R et al.,[96] with permission.)

sinus fat is diminished. The definition between the medullary and cortical portions of the kidney also become obscured. This correlates pathologically with the presence of edema and mononuclear cell infiltration, which affects the corticomedullary junction early in the course of acute rejection. A dramatic increase in the size of the renal allograft occurs, which is due to marked interstitial edema. At the same time, the graft loses its elliptic configuration and becomes spherical. Focal parenchymal abnormalities rep-

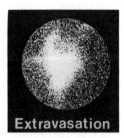

Fig. 6-3. Urine extravasation from a rejection-associated graft rupture, one of the several mechanical abnormalities easily observed in such studies. In this 20- to 24-minute image, irregular urine activity is seen deployed about the grafted kidney. (From Hattner R et al.,[96] with permission.)

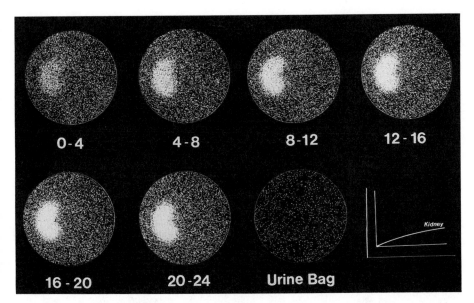

Fig. 6-4. Typical features of acute tubular necrosis (ATN) 1 day after transplantation. Uptake is slow and the transit time is prolonged. No activity is excreted by the end of the study. The physiologic explanation of these findings is that in ATN renal blood flow is disproportionately maintained compared to glomerular filtration. Thus, the radiopharmaceutical is excreted but there is no filtration to wash it out. Although ATN and acute rejection cannot be distinguished by renal scan, the time of onset of the two conditions is helpful in making a diagnosis. Acute rejection usually occurs about a week post-transplant, and the appearance of the characteristic renal scan pattern, shown here, immediately post-transplant points toward ATN. (From Hattner R et al.,[96] with permission.)

resented by sonolucent areas corresponding to edema, hemorrhage, infarcation, and necrosis have been described by numerous observers.

In one study,[62] use of all these parameters allowed a positive prediction of rejection, when compared with histopathologic findings, to be relatively high (83 to 90 percent) and the accuracy of negative prediction to be low (17 to 30 percent). Their result was influenced by the relatively high prevalence of rejection in the biopsy group. They also pointed out that baseline and serial studies were more likely to be informative because comparisons could document any change from the baseline findings.

Duplex sonography, which is real-time ultrasound coupled with pulsed doppler, is becoming popular not only because of its ability to furnish morphologic data but also because of its ability to determine the integrity of the renal blood vessels.[63–65] By analyzing the spectral characteristics of the blood flow to the kidneys, it is possible to identify renal vein thrombosis and renal artery stenosis. In patients with rejection, ATN, and CSA nephrotoxicity, the spectral pattern mimics that of high-resistance vascular beds, and diastolic flow may be absent (Fig. 6-5). This finding does not discriminate among these three clinical entities.

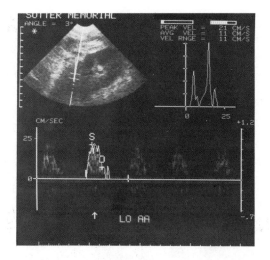

Fig. 6-5 Flow velocity pattern in a patient with rising creatinine on the tenth postoperative transplant day. Note the systolic upstroke and the absence of distolic flow, indicating a transition of the usual low-resistance renal vascular bed to a high-resistance vascular bed, indicating rejection in this clinical setting.

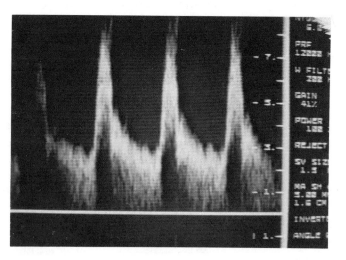

Fig. 6-6 Pulsed doppler spectral characteristics. Note frequency elevation (abscissa) and spectral broadening, indicating disturbed flow with stenosis. The spectral broadening represents the nonlamminar flow pattern as the high-velocity, high-pressure jet emanates from the stenotic portion of the lumen and spreads out into a zone of relatively low velocity and low pressure.

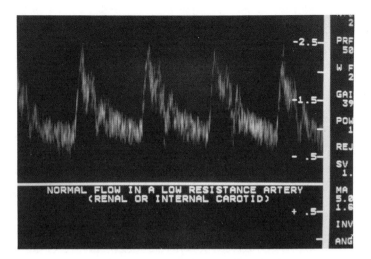

Fig. 6-7 Pulsed doppler spectral characteristics typical of low-resistance beds (kidney, brain). These are characterized by a rapid upstroke in systole and continuous forward flow in diastole. High diastolic flow is present because even the lower pressure present in diastole is enough to generate flow through an organ of low vascular resistance.

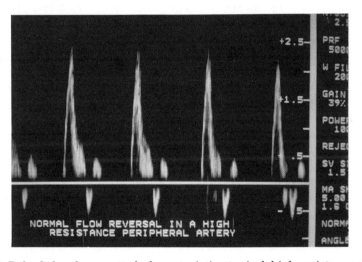

Fig. 6-8 Pulsed doppler spectral characteristics typical high-resistance vascular beds (extremities). The systolic upstroke is followed by low diastolic flow and early diastolic flow reversal.

In renal artery stenosis, spectral broadening and increase in frequency occur (Fig. 6-6). The spectral pattern of normal low- and high-resistance vascular bed are shown for comparison (Figs. 6-7 and 6-8).

Magnetic Resonance Imaging

Magnetic resonance imaging (MRI) has been found to have 98 percent accuracy in the diagnosis of acute rejection and to indicate a normal kidney in the majority of patients with ATN and CSA nephrotoxicity.[66] The parameter that was the most reliable was the percentage of corticomedullary contrast. In rejection, contrast at the corticomedullary junction is decreased where in CSA nephrotoxicity and ATN, normal contrast usually is found. The routine use of MRI as a diagnostic tool post transplant has not been well defined. Some have suggested that MRI can be used when results of ultrasound or renal scans are equivocal or contradict clinical impressions or when a biopsy cannot be performed for medical reasons.[66]

IMMUNE MONITORING

Clinical signs and symptoms of rejection and an increase in serum creatinine are late events of the process of allograft rejection. Even though it is possible to reverse the process by using various immunosuppressive regimens, sometimes the late recognition of rejection leads to the failure to reverse well-established rejections and/or to an increase in infectious complications from excessive attempts at immunosuppression. The search for a diagnostic technique with enough sensitivity and specificity to diagnose rejection early, therefore, becomes of utmost importance. Understandably, such a diagnostic tool may allow the clinician to specifically tailor the particular immunosuppressive regimen to meet the demands imposed by various complications. This may, in turn, lead to a significant improvement of allograft survival and decrease in the incidence of infection that is due to reduced immunosuppression.

The various immune-monitoring tests that are currently performed are broadly classified on Table 6-2. Most of these techniques lend themselves to criticism because of lack of (1) specificity and sensitivity, (2) reproducibility, and (3) correlation with rejection. Some of the tests become positive only after rejection is well established or become positive in a quiescent period. One recent test, however, shows promise of being a relatively sensitive and somewhat specific marker for immune system activation.

Interleukin-2 Receptor

The appearance of the receptor for interleukin-2 (IL2) is a relatively early event in immune activation. Resting T cells constitutively express an inter-

Table 6-2. Immune Monitoring of
Acute Rejection

Peripheral blood assays
    Donor-specific
        Complement-dependent antibody[61]
        Lymphocyte-dependent antibody[67]
        Lymphocyte-mediated cytotoxicity[68]
        Cell-mediated lympholysis[68]
    Donor nonspecific
        Blastogenic assays[69]
        Phenotype analysis
            T-cell subsets[70,71]
            OKT3 therapy
        NK-cell activity[72,73]
        Monocytes[74]
        Lymphokines
        Acute-phase reactants
            C-reactive protein[75]
            β_2-Microglobulin[76]
        Products of altered metabolism
            Neopterin[77]
            Urine thromboxane[78]

Intragraft assays
    Percutaneous biopsy
    Fine-needle aspiration biopsy

Abbreviation: NK, natural killer.

mediate affinity IL2 receptor (IL2-R), which is a 75-kd β-chain. Activated T cells express an additional α-chain, which is about 55 kd. The α-chain is a low-affinity receptor and is unable to internalize IL2. The functional unit that exhibits high affinity for IL2 consists of both α and β-chains.[79] On immune activation there is also a shedding or release of the IL2-receptor complex into the sera.[80] The soluble form is detected by anti CD25 antibody and is a 45-kd proteolytic product of the α-chain. A serial determination of soluble IL2-R (sIL2-R) shows that, in some uremic patients, it is slightly elevated before renal transplantation and falls to normal after transplantation.[81] A rise in the level of soluble IL2-R has been found to predict acute rejection in renal transplant patients 1 to 3 days before the elevation of serum creatinine.[82] An isolated value is less meaningful and has less predictive value when compared with serial sIL2-R measurements done before the onset of rejection. This entails a daily or every-other-day determination of IL2-R. A rise in serum sIL2-R was found to be 73 percent sensitive and 87 percent specific in the diagnosis of rejection[83] using the 90th percentile of stable patients to define a positive test. In combination with the serum creatinine, it is a new and promising approach to the diagnosis of rejection. It may be especially useful in indicating CSA toxicity where one can see stable sIL2-R levels despite a rising serum creatinine.

Attempts have also been made to use soluble IL2-R as a post-transplantation monitoring tool in other solid organ transplants. In the absence of infection, the daily determination of soluble IL2-R using flow cytometry was found to have early predictive value in liver transplantation as well.[84]

FINE-NEEDLE ASPIRATION BIOPSY

The use of fine-needle aspiration biopsy (FNAB) in renal transplantation was described by Haÿry and Von Willbrandt in 1981.[85] Compared with core biopsy, it is less traumatic and can be done daily or even twice a day with impunity.[86] This approach can reveal the dynamic nature of the rejection process in an individual allograft.[86] FNAB evaluates the presence of inflammatory cell infiltrates, parenchymal changes in the proximal and distal tubules, and endothelium. Glomeruli can also be obtained by FNAB and can be processed for histolic examination.[87] The diagnostic criteria for early renal transplant failure is displayed in Table 6-3. ATN is characterized by swelling and vacuolization of the tubular cells with minimal inflammatory cells. Acute rejection shows an increase in lymphoid blast cells and plasma cells. CSA toxicity displays isometric vacuolization of the tubular cells and endothelium with very limited inflammatory cells.

It should be emphasized that only cellular rejection can be diagnosed with certainty.[88] Vascular rejection may be inferred from endothelial changes and has to be confirmed by core needle biopsy. Moreover, FNAB can only be an adjunct rather than a replacement for needle biopsy because blood vessel histology cannot be evaluated using this procedure.

Table 6-3. Differential Diagnosis of Early Renal Transplant Failure by Fine-Needle Aspiration Biopsy

| Serum Creatinine | FNAB Cytology | | | Interpretation |
	Inflammation	Tubular Cell Morphology	IMV and CSA Deposits	
Normal	−	−	−	Well-functioning graft
Elevated	−	+ +	−	ATN
Elevated	±	+ + +	+ + +	CSA toxicity
Elevated	+ + +	+	−	Rejection
Elevated	+ + +	+ + +	+ + +	Rejection and CSA toxicity

Abbreviations: ATN, acute tubular necrosis; CSA, cyclosporine A; FNAB, fine-needle aspiration biopsy; IMV, isometric vacuolization.
(Adapted from Haÿry,[88] with permission.)

FOLLOW-UP OF THERAPY FOR REJECTION

The successful treatment of acute rejection has an obvious impact on the long-term function of the renal allograft.[89] The number of rejections and the severity of each episode strongly influence the 3-year graft outcome. Graft survival at 3 years was found to decline to 50 percent after one or two rejection episodes as compared with 78 percent in patients without rejection. For a peak serum creatinine less than 2 mg/dl at the time of rejection, graft survival approximated 70 percent. However, for a peak serum creatinine greater than 3.5 mg/dl, graft survival was only 30 percent.

The therapeutic modalities used in the treatment of acute rejection include high-dose steroid, ALG, or antithymocyte globulin (ATG) and a pan-T-cell mouse monoclonal antibody, OKT3. The latter is superior to steroids in reversing primary rejection–95 percent versus 75 percent, respectively.[90] Repeat rejection rates have also been lower in OKT3-treated patients (15 percent) compared with the steroid-treated group 33 percent.[91] Thus, OKT3 is being used with increased frequency.

Monitoring of CD3-positive T lymphocytes is recommended during OKT3 therapy. Within minutes of administering OKT3, the clearance of CD3-positive cells begins and is completed within 1 hour.[92] Opsonization of the circulating T cells with subsequent removal by the reticuloendothelial system and margination into intervascular spaces or redistribution to lymph nodes are some of the proposed mechanisms for the rapid depletion of CD3-positive cells from the circulation.[93] Subsequently, there is modulation of the CD3–TCR complex from the surface of the T cell. As therapy with OKT3 continues, CD3 marker remains very low. The target number of CD3-positive cells to be achieved by therapy is between 50 and 150/mm^3. Between days 2 to 7, the number of cells bearing the marker CD4 positive or CD8 positive increase. These cells are nonfunctional because they do not bear CD3 surface molecules.[94] After cessation of OKT3 therapy, there is rapid reappearance of CD3-positive T cells, and the return to normal is complete in about a week.

Monitoring during OKT3 treatment consists not only of measuring CD3-positive cells but also the level of antimurine OKT3 antibody and the OKT3 serum level. Before repeat therapy with OKT3, it is essential to know whether anti-OKT3 antibody has ever been formed. Patients whose antibody level 2 to 4 weeks after initial exposure is either negative or of low titer (1/100 enzyme-linked immunosorbent assay [ELISA] or 1/10 Transtat OKT3) can be successfully retreated with OKT3. Patients with high antibody titer (1/1,000 ELISA or 1/50 Transtat OKT3) or strong antibody by flow cytometry are not usually retreated because they show a low incidence of response.

The measurement of OKT3 trough levels as a guide for tailoring OKT3 therapy is very attractive. Godstein[92] showed that a mean trough level of about 902 mg/μl was achieved from days 3 to 14 following daily administration of 5 mg of OKT3 intravenously. He noted this plasma level was adequate to block cytotoxic T-cell function.

Long-Term Follow-up

Most of the preceding diagnostic techniques are applicable for long-term follow-up. Many allograft recipients are confronted with a relentless decline in renal function. Overall 5-year survival has been reported to be about 40 percent.[95] After the fifth year, chronic rejection was found to be responsible for about 22 percent of all allograft dysfunction. These patients presented with proteinuria, elevated serum creatinine, and hypertension. In this series, acute rejection constituted only 1 percent of the patients with graft dysfunction. The occurrence of late acute rejection has also been documented by others.[3] Recurrent glomerulonephritis, ureteral obstruction, and renal artery stenosis accounted for 3 percent, 4 percent, and 33 percent of the causes of graft dysfunction, respectively. Most of the graft losses were due to chronic rejection and rarely to acute rejection and recurrent pyelonephritis and perinephric abscess. The latter findings bring home the point that long-term surviving patients continue to be at risk of infection.

The widespread use of CSA since 1983 has made the concern of chronic nephrotoxicity that is due to CSA another possibly important cause of allograft dysfunction. According to Myers, [35] high-dose CSA can cause irreversible changes in the glomerular microcirculation, which can lead to glomerular sclerosis and ultimately loss of glomeruli. The reduction in the number of glomeruli might set the stage for hyperfiltration injury of the remaining glomeruli.

SUMMARY

It is evident from our discussion that the ultimate diagnostic test, which is ideally noninvasive and at the same time specific and sensitive, does not exist. It is only the combination of clinical observation and diagnostic techniques that enables one to make the diagnosis of rejection. The utility of IL2 receptor as a potentially useful diagnostic technique is certainly just the beginning of our ability to obtain a clinically meaningful analysis of the patient's immunologic status. As we continue to gain in our understanding of the immunologic basis of rejection, improved methods for the detection and treatment of rejection are bound to emerge.

ACKNOWLEDGMENTS

The authors wish to thank Cynthia Kelly for her excellent administrative and secretarial assistance. This work was supported in part by a National Institutes of Health (NIH) grant, NIH Program Project no. GM26691-12.

REFERENCES

1. U.S. Renal Data System: USRDS 1989 Annual Data Report. National Institutes of Health. National Institute of Diabetes and Digestive and Kidney Diseases. Bethesda MD. August, 1989
2. Busch GJ, Galvanek EG, Reynolds ES: Human renal allografts: analysis of lesions in long term survivors. Hum Pathol 2:253, 1971
3. Rao RV, Kassiske BC, Bloom PM: Acute graft rejection in the late survivors of renal transplant. Transplantation 47:490, 1989
4. Sibley RK, Payne W: Morphologic findings in the renal allograft biopsy. Semin Nephrol 5:294, 1985
5. Verani RR, Flechner SM, Van Buren LT et al: Acute cellular rejection or cyclosporine A nephrotoxicity? A review of transplant renal biopsies. Am J Kidney Dis 4:185, 1984
6. Matas AJ, Sibley R, Mansen M et al: The value of needle renal allograft biopsy in a retrospective study of biopsies performed during putative rejection episodes. Ann Surg 197:226, 1983
7. Siblez RK, Rynasicwicz J, Ferguson MR et al: Morphology of cyclosporine nephrotoxicity and acute rejection in patients immunosuppressed with cyclosporine and prednisone. Surgery 94:225, 1983
8. Porter KA: p. 1455. In Heptinstall RH (ed): Renal Transplantation in Pathology of the Kidney. 3rd Ed. Little, Brown, Boston, 1983
9. Lheigh JS, Stenzel KH, Susin M et al: Am J Med 57:730, 1974
10. Tilney NL, Rocha A, Strom TB, Kirkman RL: Renal artery stenosis in transplant patients. Ann Surg 199:454, 1984
11. La Combe M: Arterial stenosis complicating renal allo transplantation in man: a study of 38 cases. Ann Surg 181:283, 1975
12. Vidne BA, Leapman SB, Butt KM et al: Vascular complications in human renal transplantation. Surgery 79:77, 1976
13. Tilney NL: The early course of a patient with a kidney transplant. p. 263. In Morris P (ed): Kidney Transplantation. 3rd Ed. WB Saunders, Philadelphia, 1988
14. Jones RM, Murie JA, Ting A et al: Renal vascular thrombosis of cadaver renal allograft in patients receiving cyclosporine, azathioprine and prednisone triple therapy. Clin Transplantation 2:122, 1988
15. Meurisse M, Albert A, Defraigne JO et al: Multiple risk factor analysis of non-immunological delayed graft function after kidney transplantation. Clin Transplantation 2:312, 1988
16. Salvatierra O, Jr: Current strategy for donor-specific blood transfusions including a pre- and post transplant role for azathioprine. Transplant Proc 20:37, 1988
17. Peterson PK, Ferguson R, Fryd DS et al: Infectious diseases in hospitalized renal transplant recipients. A prospective study of a complete and evolving problem. Medicine 61:360, 1982
18. Harrison MA, DeCirolami PC, Jenkins RL, Hammer SM: Ganciclovir therapy of severe cytomegalovirus infections in solid organ transplant recipients. Transplantation 46:82, 1988
19. Rubin RH, Wolfson JS, Cosimi AB, Rubin NE: Infection in the renal transplant recipient. Am J Med 70:405, 1981
20. Rubin RH, Fang LST, Cosimi AB, et al: Usefulness of the antibody coated bac-

teria assay in the management of urinary tract infection in the renal transplant patient. Transplantation 27:18, 1978

21. Myerovitz RL, Merteiros AA, O'Brien TF: Bacterial infections in renal transplant patients. Am J Med 53:308, 1972

22. Anderson RJ, Schafer LA, Olin DB, Eickhoff TC: Septicemia in renal transplant patients. Arch Surg 106:692, 1973

23. Burleson RL, Brennan AM, Slouggs RF: Foley tip cultures: a valuable diagnostic aid in immunosuppressed patient. Am J Surg 133:723, 1977

24. Murphy JF, McDonald RD, Davison M et al: Factors influencing the frequency of infection in renal transplant recipients. Arch Intern Med 136:670, 1976

25. Tolkoff-Rubin NE, Cosimi AB, Russel PS, Rubin RH: A controlled study of trimethoprim sulfamethoxazole prophylaxis of urinary tract infection in renal transplant recipients. Rev Infect Dis 4:614, 1982

26. Mihatsch MJ, Thiel G, Ryffel B: Histopathology of cyclosporine nephrotoxicity. Transplantation Proc 20(3):759, 1988

27. Barros EJG, Biom MA, Ajzen H et al: Glomerular hemodynamics and hormonal participation on cyclosporine nephrotoxicity. Kidney Int 32:19, 1987

28. Kurtz A, Della Bruna R, Kuhn K: Cyclosporine A enhances renin secretion and production in isolated juxtaglomerular cells. Kidney Int 33:947, 1988

29. Benigni A, Uriabramilo C, Piccirelli A, et al: Increased urinary excretion of thromboxane B_2 and 2.3 donor Tx B_2 in cyclosporine A nephrotoxicity. Kidney Int 34:164, 1988

30. Rogers TS, Elzinger L, Bennett WM, Kelley VE: Selective enhancement of thromboxane in macrophages and kidneys in cyclosporine induced nephrotoxicity. Transplantation 45:153, 1988

31. Myers BD: What is cyclosporine nephrotoxicity. Transplantation Proc 21:1430, 1989

32. Mihatsch MJ, Thiel G, Spichton HP: et al: Morphologic findings in kidney transplants after treatment with cyclosporine. Transplantation Proc 15:2821, 1983

33. Mihatsch MJ, Thiel G, Bosler V et al: Morphological patterns in cyclosporine treated renal transplant recipients. Transplantation Proc 17(1):101, 1985

34. Banfi G, Tarantino A, Fogazzi GB et al: Significance of vascular lesions in cyclosporine treated renal transplants. Kidney Int 28:392, 1985

35. Myers BD, Sibley R, Newton L et al: The long term course of cyclosporine-associated chronic nephropathy. Kidney Int 33:590, 1988

36. Washwa NK, Schroeder TJ, Pesic AJ et al: Cyclosporine drug interactions: a review. Ther Drug 9:399, 1987

37. Lake KD: Cyclosporine drug interactions: a review. Cardiac Surg 2:617, 1988.39

38. Hillebrant G, Castro CA, Van Schidt W et al: Valproate for epilepsy in renal transplant recipients receiving cyclosporine. Transplantation 43:915, 1987

39. Parkin J, Lorber MK, Bia MS: Effects of H2 receptor antagonists on renal function in cyclosporine treated renal transplant patients. Transplantation 47:254, 1989

40. Camersa J, Rigby RJ, Van Deth AG, Petrie JJB: Severe tubulo-interstitial disease in a renal allograft due to cytomegalovirus infection Clin Nephrol 18:321, 1982

41. Von Willebrand E, Petterson E, Aronson T, Hayry P: CMV infection class II antigen expression and human allograft rejection. Transplantation 42:364, 1986

42. Ozarva T, Stewart JA: Immune-complex glomerulonephritis associated with cytomegalovirus infection. Am J Clin Path 72:103, 1979
43. Spector SA: Diagnosis of cytomegalovirus infection. Semin Hematol 27:11, 1990
44. Mathew TH: Recurrent disease after renal transplantation. Transplant Rev 5:31, 1991
45. Wilson CB, Dixon FJ: Anti-glomerular basement membrane antibody induced glomerulonephritis. Kidney Int. 3:74, 1973
46. Beleil OM, Coburn JW, Shinaberger JH et al: Recurrent glomerulonephritis due to anti-glomerular basement antibodies in two successive grafts. Clin Nephrol 1:371, 1973
47. Hoyer JR, Raij L, Vermis RL et al: Recurrence of idiopathic nephrotic syndrome after renal transplantation. Lancet 2:353, 1972
48. Habib R, Antignal C, Hinglow N: Glomerular lesions in the transplanted kidney in children. Am J Kidney Dis 10:198, 1987
49. Morzycka M, Crocker BP, Sieglar HF et al: Evaluation of recurrent glomerulonephritis in kidney allografts. Am J Med 72:588, 1982
50. Galle P, Hinglais N, Irosmier J: Recurrence of an original glomerular lesion in three renal allografts. Transplant Proc 3:368, 1971
51. Cameron JS: Glomerulonephritis in renal transplants. Transplantation 34:237, 1982
52. O'Meara Y, Green A, Carmody M, et al: Recurrent glomerulonephritis in renal transplants: 14 years experience. Nephrol Dial Transplant 4:730, 1989
53. Woodhall PB, McCoy RC, Gunnells JC, et al: Apparent recurrence of progressive systemic sclerosis in a renal allograft. JAMA 236:1032, 1976
54. Merino GE, Sutherland DE, Kjellstand CM et al: Renal transplantation for progressive systemic sclerosis with renal failure. Am J Surg 745:133, 1977
55. Jacobs C, Rottenourgh J, Reach I et al: Terminal renal failure due to oxalosis in 14 patients. Proc Eur Dial Transplant Assoc 11:359, 1975
56. Bohnman SO, Wilczek H, Jaremko C et al: Recurrence of diabetic nephropathy in human renal allograft. Transplant Proc. 26:649, 1984
57. Amend WJ, Vincente F, Feduska NJ et al: Recurrent systemic lupus erythermatosis involving renal allograft. Ann Intern Med 94:444, 1981
58. Berger BE, Vincenti F, Biava C et al: De novo and recurrent membranous glomerulopathy following kidney transplantaion. Transplantation 35:315, 1983
59. Cheigh JS, Mouradian J, Soliman M et al: Focal segmental glomerulosclerosis in renal transplants. Am J Kidney Dis 2:449, 1983
60. Busch GJ, Birtch AG, Luke P et al: Glomerular deposits of horse immunoglobulin G and nephritis following administration of anti lymphocyte globulin. Hum Pathol 2:299, 1971
61. Kirchner PT, Resenthall C: Renal transplant evaluation. Semin Nucl Med 30:370, 1982
62. Hoddick W, Filly RA, Gakman U et al: Renal allograft rejection: US evaluation. Radiology 161:469, 1986
63. Ward RE, Bartlett ST et al: The use of duplex scanning in evaluation of the post transplant kidney. Transplant Proc 21:1912, 1989
64. Soper WD, Birgman T et al: Use of duplex ultrasound scanning in renal transplantation. Transplant Proc 21:1903, 1989
65. Leichtman AB, Sorrel DG et al: Duplex imaging of the renal transplant. Transplant Proc 21:3607, 1989

66. Hricack H, Termier F et al: Post transplant renal rejection: comparison of quantitative scintigraphy, U.S. and MR Imaging. Radiology 162:685, 1987

67. Descamps B, Gagnon R, Van der Gaag F et al: Antibody dependent cell mediated cytotoxicity (ADCC) and complement dependent cytotoxicity (CDC) in 229 sera from human renal allograft recipients. J Clin Lab Immunol 2:303, 1979

68. Thomas FT, Lee HM, Lower RR, Thomas JM: Immunological monitoring as a guide to the managment of transplant recipients. Surg Clin North Am 59:253, 1979

69. Hersh EM, Butler WJ, Rosen RD et al: In vitro studies of the human response to organ allografts: appearance and detection of circulating activation lymphocytes. J Immunol 107:571, 1971

70. Carter NP, Cullen PR, Thompson JF, et al: Monitoring lymphocyte subpopulation in renal allograft recipients. Transplant Proc 15:1157, 1983

71. Von Willebrandt E: OKT4/OKT8 ratio in the blood and in the graft during episodes of human renal allograft rejection. Cell Immunol 77:196, 1983

72. Ellis TM, Mokana Kumar T, Mendez-Ricon G et al: Post transplant monitoring of circulating K cells, NK-cell and total T-cell levels: lack of association with renal allograft rejection. Transplant Proc 15:1830, 1983

73. Waltzer WC, BachVaroff RJ, Anaise D, Rapport, FT: Natural killer cell activity after renal transplantation. Transplant Proc 16:1527 1984

74. Smith WJ, Burdick TF, Williams GM: Fluorescent and light microscopic analysis of peripheral blood leukocytes from human renal allograft recipients. Transplant Proc 16:1546, 1984

75. Freed B, Walsh A, Pietrocia D et al: Early detection of renal allograft rejection by serum monitoring of serum reactive protein. Transplantation 37:215, 1984

76. Barnes RM, Alexander LC, West CK: Beta 2 microglobulin and renal allograft rejection: relationship to plasma creatinine during stable transplant function and graft rejection. Transplant Proc 16:1613, 1984

77. Margteiter R, Fuchs D, Hansen A et al: Neopterin as a new biochemical marker for diagnosis of allograft rejection. Transplantation 36:650, 1987

78. Foegh ML, Alijami M, Helfrich GI et al: Urine thomboxane as an immunologic monitor in kidney transplant patients. Transplantation Proc 16:1603, 1984

79. Smith KA: Interleukin-2: inception, impact and implications. Science 240:1169, 1988

80. Rubin LA, Kurman, CC, Fritz ME et al: Soluble interleukin-2 receptors are released from activated human lympoid cells in vitro. J Immunol 135:3172, 1985

81. Colvin B, Fuller TC, Mackeen L et al: Plasma interleukin 2 receptor levels in renal allograft recipients. Clin Immunol Immunopathol 43:273, 1987

82. Simpson MA, Madras PN, Cornaby AJ et al: Sequential determination of urinary cytology and plasma and urinary lymphokines in the management of renal allograft recipients. Transplantation 47:218, 1987

83. Colvin RB, Preffer DI, Fuller TC, et al: A critical analysis of serum and urine interleukin 2 receptor assays in renal allograft recipients. Transplantation 48:800, 1989

84. Cohen N, Gumbert, M Birnbaum J et al: An improved method for the detection of soluble interleukin 2 receptors in liver transplant recipients by flow cytometry. Transplantation 51:417, 1991

85. Hayry P, Von Willebrandt F: Monitoring of human renal allograft rejection with fine needle aspiration cytology. Scand J Immunol 13:87, 1981

86. Ahonen J: Clinical use of FNAB in renal transplantation in renal transplant cytology. p. 31. In Kreis H, Droz D, Milan, Wilking (eds.): 1984

87. Miller SM, Belitsky P, Compta R: Glomeruli in kidney transplant collected by fine needle aspiration biopsy. Transplant Proc 20:584, 1988

88. Haÿry PJ: Fine needle aspiration biopsy in renal transplantation. Kidney Int 36:130, 1984

89. Terasaki PI, Cecka JM, Takemoto S et al: Overview. p. 409. In Terasaki P (ed): Clinical Transplants. UCLA Tissue typing laboratory, Los Angeles, CA. 1988

90. Ortho Multicenter Transplant Study Group: A randomized clinical trial of OKT3 monoclonal antibody for acute rejection of cadaveric renal transplants. N Engl J Med 313:337, 1985

91. Deierhoi MH, Barber WH, Curtis, GG et al: A comparison of OKT3 monoclonal antibody and corticosteroids in the treatment of acute renal allograft rejection. Am J Kidney Dis 11:86, 1988

92. Goldstein G: Overview of the development of Orthoclone OKT3 monoclonal antibody for therapeutic use in transplantation. Transplant Proc 19:1, 1987

93. Miller RA, Maloney DG, McKillop J, Levy R: In vitro effects of murine hybridoma monoclonal antibody in a patient with T cell leukemia. Blood 58:78, 1981

94. Chatenaud L, Baudrihaye MF, Kreis H et al: Human in vivo antigenic modulation induced by the anti-T cell OKT3 monoclonal antibody. Eur J Immunol 12:979, 1982

95. Kirkman RL, Strom TB, Mathew et al: Late mortality and morbidity in recipients of long term renal allografts. Transplantation 34:340, 1982

96. Hattner R et al: Radionuclitide evalution of renal transplants. In Freeman LM, Weissmann HS (eds): Nuclear Medicine Annual. Raven Press, New York, 1984

7

Diagnostic Approaches to Renal Osteodystrophy and Divalent Ion Metabolism

Francisco Llach
Bijan Nikakhtar

PLASMA ALUMINUM LEVELS AND THE DEFEROXAMINE INFUSION TEST

SPECIAL DIAGNOSTIC TECHNIQUES
    Bone Biopsy
      Techniques for Bone Biopsy
    Osteitis Fibrosa
    Osteomalacia
    Aplastic Bone Disease
    Mixed Skeletal Lesion

RADIOGRAPHIC FEATURES OF RENAL OSTEODYSTROPHY
    Secondary Hyperparathyroidism
      Subperiosteal Erosions
      Periosteal Neostosis
      Osteosclerosis
    Osteomalacia
      Protusio Acetabuli

QUANTITATIVE MEASUREMENTS OF BONE MINERAL

PHOTON ABSORPTIOMETRY

NEUTRON ACTIVATION

SCINTISCAN

COMPUTED TOMOGRAPHY

INTRODUCTION

The lives of patients with end stage renal failure are now prolonged by better conservative therapy, maintenance dialysis, and successful renal transplantation; consequently, the morbidity resulting from disordered divalent ion metabolism, soft tissue calcification, and osseous pathology has become clinically more significant. The clinical features of renal osteodystrophy are well defined, and rational approaches to the diagnosis of renal osteodystrophy have been developed. The term *renal osteodystrophy* is used here to include various skeletal diseases reported in patients with renal failure, i.e., retardation of growth, osteomalacia, osteitis fibrosa, and aplastic bone disease. With the routine measurements of serum aluminum, the advent of the immunoradiometric assay of parathyroid hormone (PTH), and more widespread use of bone biopsy, a specific diagnosis of the type of bone lesion can be made and a more appropriate therapy can be instituted. In this chapter, we discuss *(1) clinical signs and symptoms of osteodystrophy, (2) biochemical features*, and *(3) special diagnostic techniques.*

CLINICAL SIGNS AND SYMPTOMS OF OSTEODYSTROPHY

Bone Pain

The symptoms that appear in association with osteodystrophy may be quite subtle and insidious in their onset. Although fortunately not common, bone pain may develop and slowly progress to produce total disability. This can occur independent of skeletal pathology, whether primarily osteitis fibrosa, osteomalacia, or a mixture of both. The most common cause of bone pain, however, is aluminum bone disease. The pain is generally vague and deep-seated, and it may be located in the low back, hips, knees, or legs. Pain is not relieved by massage or local heat, and the patient usually perceives the pain as being more deeply seated than in the joints or muscles.

Physical findings are frequently lacking; occasionally, localized tenderness may be apparent with pressure on the chest wall or lateral compression of the pelvis; tenderness may also be localized over the vertebral spines or ribs.

Muscular Weakness

Muscular weakness, largely limited to the proximal musculature, can be a serious and debilitating problem. This myopathy resembles in many ways the muscle weakness reported in vitamin D deficiency. In both forms of myopathy, plasma levels of muscle enzymes, such as creatine phosphokinase, are usually normal and electromyographic abnormalities are either absent or nonspecific. The muscle weakness appears slowly, with the patient unable to climb stairs easily or rise from a sitting position without help.

Striking improvement in muscle weakness has been observed in some uremic patients following the administration of calcitriol.[1] Muscle biopsy, carried out in selected patients, has revealed mild, nonspecific myopathic alterations by light microscopy and severe degenerative changes by electron microscopic examination. In patients with mild to severe muscle weakness, electron micrographs revealed localized areas of severe disorganization of the myofibrils, with dispersion of Z-brand materials; the latter reverted to normal following treatment with 25-hydroxy vitamin D_3 (25-OH-D_3).[2] However, muscle weakness may also be profound in patients with aluminum-related osteomalacia. Striking improvement has occurred in this latter setting after aluminum removal with deferoxamine.[3]

Pruritus

Pruritus, a common symptom in patients with advanced renal failure, often improves and may disappear following initiation of regular hemodialysis. It usually reflects the presence of high PTH levels. Pruritus sometimes is of such intensity that it prevents sleep and interferes with a patient's normal activities. Pruritus may be severe in patients with clinically evident secondary hyperparathyroidism (2°HPTH) and may improve or, indeed, totally disappear within a few days after partial parathyroidectomy.[4] In the absence of specific evidence of 2°HPTH—i.e., very high levels of PTH, radiographic evidence of bony erosions, and/or bone biopsy features of osteitis fibrosa—parathyroid surgery is not indicated. The presence of refractory pruritus, however, should direct a clinician to seek evidence of overt and severe 2°HPTH.

Calciphylaxis

Calciphylaxis, typified by peripheral ischemic necrosis, vascular calcification, and cutaneous ulcerations, has been noted for many years in isolated patients with chronic renal failure.[5] This syndrome usually appears in patients with end stage renal disease and is usually associated with a longstanding history of renal failure, although patients have developed the syndrome following successful renal transplantation. The syndrome has been observed in association with renal diseases of varying causes; there has been no predilection for a specific age or sex.

The skin lesions make their appearances as superficial violacious discolorations in a mottled, circumscribed pattern involving the tips of the toes or fingers or occurring about the ankles, thighs, or buttocks. The lesions are often accompanied by pain. As the lesions progress, they become hemorrhagic with ischemic, "dry" necrosis. Biopsy specimens fail to show fibrinoid necrosis or granulomatous inflammation. All patients with these lesions have demonstrated evidence of medial calcinosis of small- and medium-sized arteries; skin biopsies generally reveal the presence of medial calcification and intimal thickening.

Current or historical evidence of overt 2°HPTH is present in most uremic patients presenting with this syndrome.[5] Substantial improvement usually follows partial parathyroidectomy. Without treatment, the lesions often progress with varying degrees of rapidity; many patients have died, usually from secondary infection.[5] Because of the poor prognosis, partial parathyroidectomy is recommended when such lesions appear in conjunction with evidence of 2°HPTH.[5]

Periarthritis

Periarthritis manifested by acute pain, redness, and swelling around one or more joints can develop as a result of altered metabolism of calcium and phosphorus in uremia. Rarely, pain may occur in the ankle or foot without local signs except for vague tenderness and can be associated with radiographic changes of subperiosteal resorption.[6] This syndrome probably reflects over 2°HPTH; the affected patients have high levels of serum alkaline phosphatase activity, calcium-phosphorus product, and PTH levels when compared with other dialysis patients.[7] Further evidence favoring the relationship between the symptoms and 2°HPTH is provided by the observation that such discomfort can disappear completely within 1 or 2 weeks following parathyroidectomy.

Occasionally, calcium deposits may be observed radiographically about the affected joints. Synovial biopsy may reveal crystals that, when studied by x-ray diffraction, are characteristic of hydroxyapatite. This syndrome must be differentiated from pseudogout or gouty arthritis, which are characterized by a true monoarticular arthritis and can be differentiated by the identification of specific crystals of either urate or calcium pyrophosphate within the synovial fluid.[8] In general, this syndrome responds well to treatment with anti-inflammatory agents such as indomethacin; parathyroidectomy, as mentioned, may lead to marked improvement.

Spontaneous Tendon Rupture

Spontaneous tendon rupture also occurs in patients with long-standing renal failure and is usually associated with evidence of marked 2°HPTH.[9] The syndrome has been reported in association with primary HPTH and other causes of 2°HPTH.[10,11]

Rupture occurs most commonly in the quadriceps tendons, triceps tendons, or in extensor tendons of the fingers. Typically, the quadriceps tendon ruptures while the patient is walking or descending stairs, or after stumbling. Patients are usually unable to extend the affected leg; a palpable gap and ecchymoses above the tendon are characteristic signs. Surgical treatment with slow rehabilitation has had satisfactory results.[11]

Skeletal Deformities

Skeletal deformities of bone are quite common in uremic children, in whom the bone undergoes growth, modeling, and remodeling. Skeletal deformities can and occasionally do occur in adults; such deformities arise from abnormalities of skeletal remodeling and from recurrent fractures.

Slipped Epiphyses

The deformities commonly observed in children include bowing of the tibia and femur and defects arising from slipped epiphyses.[12] Most commonly, slipped epiphyses become manifest in preadolescence. The hip is the most commonly afflicted site, followed by the radius and ulna; lower humeral, lower femoral, and lower tibial sites are more rarely involved.[13] With hip involvement, a limp is common, and pain is often absent. When the radius and ulna are involved, local swelling and ulnar deviation of the hands appear. The histologic abnormalities associated with slipped epiphyses are those of osteitis fibrosa (2°PHTH).

Growth Retardation

Growth retardation is a common feature in children with renal insufficiency; growth retardation occurs both before and during treatment with maintenance hemodialysis.[14] Growth can also be impaired when there is no evidence of renal osteodystrophy. Before dialysis, one-third to one-half of children with a "preterminal" stage of chronic renal failure in one study had body heights below the third percentile[15]; growth velocity is below normal limits for age in two-thirds of children treated with dialysis.[16] Providing caloric supplements has been reported to improve growth,[17] although this is not always successful.[18] Studies have shown that correction of acidosis can improve growth in children with renal tubular acidosis, thereby, suggesting that long-standing acidosis in azotemic children could also have a deleterious effect on growth.[19] Improved or even "catch-up" growth has also been reported during treatment with calcitriol[20]; subsequent observations, however, have not confirmed the improvement.[21] During treatment with calcitriol, catch-up growth did not occur during the early period of treatment when the serum PTH levels were still elevated and renal osteodystrophy was still evident, but catch-up growth did begin after the apparent "healing" of the marked 2°HPTH.

BIOCHEMICAL FEATURES OF RENAL OSTEODYSTROPHY

Despite evidence that the pathophysiologic alterations develop early in the course of renal insufficiency, signs and symptoms of altered calcium homeostasis generally appear only in patients with advanced uremia. In part, this may occur because some symptoms, such as muscle weakness, are so insidious in their appearance that they are not even noticed by the patient. The evaluation of osteodystrophy is often made from biochemical measurements.

Serum Phosphorus

Serum phosphorus (Pi) levels are usually slightly lower than normal[22] or normal in the early stages of renal failure.[23] Hyperphosphatemia is generally absent until renal function falls to 20 to 30 percent of normal.[24] In patients with creatinine clearance rates below 20 ml/min, serum Pi levels show wide variation, ranging from 2.5 to 15 mg/dl in individual patients. Serum Pi can be sharply affected by dietary intake of the mineral.

Some factors that can affect the serum Pi level in patients with renal insufficiency are shown in Table 7-1. The dietary content of Pi is a major determinant of its serum levels in patients with renal failure. The intake of Pi, however, varies considerably in different parts of the world. In the United States, for example, dietary intake of Pi is higher than in many other parts of the world, and it is not uncommon for normal individuals to ingest 1,500 to 2,000 mg of Pi/d. In dialysis patients, this quantity may fall to 500 to 1,000 mg/d with dietary restriction. Very low protein diets may provide only 300 to 400 mg/d.[25]

The aluminum-containing gels and calcium carbonate, which bind Pi in the intestine and render it nonabsorbable, are commonly employed to reduce the absorption of Pi in uremia. In general, the appropriate dose of aluminum (Al) hydroxide or calcium carbonate for satisfactory control of serum Pi

Table 7-1. Serum Phosphorus (Pi) in Renal Failure:
Modifying Factors

Nutritional/Enteral
    Dietary Pi intake
    Pi-containing enemas
    Parenteral alimentation
    Pi-binding compounds
    Calcium supplementation

Renal/Dialysis
    Residual renal function
    Dialysis: frequency, duration, efficiency

Hormonal
    PTH: Secretion and skeletal responsiveness
    Vitamin D: Balance of deficiency and replacement
        therapy

Miscellaneous
    Hypomagnesemia
    Balance of anabolism/catabolism
    Rate of skeletal accretion

Abbreviations: Pi, phosphorus; PTH, parathyroid hormone.

levels is determined by empirically adjusting the dosage. When dietary Pi intake is below 1.0 g/d, fecal Pi loss exceeds dietary intake as Al hydroxide is added. With dietary Pi intake above 2.0 g/day, however, fecal Pi excretion is less than dietary intake despite ingestion of Al hydroxide gel. Thus, intake of a diet high in Pi content can overcome the effect of ingesting substantial amounts of Al hydroxide or Al carbonate. Serum Pi levels are often higher in uremic patients with over 2°HPTH than in other patients with equal degrees of renal insufficiency but lacking overt 2°HPTH.[26] It is evident that serum Pi levels can be markedly altered in patients with little or no residual renal function by events that lead to a change in the balance between bone formation and bone resorption. The initial healing of osteomalacia or osteitis fibrosa is sometimes associated with a fall in serum Pi concentration, presumably because bone formation and the deposition of calcium and Pi in the skeleton are increased out of proportion to the rate of bone resorption. Because a major action of vitamin D is to enhance Pi absorption, one might anticipate that levels of the anion would serum increase following the administration of calcitriol to uremic patients, especially to those with overt 2°HPTH. However, the intravenous administration of calcitriol to these patients suppresses 2°HPTH, which, in turn reduces bone resorption and increases the net osseous deposition of calcium and Pi. It thereby follows that serum Pi levels often decreases. In patients with mild HPTH, serum Pi concentration sometimes decrease, thereby diminishing the need for phosphate binders during the first 2 to 3 months of treatment with calcitriol. In time, serum Pi levels may increase, once remineralization is complete.[27]

Hypocalcemia

Hypocalcemia is a common but not invariable finding in patients with advanced renal failure. Although both the mean serum calcium (Ca) level and the Ca clearance rate of 5 to 20 ml/min are significantly lower in patients with advanced renal failure than in normal subjects, total serum Ca levels are below normal (less than the lower limits of the 95 percent confidence interval) in only 40 percent of uremic patients.[28] Moreover, levels below 7.5 mg/dl are observed infrequently.

The initiation of regular hemodialysis is often associated with an increase in total serum Ca concentration toward normal.[29] Moreover, this increase in serum Ca concentration has been observed despite persistent hyperphosphatemia, and the use of low levels of dialysate Ca.[30] Such an observation, made several years ago when the control of hyperphosphatemia was poor, points to the existence of some unknown factor related to dialysis per se, which aids the correction of uremic hypocalcemia.

Hypercalcemia

Hypercalcemia can also occur in patients with renal failure, particularly those undergoing hemodialysis. Some of the causes of hypercalcemia in patients with advanced renal failure are listed in Table 7-2. Symptoms of hypercalcemia are sometimes greater in uremic patients than in patients with normal renal function and elevated serum calcium levels. Thus, the cause of hypercalcemia in a patient with renal insufficiency should be delineated; in particular, aluminum-related bone disease must be separated from overt 2°HPTH because their treatments are so different.

Transient hypercalcemia can occur in uremic patients who ingest large quantities of Ca carbonate or other Ca salts, during treatment with calcitriol, and in some but not all dialysis patients after the prolonged use of dialysate with a Ca concentration of 7 to 8 mg/dl. Hypercalcemia can also occur in patients with severe or "overt" 2°HPTH; such hypercalcemia may appear within weeks to months after hemodialysis has been initiated.

In the absence of high serum PTH levels or radiographic or histologic evidence of osteitis fibrosa, 2°HPTH cannot be assumed to be responsible for hypercalcemia. Persistent elevation of serum Ca levels has been observed among dialysis patients with Al accumulation and Al-related bone disease. For example, radiographs may show only "osteopenia," although subperiosteal erosions may persist from earlier hyperparathyroidism that failed to mineralize as the PTH levels were reduced because of Al accumulation.[31] The hypercalcemia associated with Al accumulation may first appear or become aggravated under the following conditions: administration of oral Ca supplements and/or small doses of vitamin D sterols; treatment with dialysate containing a high Ca concentration; or immobilization.[32–33]

Table 7-2. Hypercalcemia in Renal Failure: Associated Conditions

Dietary
    High calcium intake
    Pi restriction and hypophosphatemia
    Low protein or amino acid diet
Renal
    High dialysate calcium
    Recovery from acute renal failure
    Postrenal transplantation
Hormonal
    Severe 2°HPTH
    Therapy with vitamin D sterols
Drugs
    Thiazides
    Calcium-cycle ion-exchange resins
Miscellaneous
    Al-related bone disease
    Immobilization (with Al bone disease or 2°HPTH)
    Associated diseases
        Myeloma, jarcoid, malignancy

Abbreviations: Aluminum, Al; 2°HPTH, secondary hyperparathyroidism; Pi, phosphorus.

Hypercalcemia also has been reported with the use of a calcium-containing exchange resin,[34] in association with marked phosphate restriction and hypophosphatemia,[35] in conjunction with immobilization, and during the ingestion of thiazide diuretics.[36] Uremic patients may also develop hypercalcemia from associated illnesses, e.g., multiple myeloma or sarcoidosis.[37] The hypercalcemia may also be prolonged and more marked in uremic patients because the loss of renal function eliminates the body's ability to excrete the calcium mobilized from bone or absorbed through the intestine.

Serum Alkaline Phosphatase

Serum alkaline phosphatase is made up of isoenzymes that arise from the intestine, liver, kidney, and bone. Despite the heterogeneity of this enzyme, the measurement of alkaline phosphatase activity can provide a rough indication of increased osteoblastic activity; moreover, studies of isoenzymes have shown that the increased amount of alkaline phosphatase in uremia arises primarily from bone.[38] Serum total enzyme levels are commonly increased in association with osteitis fibrosa, or mixed lesions, although markedly elevated levels are more characteristic of osteitis fibrosa.[39] Nonetheless, serial measurement of plasma alkaline phosphatase activity may provide a useful clinical guide for monitoring the therapy of skeletal disease with Ca compounds and/or calcitriol. Serial measurements can identify the slow progression of skeletal disease in a uremic patient. It should be kept in mind that uremic patients can exhibit significant and overt skeletal disease and yet have normal levels of plasma alkaline phosphatase activity. Plasma alkaline phosphatase levels in patients with Al-related bone disease (osteomalacia or aplastic bone disease) are usually not elevated despite the presence of severe disease.[40] Others have reported elevated alkaline phosphatase activity levels[41]; thus, this measurement may not discriminate between Al-related bone disease and osteitis fibrosa.

Serum PTH

Serum PTH levels, as noted earlier, are commonly elevated in patients with renal insufficiency, and the degree of elevation may be striking. Serum levels are dramatically elevated when measured with an antiserum directed primarily toward the midregion or the carboxy-terminus of the PTH molecule, while the degree of elevation is far less when PTH concentration is measured with an antiserum directed toward the amino-terminus.[42] As mentioned earlier, with the advent of sensitive immunoradiometric assays (IRMA) for the secreted intact PTH molecule, the evaluation of dialysis patients with 2°HPTH is easier, and in many instances the performance of bone biopsy may be avoided. In the past, the conventional radioimmunoassay of PTH was limited by the measurement of biologically inactive fragments generated by the metabolism of the hormone; this is even more so in patients with renal insufficiency because these fragments are cleared via the kidney. The IRMA assays for PTH have high specificity and sensitivity as well as excellent precision allowing measurement within and below the normal range. In addition to its diagnostic value, the IRMA assay has helped in the evaluation of parathyroid function of dialysis patients.[43] Furthermore, a large number of commercially available conventional PTH radioimmunoassays (RIA) are of no value in predicting or assessing the severity of the osteitis fibrosa present. Fortunately, the IRMA assay provide correlative data between serum PTH levels and histologic features of bone disease in uremic patients.[44] This assay allows the diagnosis of HPTH to be made without difficulty. Provided that Al toxicity is excluded, the presence of high PTH levels (by IRMA) is sufficient for the diagnosis of osteitis fibrosa and bone biopsy is not necessary. In addition, the therapeutic response to calcitriol therapy can be easily monitored with this assay.

PLASMA ALUMINUM LEVELS AND THE DEFEROXAMINE INFUSION TEST

Endothermal atomic absorption spectroscopy provides an accurate means to measure plasma Al levels. Tissue and plasma Al levels are substantially above normal in most patients with end stage renal disease, particularly those who have taken Pi binders containing Al.[45] Plasma Al concentration largely reflects the recent "load" of the metal concentrations, however, do not correlate very well with tissue stores.[46] However, most patients with Al-related bone disease have markedly elevated plasma Al concentrations (e.g., greater than 75 to 100 μg/L, compared to levels of 2 to 8 μg/L in normal patients) (Fig. 7-1). Also, patients with markedly elevated plasma Al levels (e.g., values above 150 to 200 μg/L) are very likely to develop Al-related bone disease and/or encephalopathy if the exposure to Al continues.[47] There has been some uncertainty about the value of monitoring plasma Al concentrations at regular intervals in dialysis patients. Measuring plasma Al every 3 to 4 months has been recommended by some.[48] Marked elevation of plasma Al (e.g., above 75 to 100 μg/L) in the majority of patients in a dialysis unit indicates that there has been exposure to unacceptably high concentrations of Al in the dialysate. This could indicate that the water treatment system has malfunctioned at some time in the recent past. Because contamination varies over time, the concentration of Al in water or dialysate may be normal at any given moment. If only a few patients exhibit plasma Al levels above 75 to 100 μg/L, those ingesting excessive amounts of Al-containing gels or absorbing excess Al from the Pi-binders may be identified.

Measurement of the increment in plasma Al concentration following a standardized infusion of the chelating agent *deferoxamine (DFO)* has been proposed as a method to recognize dialysis patients with increased Al stores and a greater risk of Al-related bone disease[49] (Fig. 7-2). The relationship

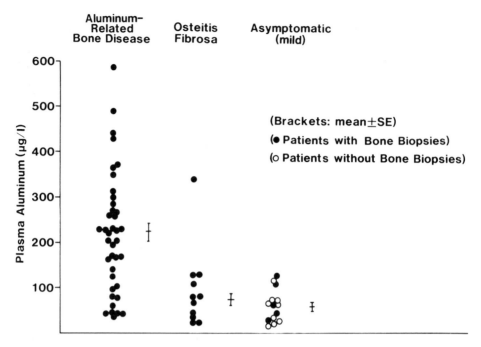

Fig. 7-1. Plasma aluminum levels in individual dialysis patients with aluminum-related bone disease or osteitis fibrosa and in asymptomatic patients (with no bone biopsy or a bone biopsy showing a "mild" lesion). Plasma aluminum levels in the aluminum group were significantly higher than those in both the osteitis fibrosa and the asymptomatic groups ($P < 0.01$), but the mean values of the latter two groups did not differ. (Adapted from Norris et al.,[101] with permission.)

between the increment in plasma Al levels following an infusion of DFO and the total Al content in bone is closer than that between the basal plasma Al and the bone Al content. Not all patients with elevated tissue levels of Al have evidence of Al-related bone disease[50]; Al may not be similarly distributed in tissues in all patients or a certain quantity of tissue Al may not always be pathogenic. Testing plasma Al concentrations may be a useful screening procedure, but it is not specific in all cases, as is shown in Figure 7-3.[49] Once patients are protected from any Al source for several months, serum levels, i.e., both basal and the increment induced by DFO, may decrease substantially. This reduction in circulating levels occurs even though some patients retain significant bone surface staining for Al. These observations suggest that in certain patients removal of bone Al may be more difficult than others. In addition, we have recently shown that in patients with a mild Al burden, the increment of plasma Al after DFO correlated with bone Al, but it is not a good predictor of bone histology.[50] Nevertheless, it is becoming, more clear that Al bone disease is decreasing in its frequency and severity. Thus, patients with significant Al bone disease are fewer, in number and becoming more difficult to detect. Noninvasive strategies for identi-

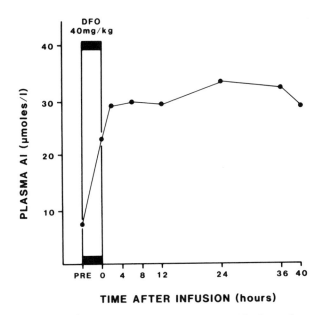

Fig. 7-2. Changes in plasma aluminum concentration with time after a standardized infusion of deferoxamine (DFO), 40 mg/kg body weight, given after hemodialysis to patients with proven aluminum-related bone disease. Values are expressed as percentage of maximum value; peak levels occurred by 24 hours. (Adapted from Milliner et al.,[49] with permission.)

fying and monitoring these patients have used a combination of the increment is serum Al after DFO administration and measurement of intact PTH (IRMA). Thus, an Al increment of 150 μg/L and a low PTH (less than 160 pg/ml) identifies those at high risk of Al bone disease with 95 percent probability.[51]

Finally, recent data have shown that the iron stores of any given patient may influence the DFO test.[52] Patients with iron depletion are more able to increase their serum Al, while those with iron overload are less able to mobilize Al from tissues; this may occur because DFO also binds iron and the more iron available, the lesser the increment in serum Al. This may explain some of the false-negative responses observed in patients with obvious Al bone disease. Thus, iron status may have to be considered in the interpretation of this test.

SPECIAL DIAGNOSTIC TECHNIQUES

Bone Biopsy

With the advent of the IRMA assay for PTH and with the DFO test, many bone disorders may be diagnosed noninvasively. In certain clinical settings, however, these noninvasive tests may not be adequate and a bone biopsy is

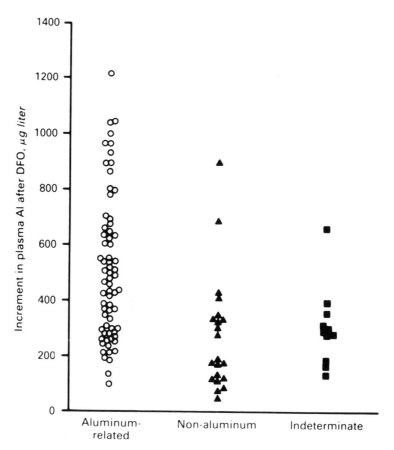

Fig. 7-3. Increment in plasma aluminum after a standardized infusion of deferoxamine (DFO) (40 mg/kg of body weight) for dialysis patients with aluminum-related bone disease, those without aluminum bone disease, and others considered indeterminate.

required to establish a definitive diagnosis. This is of critical importance because the therapy for Al bone disease, i.e., DFO and cessation of Al-containing gels, differs from that of osteitis fibrosa, i.e., calcitriol therapy. Bone biopsy is sometimes required in the presence of severe HPTH, in which parathyroidectomy may be needed. In this setting, a bone biopsy is mandatory to exclude significant bone Al deposits.

Techniques for Bone Biopsy

The study of bone itself has evolved into a clinically useful tool for understanding the pathophysiologic processes involved and as a guide to the management of renal osteodystrophy. Under local anesthesia, a bone biopsy can easily and safely be obtained from the iliac crest. The sample, 5 × 20 mm, containing trabecular bone and both tables of cortices,[53] is fixed in neutral formalin, transferred to alcohol to prevent Ca loss, and embedded in a hard plastic, such as methacrylate. Thin sections of the undecalcified bone can be cut with a special microtome having a heavy steel blade. Uncalcified osteoid and calcified bone can be readily identified with such methods, unlike the specimen of bone prepared with the usual decalcification.

In addition to the qualitative interpretation of bone histology, quantification of various features and bone dynamics with tetracycline labeling can increase the sensitivity of the method and aid in comparison of biopsy samples. One method use a grid eye-piece to microscopically view the bone.[54] The surfaces of trabecular bone that intersect the grid markings are identified as forming bone (i.e., with osteoblasts and osteoid); resorbing bone (i.e., with osteoclasts and Howship's lacunae); or resting bone (i.e., surfaces are without cellular activity). With another method, the microscopic image of bone is projected on to a screen, and each specific type of bone surface is traced with an electrical pencil attached to a computer and X–Y plotter.[54] Quantitation of the surfaces occupied by active resorption, formation, or by inactive bone can provide static information, but they may not provide data on the dynamics of bone formation, mineralization, or resorption. Errors in static data may occur if the rate of metabolic activity varies[53]; thus, the forming and resorbing surfaces could be twice normal and yet skeletal dynamics can be normal if the activity of the osteoclasts and osteoblasts is reduced to half of normal. To obviate this problem, tetracycline, a fluorescent marker that is rapidly incorporated into newly forming bone, is given on two separate occasions; this permits a measure of bone formation rate.[55] In practice, the dynamics of trabecular bone are assessed after giving two separate doses of tetracycline, with the bone formation rate quantitated as the distance between the two lines of fluorescence divided by the time between doses.

The dynamics of trabecular bone turnover differ from those of cortical bone, which is organized into units called *osteons*, which surround a Haversian canal. Cortical bone turnover involves sequential osteoclastic resorption within the Haversian canal; this is followed by osteoblastic formation; also, the numerous osteocytes, which are buried within the osteon, can participate in bone resorption through an "osteocytic osteolysis."

Osteitis Fibrosa

Osteitis fibrosa, which presumably arises due to the high levels of PTH, is characterized by increased bone resorption and formation with a progressive increase in peritrabecular fibrosis (Fig. 7-4). A greater fraction of trabecular bone surface is occupied by resorption cavities filled with osteoclasts (Howships's lacunae); also, increased numbers of osteoblasts overlie the newly formed unminerlized matrix of bone. As this process becomes severe, the narrow space is filled with fibrous tissue, creating typical osteitis fibrosa.[56] Double tetracycline labeling often reveals normal or increased bone turnover[57] in patients with osteitis fibrosa (Fig. 7-5).

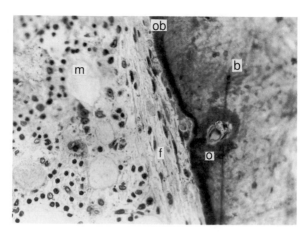

Fig. 7-4. Peritrabecular fibrosis in a chronic renal failure patient. Endosteal fibrosis (f) visible adjacent to trabecular bone (b) and osteoid (o) with overlying osteoblasts (ob); normal marrow (m) is also present. (× 375). (From Felsenfeld and Llach,[57] with permission.)

Another feature of osteitis fibrosa is the alignment of collagen strands in an irregular, haphazard "woven" pattern; this contrasts to the normal parallel alignment of strands of collagen in a lamellar manner. This disorganized structure of collagen in woven bone may lead to defective physical properties of bone in response to stress, and a greater amount of inferior, woven bone may be required to maintain mechanical stability.[58] Also, increased mineralization of large quantities of woven bone may contribute to the osteosclerosis seen in uremia.

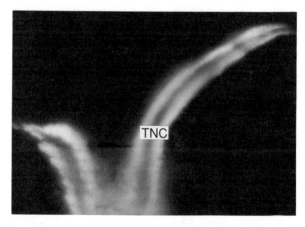

Fig. 7-5. Mineralization in osteitis fibrosa as assessed by double tetracycline label (TNC). Extent of mineralization and bone appositional rate (distance between labels divided by time) are normal. (× 375). (From Felsenfeld and Llach,[57] with permission.)

Osteomalacia

Osteomalacia is characterized by an excess of unmineralized osteoid tissue; this arises from impaired mineralization of the protein matrix of bone. The major feature of osteomalacia is an increase in the width of unmineralized osteoid (Fig. 7-6). This is also found, to a certain extent, in osteitis fibrosa, which is due to the delay of osteoid mineralization that is formed so rapidly. Therefore, the use of tetracycline labeling to identify impaired mineralization rate is useful in the identification of osteomalacia (Fig. 7-7). Nonetheless, the criteria employed in the recognition of osteomalacia include (1) the measurement of the width of osteoid seams; (2) the specific number of osteoid lamellae in these seams; (3) the extent to which bone surface is covered with osteoid; (4) the volume of osteoid expressed as a fraction of total bone surface; and (5) a delayed rate of mineralization by tetracycline labeling.[57]

The frequency of osteomalacia appears to have a marked geographic variation. Osteomalacia was initially noted in patients receiving maintenance dialysis.[58] Recently, osteomalacia has been observed in patients before the initiation of dialysis.[59] Epidemiologic evidence has implicated the presence of Al in the water because the incidence of osteomalacia is increased greatly in areas of high Al water content. Pretreatment of the water with reverse osmosis has decreased the incidence of osteomalacia.[60] With the advent of the Maloney stain for Al, it has been shown that the great majority of osteomalacic dialysis patients have large deposits of Al in the bone.[61] The characteristic pattern is a linear deposition of Al along the interface between trabecular bone and osteoid.[62] The degree of osteomalacia has correlated closely with bone Al content, whether analyzed biochemically or histologically.[63]

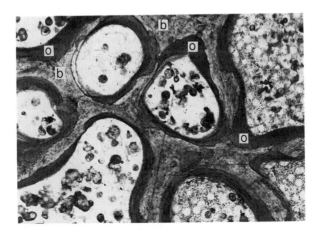

Fig. 7-6. Osteomalacia of renal failure. Large irregular deposits of osteoid (o) cover almost the entire surface of trabecular bone (b). Osteoblasts, osteoclasts, and endosteal fibrosis are absent. (× 150).

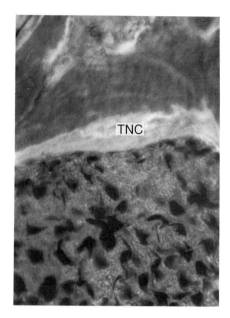

Fig. 7-7. Osteomalacia of renal failure. Marked decrease in bone mineralization with almost absence of double tetracycline label (TNC).

Aplastic Bone Disease

Aplastic bone disease is also observed in dialysis patients.[64] This entity most likely is the result of Al toxicity. It is characterized by features similar to those of osteomalacia; the major difference between them is the absence of large osteoid seams. These patients also have a deficiency of cellular activity and absence of endosteal fibrosis; aluminum deposits are present in both the osteoid–bone interface and on the surface of trabecular bone. It seems that Al may be toxic to bone by simultaneously affecting bone formation and remodeling. Thus, aplastic bone may be a variant of osteomalacia; both are caused by Al accumulation. As mentioned previously, in the absence of PTH, Al toxicity may be more likely to result in aplastic bone disease rather than osteomalacia.[65] Because the incidence of Al-induced bone disease is steadily decreasing, a new form of aplastic or adynamic bone disease has surfaced. The histologic features of this entity are similar to that previously mentioned; however, Al deposits are not present. This lesion has been observed with increasing frequency in diabetic patients as well as continuous ambulatory peritoneal dialysis (CAPD) patients.[66]

Mixed Skeletal Lesion

Mixed skeletal lesion includes wide osteoid seams combined with typical features of osteitis fibrosa. Such skeletal lesions are somewhat more common in young patients, in those with hypocalcemia, and in patients who have not undergone dialysis or treatment with vitamin D.[67] These histologic features may be characteristic of vitamin D deficiency itself, with components of both 2°HPTH, which commonly occurs with vitamin D deficiency, and osteomalacia. Serum PTH levels are significantly elevated in these patients.[68]

There is disagreement as to whether dialysis treatment can lead to specific qualitative differences in skeletal disease or whether dialysis merely prolongs the lives of patients with end stage uremia, thereby exposing them to the various pathogenic factors for a longer period of time. Certain incriminating factors unique to dialysis patients include the administration of heparin,[69] exposure to fluoridated water, exposure to high concentrations of acetate, periodic removal of bicarbonate, exposure to varying concentrations of Ca and Mg in dialysate, and the presence of Al, trace elements, and other substances in dialysate. From their observations on patients studied in Heidelberg, Ritz et al.[70] concluded that there are no qualitative differences between the findings in bones of patients undergoing dialysis compared with those of patients with stable advanced uremia.

RADIOGRAPHIC FEATURES OF RENAL OSTEODYSTROPHY

In general, radiographic evaluation of renal bone disease is not rewarding. First, radiographically observed abnormalities occur late in the course of renal osteodystrophy, and second, they do not specifically identify the type of bone lesion present. The major value of radiographic evaluation may be in the follow-up of the patient after specific therapeutic maneuvers have been instituted. In the following sections, we review the radiographic findings of 2°HPTH as well as those of osteomalacia.

Secondary Hyperparathyroidism

One of the principal radiographic features of 2°HPTH is the presence of *resorption or erosions,* which may occur on the subperiosteal, intracortical, and endosteal surfaces of cortical bone. Another radiographic feature of excess parathyroid activity in azotemic patients is new bone formation at the periosteal surface, a process termed *periosteal neostosis* by Meema et al.[71] Alterations of the trabecular volume of spongy bone may lead to osteosclerosis or osteopenia.

Erosions occurring in conjunction with new bone formation may take the form of *cysts* or osteoclastomas (brown tumors), although these occur less commonly in 2°HPTH than in 1°HPTH.[72]

Subperiosteal Erosions

Subperiosteal erosions of the phalanges identified with the use of fine-grain radiographs of the hands are the most sensitive radiographic sign of 2°HPTH.[73] Abnormalities have been found on radiographs in approximately

40 to 50 percent of the patients who show increased resorptive surfaces on bone biopsy.[74]

The earliest lesions usually appear on the *radial surface* of the *middle phalanges* of the *second or third digits* of the *dominant hand*. These erosions first appear as slight irregularities near either the proximal or distal shoulder formed by the metaphysis of the phalanx.[75] As the lesions progress, the erosions extend along a greater length of the radial surface of the phalanx and involve other digits and adjacent proximal and distal phalanges. Erosions eventually appear on the ulnar border. When Al overload occurs in conjunction with the presence of significant subperiosteal erosions, remineralization and normalization of radiographs may not occur when 2°HPTH is reversed by treatment with calcitriol or by parathyroidectomy.[31] Thus, some caution must be exercised in interpreting the presence of subperiosteal erosions as specific radiologic signs of osteitis fibrosa on 2°HPTH.

Other skeletal sites commonly showing subperiosteal erosions include the upper end of the tibia, the neck of the femur and humerus, the lower end of the radius and ulna, and the lower surface of the medial end of the clavical. Resorption can be seen in the skull, leading to a mottled, lucent appearance; this is commonly associated with areas of osteosclerosis. These abnormalities of the skull may disappear after appropriate treatment (Fig. 7-8).

Periosteal Neostosis

New woven bone arising within fibrous tissue overlying the periosteum is separated from existing bone by a radiolucent area, which represents the interposed area of fibrous tissue.[71] As the process progresses, the fibrous tissue may calcify and the lucent zone disappear, and the existence of such new bone formation may be distinguished from an increased outer bone diameter.

Osteosclerosis

Osteosclerosis arises as a result of an increase in the thickness and number of trabeculae in spongy bone. It is generally apparent only in skeletal areas composed largely of cancellous bone with little contribution of compact bone; these areas include the vertebrae, pelvis, skull, clavicle, proximal humerus, and proximal and distal femur and tibia. In the spine, osteosclerosis may lead to a characteristic "rugger jersey" appearance.

Osteomalacia

The radiographic features of osteomalacia are far less distinctive than those of 2°HPTH. Once the epiphyses have closed, the typical radiographic findings of rickets, i.e., widening and splaying of the epiphyseal growth plate, do not occur. The only pathognomonic finding of osteomalacia present in adults is the *Looser zone* or *pseudofracture*. The Looser zone is a straight,

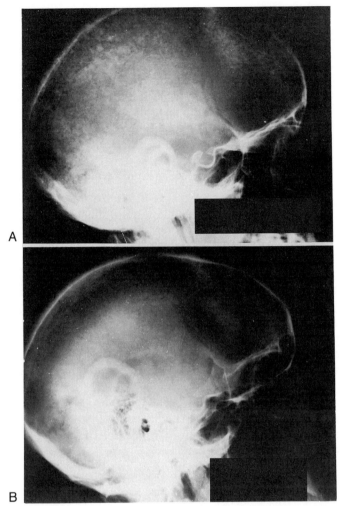

Fig. 7-8. Radiographs of the skull in patients with overt renal osteodystrophy. **(A)**, Areas of modeling, granularity, and increased sclerosis; **(B)**, appearance after 10 months of treatment with 1,25-(OH)$_2$D$_3$ (From Coburn and Llach,[102] with permission.)

wide band of radiolucency that abuts the cortex and is usually perpendicular to the long axis of the bone; it may be bilateral and symmetric and may or may not be accompanied by a narrow area of sclerosis or a small, poorly mineralized callus.[76–78] Healing or callus formation is usually minimal unless specific treatment is given. Looser zones have appeared remarkably infrequently in our experience. They can occur with osteomalacia due to Al accumulation but are infrequent; true fractures may be seen more commonly.

Protusio Acetabuli

Identified as a convex bulging into the pelvis over the acetabulum, protrusio acetabuli may be a specific feature of osteomalacia.[79] Skeletal demineralization occurs with osteomalacia but is nonspecific. Features such as increased haziness or coarsening of the trabeculae, biconcavity of the vertebral bodies, particularly in association with normal bone density, and bending deformities of long bones are said to be typical of osteomalacia; however, few radiologists can make such distinctions.[80] Uremic patients with osteomalacia may also have secondary hyperparathyroidism, and bone erosions commonly coexist. Thus, the features of osteomalacia are predominantly microscopic, and this diagnosis can only be verified by bone histology.

QUANTITATIVE MEASUREMENTS OF BONE MINERAL

The metacarpal index can be obtained by measuring the dimensions of the cortex of a metacarpal bone on x-ray film using magnification and a special caliper.[81] Normal data are available for the second left metacarpal, and the metacarpal index is the ratio of cortical to total bone width. On the basis of the assumption that this bone is a perfect cylinder, the ratio of cross-sectional cortical area to total cross section can be calculated.[82] The metacarpal index has been validated by direct comparison to measurement of bone ash.[82] Observations in patients with 1°HPTH have suggested that total bone area is increased while the cortical area is reduced.[83] In patients with chronic renal failure not treated with dialysis, the metacarpal index was found to be reduced in 20 to 40 percent.[84] One study suggested that the metacarpal index progressively decreases with the duration of dialysis.[85]

PHOTON ABSORPTIOMETRY

Another noninvasive method for the serial evaluation of the skeleton is photon absorptiometry, in which the absorption of photons emitted from an isotopic source is used to assess the mineral content of bone. The isotopes employed, either ^{125}I or ^{241}Am, emit photons of specific, narrow wavelengths and low energy.[86] Such measurements are taken over the phalanges, the radius and ulna, and the femur. Hahn and Hahn measured both the distal radius, which comprises primarily trabecular bone, and the midshaft of the radius, which represents compact bone; this has enabled them to evaluate the ratio of these two types of bone, which have different turnover rates.[87] Griffiths et al. found the mineral content of the midradius and ulna to be lower in dialysis patients than in age-matched controls; they also observed a progressive loss of bone with increasing duration of treatment in a dialysis center using a dialysate Ca level of 5.3 mg/dl.[88] In a subsequent study, they reported that most women on dialysis maintained a stable bone mineral content, whereas 44 percent of males lost bone mass.[89] Photon absorptiometry appears to be more accurate than the methods that measure bone density from radiographs; however, the measurements are limited to certain sites of the skeleton that primarily comprise cortical bone.

It should be noted that bone mineral content can be reduced as a result of several causes: (1) primary reduction in volume of bone tissue, (2) increase in intracortical porosity as a consequence of enlarged Haversian canals, or (3) replacement of normally mineralized bone by unmineralized osteoid or poorly mineralized woven bone. The measurement of bone density by photon absorptiometry does not allow distinction between these causes; the technique is best used when serial measurements are obtained for quantifying bone mineral and when the results are evaluated in conjunction with findings on fine-detail radiographs.

Dual-beam photon absorptiometry uses two separate isotopes, permitting the subtraction of overlying soft tissue mass from that of bone. The technique can thus be used to measure the mineral content of sites of the skeleton lying deep within tissues; it is useful for assessing the mineral content of vertebral bodies and the femoral neck.[90,91] With the advent of dual-energy x-ray bone absorptiometry, a more precise and complete evaluation of bone mineral content can be obtained. Preliminary observations with this more advanced technique suggest that it may be valuable in the follow-up of dialysis patients with bone disease.[92]

NEUTRON ACTIVATION

Neutron activation provides a more accurate method for measuring total Ca or bone mineral content in either the entire body or in isolated parts of the skeleton. This technique requires the availability of a neutron source for the activation of Ca and other elements in the skeleton and immediate access to a whole-body counter for measuring the short-lived radionuclides. This technique has proved useful in research studies of bone mineral content in uremic patients, and it may be particularly useful when serial measurements are used to evaluate the effects of a specific treatment modality.[93]

SCINTISCAN

Skeletal scintigraphy using ^{99m}Tc pyrophosphate provides a sensitive method for the detection of skeletal alterations in patients with renal failure. The technique allows for noninvasive follow-up evaluation of the response to treatment. Although the mechanism responsible for the accumulation of pyrophosphates in bone has not been elucidated, evidence indicates that the pyrophosphate accumulates in areas of increased bone turnover.[94] Kaye et al. suggested that pyrophosphate accumulates in skeletal areas with ab-

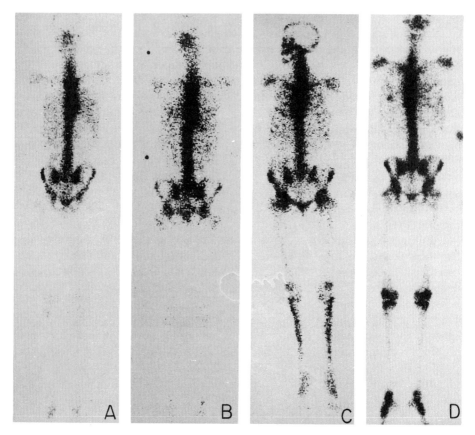

Fig. 7-9. Bone scintigrams with technetium-labeled pyrophosphate in a normal subject (A) and in patients with renal failure (B–D). Grading of severity of abnormality: **(A),** grade 0, normal scintigram; **(B)** grade 1, scintigram showing normal uptake in femoral heads with extension into femoral neck and trochanter region; **(C)** grade 2, scintigram showing abnormal uptake in femoral head and neck and in proximal half of the tibial shaft; **(D)** grade 3, scintigram showing extensive uptake in the femoral head and marked uptake in the femoral and tibial condyles, tarsis, and proximal part of the metatarsis. (From Olgaard et al,[98] with permission.)

normal collagen metabolism, including either osteitis fibrosa or osteomalacia.[95] From evaluation of the uptake of the isotopes over the distal femur, Lien et al. calculated the bone/soft tissue ratio of isotope uptake.[96] Abnormal uptake was found in 78 percent of long-term dialysis patients and a similar proportion of patients with chronic renal failure who were not undergoing regular dialysis. On the basis of the correlation between bone uptake of ^{99m}Tc pyrophosphate and urinary excretion of hydroxyproline, Lien et al. concluded that increased skeletal uptake in uremia is related to the presence of immature collagen.[96] Others have found abnormal scintiscans in 13 of 14 patients undergoing dialysis.[97] Symmetrically increased activity was noted over the skull, mandible, sternum, shoulders, vertebrae, and distal aspects of the femur and tibia. Uptake of the labeled pyrophosphate over certain areas, such as the mandible, was pronounced and appeared before radiographic abnormalities. Olgaard et al. found that 90 percent of patients undergoing regular dialysis had pathologic pyrophosphate accumulation on scintigrams, while radiographic abnormalities were present in only one-third[98] (Fig. 7-9). In the presence of osteomalacia or aluminum-related bone disease, bone scintiscans may reveal increased uptake at sites of either true fractures or pseudofractures, particularly the ribs, pelvis, and scapulae; these may be seen on scintiscans at a time when they cannot be detected by radiography. In general, however, pyrophosphate uptake may be reduced in patients with aluminum-related osteomalacia, and uptake can increase strikingly during chelation therapy.

Abnormal scintigrams are more common in dialysis patients who previously received renal homografts. Intensive glucocorticoid treatment may aggravate the abnormalities responsible for an abnormal scintiscan. The diphosphate scintiscan can be used to detect soft tissue calcification, particularly in the lungs.[99]

COMPUTED TOMOGRAPHY

Computed tomography has been applied to measure the mineral content of the lumbar vertebral bodies.[100] It is of value in conditions such as osteoporosis that primarily affect the trabecular bone and axial skeleton. It has not been applied widely to renal osteodystrophy, and results with this technique have not been correlated with other methods, particularly bone histology.

REFERENCES

1. Brickman AS et al: Action of 1,25-dihydroxycholecalciferol, a potent, kidney-produced metabolite of vitamin D_3, in uremic man. N Engl J Med 287:891, 1972
2. Schoenfeld PJ et al: Amelioration of myopathy with 25-hydroxyvitamin D_3 therapy (25(OH)D_3) in patients on chronic hemodialysis. p. 160. In Third Workshop on Vitamin D, Book of Abstracts, University of California Riverside Press, Asilomar, Riverside, CA, 1977
3. Nebecker HG et al: Clinical response of aluminum-related osteomalacia to desferrioxamine, p. 115A. abstracted. Abstracts IXth International Congress Nephrology, Los Angeles, 1984
4. Massry SG et al: Intractable pruritus as a manifestation of secondary hyperparathyroidism in uremia: disappearance of itching following subtotal parathyroidectomy. N Engl J Med 279:697, 1968
5. Gokal R et al: Histological renal osteodystrophy and 25 hydroxycholecalciferol

and aluminum levels in patients on continuous ambulatory perioneal dialysis. Kidney Int 23:1521, 1983

6. Mirahmadi KS et al: Calcific periarthritis and hemodialysis. JAMA 223:548, 1973

7. Llach F et al: Skeletal resistance of endogenous parathyroid hormone in patients with early renal failure: a possible cause for secondary hyperparathyroidism. J Clin Endocrinol Metab 41:338, 1975

8. Massry SG et al: Abnormalities of the musculoskeletal system in hemodialysis patients. Semin Arthritis Rheum 4:321, 1975

9. Lotem M et al: Spontaneous rupture of tendons: A complication of hemodialyzed patients treated for renal failure. Nephron 21:201, 1978

10. Preston FS, Adicoff A: Hyperparathyroidism with avulsion of three major tendons. N Engl J Med 266:968, 1962

11. Preston ET: Avulsion of both quadriceps tendons in hyperparathyroidism. JAMA 221:406, 1972

12. Mehls O et al: Slipped epiphysis in renal osteodystrophy. Arch Dis Child 50:545, 1975

13. Mehls O et al; Roentgenological signs in the skeleton of uremic children. Pediatr Radiol 1:183, 1973

14. Potter DE et al: Hyperparathyroid bone disease in children undergoing long-term hemodialysis: treatment with vitamin D. J Pediatr 85:60, 1974

15. Scharer K: Growth in children with chronic renal failure. Kidney Int 13(suppl 8):S68, 1978

16. Chantler C et al: Combined report on regular dialysis and transplantation of children in Europe, 1976. Proc Eur Dial Transplant Assoc 14:70, 1977

17. Simmons JM et al: Relation of calorie deficiency to growth failure in children on hemodialysis and the growth response to calorie supplementation. N Engl J Med 285:653, 1971

18. Betts PR, Magrath G: Growth pattern and dietary intake of children with chronic renal insufficiency. Br Med J 2:189, 1974

19. McSherry E, Morris RC: Attainment and maintenance of normal stature with alkali therapy in infants and children with classic renal tubular acidosis (RTA). J Clin Invest 61:509, 1978

20. Chesney RW et al: Increased growth after long-term oral 1, 25-vitamin D_3 in childhood renal osteodystrophy. N Engl J Med 298:238, 1978

21. Chesney RW et al: Influence of long-term oral 1,25 dihydroxyvitamin D in childhood renal osteodystrophy. Contrib Nephrol 18:55, 1980

22. Coburn JW et al: Study of intestinal absorption of calcium in patients with renal failure. Kidney Int 3:264, 1973

23. Goldman R, Bassett SH: Phosphorus excretion in renal failure. J Clin Invest 33:1623, 1954

24. Weeke E, Friis TH: Serum fractions of calcium and phosphorus in uremia. Acta Med Scand 189:79, 1971

25. Kopple JD, Coburn JW: Metabolic studies of low protein diets in uremia: II. Calcium, phosphorus and magnesium. Medicine 52:597, 1973

26. Massry SG et al: Secondary hyperparathyroidism in chronic renal failure: the clinical spectrum in uremia, during hemodialysis and after renal transplantation. Arch Intern Med 124:431, 1969

27. Coburn JW et al: Clinical efficacy of 1,25-di-hydroxyvitamin D_3 in renal osteo-

dystrophy. p. 657. In Norman AW et al (eds): Vitamin D: Biochemical, Chemical and Clinical Aspects Related to Calcium Metabolism. Walter de Gruyter, Berlin, 1977

28. Coburn JW et al: The physiocochemical state and renal handling of divalent ions in chronic renal failure. Arch Intern Med 124:302, 1969

29. Wing AJ et al: Transient and persistent hypercalcaemia in patients treated by maintenance haemodialysis. Br Med J 4:150, 1968

30. Coburn JW et al: Medical treatment in primary and secondary hyperparathyroidism. Semin Drug Treat 2:117, 1972

31. Shimada H et al: Influence of aluminum on the effect of 1 (OH)D on renal osteodystrophy. Nephron 35:163, 1983

32. Boyce BF et al: Hypercalcemic osteomalacia due to aluminum toxicity. Lancet 2:1009, 1982

33. Llach F et al: Prevalence of various types of bone disease in dialysis patients. p. 1374. In Robinson RR (ed): Nephrology. Vol. 2. Springer-Verlag, New York, 1984

34. Papadimitriou M et al: Hypercalcemia from calcium ion-exchange resins in patients on regular hemodialysis. Lancet 2:948, 1968

35. Papapoulos SE et al: Hyperparathyroidism in chronic renal failure. Clin Endocrinol 7(suppl):59S, 1977

36. Koppel MH et al: Thiazide induced rise in serum calcium and magnesium in patients on maintenance hemodialysis. Ann Intern Med 72:895, 1970

37. Barbour GL et al: Extrarenal production of 1,25-dihydroxyvitamin D in an anephric patient with sarcoidosis. N Engl J Med 305:440, 1981

38. Skillen AW, Pierides AM: Serum alkaline phosphatase isoenzyme patterns in patients with chronic renal failure. Clin Chim Acta 80:339, 1977

39. Alvarez-Ude F et al: Hemodialysis bone disease: correlation between chemical, histologic, and other findings. Kidney Int 14:68, 1978

40. Pierides AM et al: Hemodialysis encephalopathy with osteomalacia fractures and muscle weakness. Kidney Int 18:115, 1980

41. Hodsman AB et al: Bone aluminum and histomorphometric features of renal osteodystrophy. J Clin Endocrinol Metab 54:539, 1982

42. Slatopolsky E et al: Parathyroid hormone: alterations in chronic renal failure. p. 1292. In Robinson RR (ed): Nephrology. Vol. 2. Proceedings IXth International Congress Nephrology. Springer-Verlag, New York, 1984

43. Dunlay R, Rodriquez M, Felsenfeld AJ, LLach, F: Direct inhibitory effect of calcitriol on parathyroid function (sigmoidal curve) in dialysis patients. Kidney Int 36:1093, 1989

44. Murphy G, Quarles LD: Intact parathyroid hormone: an index of the presence/severity of osteitis fibrosa. Kidney Int 37:450, 1990

45. Alfrey AC et al: Metabolism and toxicity of aluminum in renal failure. Am J Clin Nutr 33:1509, 1980

46. Alfrey AC: Aluminum. Adv Clin Chem 21:69, 1983

47. Llach F et al: The natural course of dialysis osteomalacia. Kidney Int 28:574, 1986

48. Winney RJ et al: The role of plasma aluminum in the detection and prevention of aluminum toxicity. Kidney Int 28:591, 1986

49. Milliner DS et al: Deferoxamine infusion test for diagnosis of aluminum-related osteomalacia. Ann Intern Med 101:775, 1984

50. de Vernejoul MC, Marchais S, London G et al: Deferoxamine test and bone disease in dialysis patients with mild aluminum accumulation. Am J Kidney Dis 14:124, 1989

51. Hercz G et al: Low turnover bone disease without aluminum in dialysis patients. Kidney Int 35:378, 1989

52. Cannata TB et al: Interpreting the deferroxamine test: effect of iron status. p. 17. In Renal Bone Disease, Parathyroid Hormone and vitamin D. Singapore, 1990

53. Eastwood JB et al: Biochemical and histological effects of 1,25-dihydroxychole-calciferol in the osteomalacia of chronic renal failure. p. 595. In Norman AW et al (eds): Vitamin D and problems related to uremic bone disease. Walter de Gruyter, Berlin, 1975

54. Eastwood JB et al: The effect of 25-hydroxyvitamin D_3 in osteomalacia of chronic renal failure. Clin Sci 52:499, 1977

55. Eisman JA et al: 1,25-Dihydroxyvitamin D in biological fluids: a simplified and sensitive assay. Science 193:1021, 1976

56. Sherrard DJ, Baylink DJ, Wergedal JE, Maloney N: Quantitative histological studies on the pathogenesis of uremic bone disease. J Clin Endocrinol 39:119, 1974

57. Felsenfeld AJ, Llach F: Vitamin D and metabolic bone disease: a clinicopatho-logic overview. Pathol Annu 17:383, 1982

58. Ellis HA, Peart KM: Azotaemic renal osteodystrophy, quantitative study on iliac bone. J Clin Pathol 26:83, 1973

59. Felsenfeld AJ et al: Osteomalacia in chronic renal failure: a syndrome pre-viously reported only with maintenance dialysis. Am J Nephrol 2:147, 1982

60. Platts MM, Owen G, Smith S: Water purification and the incidence of fractures in patients receiving home dialysis supervised by a single centre: Evidence for "safe" upper limit of aluminum in water. Br Med J 288:969, 1984

61. Maloney NA, Ott SM, Alfrey AC et al: Histologic quantitation of aluminum in iliac bone from patients with renal failure. J Lab Clin Med 99:206, 1981

62. Ott SM, Maloney NA, Coburn JW et al: The prevalence of bone aluminum deposition in renal osteodystrophy and its relation to the response to calcitriol therapy. N Engl J Med 307:709, 1982

63. Cournot-Witmer G, Zingraff J, Plachot JJ: Aluminum localization in bone from hemodialyzed patients: relationship to matrix mineralization. Kidney Int 20:375, 1981

64. Sherrard DJ et al: Uremic osteodystrophy: classification, cause and treatment. p. 254. In Frame B, Potts JT, Jr (eds): Proceedings of the Symposium on Clinical Disordors of Bone and Mineral Metabolism. Excerpta Medica, Am-sterdam, 1984

65. Rodriquez M, Lorenzo V, Felsenfeld AJ, Llach F: The effect of parathyroidec-tomy on aluminum toxicity and azotemic bone disease in the rat. J Bone Min Res 5:379, 1990

66. Pei Y et al: Predicting aluminum bone disease in unselected dialysis patients. Am Int Med, in press

67. Parfitt AM: The quantitative approach to bone morphology. A critique of cur-rent methods and their interpretation. p. 86. In Frame B et al (eds.): Clinical Aspects of Metabolic Bone Disease. Excerpta Medica, Amsterdam, 1973

68. Andress DL, Felsenfeld AJ, Voigts A, Llach F: Parathyroid hormone response to hypocalcemia in hemodialysis patients with osteomalacia. Kidney Int 24:364, 1983

69. Jaffe MD, Wellis PW III: Multiple fractures associated with long-term sodium heparin therapy. JAMA 193:152, 196

70. Ritz E, Malluche HH, Krempien B, Mehls O: Bone histology in renal insufficiency. p. 197. In David DS (eds.): Perspectives in Nephrology and Hypertension. John Wiley & Son, New York, 1977

71. Meema HE et al: Periosteal new bone formation (periosteal neostasis) in renal osteodystrophy. Radiology 110:513, 1974

72. Parfitt AM: Clinical and radiographic manifestations of renal osteodystrophy. p. 150. In David DS (ed): Calcium Metabolism in Renal Failure and Nephrolithiasis. John Wiley & Sons, New York, 1977

73. Dent CE, Hodson CJ: Radiological changes associated with certain metabolic bone diseases. Br J Radiol 27:605, 1954

74. Doyle FH et al: Bone resorption in chronic renal failure: a comparison of radiological and histological assessments. Br Med Bull 28:225, 1972

75. Doyle FH: Radiological patterns of bone disease associated with renal glomerular failure in adults. Br Med Bull 28:220, 1972

76. Chalmers J et al: Osteomalacia: a common disease in elderly women. J Bone Joint Surg 49-B:403, 1967

77. Sherrard DJ et al: Skeletal response to treatment with 1,25-dihydroxy-vitam D in renal failure. Contrib Nephrol 18:92, 1980

78. Ellis HA: Aluminum and osteomalacia after parathyroidectomy. Ann Intern Med 96:533, 1982

79. Norfray J et al: Renal osteodystrophy in patients on hemodialysis as reflected in the bony pelvis. Am J Roentgenol Radium Ther Nucl Med 125:352, 1975.

80. Meema HE et al: Improved radiological diagnosis of azotemic osteodystrophy. Radiology 102:1, 1972.

81. Nordin BEC et al: The incidence of osteoporosis in normal women: Its relation to age and menopause. Q J Med 35:25, 1966.

82. Gryfe CI et al: Determination of the amount of bone in the metacarpal. Age Ageing 1:213, 1972.

83. Parfitt AM: The actions of parathyroid hormone on bone: relation to bone remodeling and turnover, calcium homeostasis and metabolic bone disease. Part II of IV parts: PTH and osteoblasts, the relationship between bone turnover and bone loss, and the state of the bones in primary hyperparathyroidism. Metabolism 25:1033, 1976.

84. Cochran M et al: Hypocalcemia and bone disease in chronic renal failure. Nephron 10:113, 1973.

85. Bone JM et al: Role of dialysate calcium concentration in osteoporosis in patients on hemodialysis. Lancet 1:1047, 1972.

86. Cameron JR et al: Precision and accuracy of bone mineral determination by direct photon absorptiometry. Invest Radiol 3:9, 1968.

87. Hahn TJ, Hahn BH: Osteopenia in patients with rheumatic diseases: Principles of diagnosis and therapy. Semin Arthritis Rheum 6:165, 1976.

88. Griffiths HJ et al: The use of photon absorptiometry in the diagnosis of renal osteodystrophy. Radiology 109:277, 1973.

89. Griffiths HJ et al: The long-term follow-up of 195 patients with renal failure: A preliminary report. Radiology 122:643, 1977.

90. Mazess RB et al: Total body mineral and lead body mass by dual photon absorptiometry. Calcif Tissue Int 33:361, 1981.

91. Cohn SH: Techniques for determining the efficacy of treatment of osteoporosis. Calcif Tissue Int 34:433, 1982.

92. Zandetta et al: Bone mineral content in renal transplant patients. p. 92. In Llach F (ed): Renal Bone Disease, Parathyroid Hormone and Vitamin D. Abstract Book, Singapore, 1990

93. Denney JD et al: Total calcium and long term calcium balance in chronic renal disease. J Lab Clin Med 82:226, 1973.

94. Fleisch H, Russel RGG: Experimental clinical studies with pyrophosphate and diphosphonates. p. 293. In David DSD (ed): Calcium Metabolism in Renal Failure and Nephrolithiasis. John Wiley & Sons, New York, 1977

95. Kaye M et al: A study of vertebral bone powder from patients with chronic renal failure. J Clin Invest 49:442, 1970.

96. Lien JWK et al: Abnormal [99m]technetium-tinpyrophosphate bone scans in chronic renal failure. Clin Nephrol 6:509, 1976.

97. Sy WM, Mittal AK: Bone scan in chronic dialysis patients with evidence of secondary hyperparathyroidism and renal osteodystrophy. Br J Radiol 48:878, 1975.

98. Olgaard K et al: Scintigraphic skeletal changes in uremic patients on regular hemodialysis. Nephron 17:325, 1976.

99. Davis BA et al: Scanning for uremic pulmonary calcifications. Ann Intern Med 85:132, 1976.

100. Cann CE et al: Spinal mineral losses in oophorectomized women. JAMA 244:2056, 1980.

101. Norris KC, Crooks PW, Nebeker HG, et al: Clinical and laboratory features of aluminum-related bone disease: differences between sporadic and "epidemic" forms of the syndrome. Am J Kidney Dis 6:342, 1985

102. Coburn JW, Llach F: Renal osteodystrophy. Ch. 4. In Maxwell MH et al (eds): Clinical Disorders of Fluid and Electrolyte Metabolism. 4th Ed. McGraw-Hill, New York, 1987

8

Diagnostic Approach to the Patient With Nephrolithiasis

Mohammed A. J. Sikder
Stanley Goldfarb

Therapy of Hyperoxaluria
Therapy of Uric Acid Stones
Therapy of Struvite Stones
Therapy of Cystine Stones
Lithotripsy

FOLLOW-UP OF PATIENTS WITH RECURRENT NEPHROLITHIASIS

INTRODUCTION

Four to five percent of all Americans have experienced at least one episode of nephrolithiasis, yielding an incidence of approximately 16 cases per 1,000 per year.[1] The overall hospitalization rate is about 20 percent of those affected and is due to the complications of obstruction, infection, and pain.[2] The strategies required to prevent this very common clinical entity have not received adequate attention lately, in part because of the erroneous impression that the advent of extracorporeal shock wave lithotripsy has obviated the need for diligent attempts at preventing stone formation. Rather, the continued morbidity and expense of the therapy requires that an investigative approach to the patient be adopted that allows for an etiologic diagnosis to be made, which, in turn suggests options for prevention. This diagnostic approach rests on a careful history, physical examination, and analysis of laboratory data and will be the focus of this review.

DIAGNOSIS AND MANAGEMENT OF NEPHROLITHIASIS

Acute Stone Passage

Clinical Presentation

Patients with acute stone passage generally present with abdominal pain and hematuria. The pain is usually abrupt in onset, localized to the flank with or without radiation. It is typically constant rather than colicky and is classically severe in nature. Abdominal pain may be associated with nausea, vomiting, and fever. Anterior abdominal pain, however, is a rare clinical presentation of stone passage and should prompt a careful search for other etiologies. Although fever is usually associated with superimposed infection, it can be one of the most common presenting signs of acute stone passage in children.[3]

Localization of pain depends on the site of obstruction. As a general rule, when the stone is located at the renal pelvis or upper part of the ureter, patients usually complain of flank pain. Radiation of pain to the groin and testicle in males and groin and labium in females localizes the stone to the mid- or lower part of the ureter. Obstruction at the terminal ureter usually evokes signs and symptoms of cystitis superimposed on abdominal pain. Pain typically ceases with passage of an obstructing stone. However, when obstruction is continued over many days, pain also diminishes and eventually resolves leading to a situation in which the kidney is irreversibly damaged by the now-painless obstruction.

Passage of a sloughed papilla, clot, or fungal ball can produce symptoms similar to the passage of a stone and should also be considered as potential causes of renal colic. Occasionally, a symptomatic abdominal aortic aneurysm may also present with some of the clinical features of an obstructing renal stone.[4]

Hematuria is typically found and may be microscopic or macroscopic. Hematuria can be caused by direct irritation of the urothelial lining by the crystals or erosion caused by the presence of large stone in the collecting system. Hypercalciuria per se, through unknown mechanisms, may be associated with hematuria in children.[5]

Occasionally, patients may present with volume depletion as a result of vomiting associated with orthostasis. Finally, presentation may be atypical, with silent obstruction with progressive renal failure, adynamic paralytic ileus suggesting a primary gastrointestinal disorder, or as urosepsis.

History and Physical Examination

The medical/surgical history, social, family, drug, and dietary history may provide important hints to the possible cause of the urolithiasis.[6] Physical examination may reveal clinical evidence of extracellular volume depletion secondary to vomiting, adynamic paralytic ileus, and rarely, clinical evidence of urinary tract obstruction such as a palpable, hydronephrotic kidney.[7]

Laboratory Studies

A careful urinalysis using a freshly voided sample is advisable because crystal formation may result from the cooling and spontaneous alkalinization that occurs with prolonged standing. Diagnostically important crystalluria may frequently be found during acute stone passage when freshly voided, warm urine is examined. Stone-associated crystals are shown in Table 8-1. Mild degrees of glycosuria and proteinuria may be seen because of tubular dysfunction induced by obstruction to the urinary tract.

Urine specimens should be sent for culture in all cases of urolithiasis because the co-existence of unsuspected infection and obstruction could be associated with a devastating outcome. Infection is, of course, of paramount etiologic importance in struvite nephrolithiasis. All voided urine during an acute stone passage should be filtered to recover stones or gravel, which is of vital diagnostic importance. Stones are best analyzed by x-ray diffraction, the "gold-standard," with infrared spectroscopy being an acceptable alternative.[8]

Leukocytosis may indicate concurrent infection but may also result from stress-induced demargination. Serum total CO_2 may be low or high, depending on whether acute respiratory alkalosis, resulting from associated pain or anxiety, or metabolic alkalosis resulting from vomiting, are present. A syndrome of type IV renal tubular acidosis (RTA) (hyperkalemia, urine pH less than 5.5, and hyperchloremic acidosis resulting from reduced ammonia production) has been described in association with bilateral ureteral obstruction but is typically seen in conjunction with bladder-outlet obstruction associated with chronic prostatism.[9] Rarely, patients may present with metabolic acidosis associated with renal failure that is due to bilateral obstruction or to concurrent sepsis.

Table 8-1. Composition, Clinical Frequency, and Urinary and Radiographic Appearance of Stone-Forming Components

Stone Type and Composition	Frequency (%)	Urinary and Radiographic Appearance
Calcium oxalate $Ca(COO)_2 \cdot H_2O$ $Ca(COO)_2 \cdot 2H_2O$ Calcium apatite $Ca_{10}(PO_4)_6(OH)_2$	70	"Dumbbells and octahedrons"; radiopaque
Monohydrogen phosphate (brushite) $CaHPO_4 \cdot H_2O$	1–2	Amorphous crystals; radiopaque,
Magnesium ammonium phosphate (struvite) $MgNH_4PO_4 \cdot 6H_2O$	10–15	
Uric acid	10–20	"Coffin lids"; radiopaque
Cystine	<1	"Pears and diamonds"; radiolucent Hexagonal; radiopaque

It is generally not useful to perform extensive biochemical screening tests of calcium metabolism during acute stone passage for several reasons. First, serum calcium levels could be falsely elevated as a result of concurrent volume depletion. Second, abnormalities in urinary calcium, phosphate, citrate, and pH may be induced by acute obstruction and may therefore falsely modify true, steady-state values. One should usually delay such metabolic evaluations until at least 3 months after an acute stone episode.

Radiologic Studies

Radiologic studies are also important tools in the initial evaluation of acute stone passage. A flat film of the abdomen may show the location of a radio-opaque stone and may also provide evidence of ileus, however, a solitary flat plate of the abdomen often is not diagnostic during acute stone passage and may be an unnecessary expense. It is often impossible to detect small stone fragments especially if fecal matter is present throughout the colon.[10–12] Ultrasound examination may be a useful first step, because it may also detect nonradio-opaque stones and can identify the presence of urinary tract obstruction. In one study 79 percent of patients with ureteral obstruction were correctly diagnosed with ultrasound.[13] However, intravenous urography (IVU) remains the standard method for evaluating the obstructed urinary tract. A diagnosis should be sought by promptly performing an IVU unless the patient is truly allergic to contrast media or is at substantial risk for contrast-induced renal failure.[12] Some have recently suggested that IVU can no longer be justified as the primary investigative tool for acute stone passage.[13–15] Ultrasonography has been promoted as a better choice, but it may fail to identify very small stones (less than 5 mm) and cannot define the degree of obstruction. We thus favor the use of IVU in each case of renal colic with possible obstruction.

Therapy

Most kidney stones less than 5 mm in maximum diameter will pass into the urine within 48 hours after the onset of an acute attack. However, the morbidity from a single stone is relatively high, with up to 20 percent requiring some form of intervention to effect passage of the stone. Generally, patients require supportive treatment for pain and extracellular fluid (ECF) volume depletion or dehydration. The majority of patients do not require hospitalization unless they have infection, intractable vomiting, or a poor home situation. The goal of intravenous fluid replacement is to maintain high urine flow rate (100 ml or more per hour). Agents that induce ureteral smooth muscle dilation such as nonsteroidal antiinflammatory drugs (NSAIDs) or calcium channel blockers have been recommended, but the evidence in support of their use is largely anecdotal. In practice, the majority of the cases require narcotic analgesics.

If a totally obstructing stone does not pass, active intervention is needed. Urgent nephrostomy relieves the obstruction and can be followed by extracorporeal shock wave lithotripsy, percutaneous lithotripsy, or rarely, surgical intervention (vide infra). Patients should be considered for metabolic evaluation no sooner than 6 weeks after the acute stone event.[16] An algorithm for the approach to the patient with acute stone passage is provided in Figure 8-1.

CHRONIC AND RECURRENT NEPHROLITHIASIS

Diagnostic Approach to the Patient

Although the approach to patients with chronic or recurrent urolithiasis differs from the approach to acute stone passage, the emphasis of careful history and physical examination remains the same. However, reports of crystallographic analysis are usually available, allowing the diagnosis and therapeutic approaches to be tailored to the specific stone constituents.

It is controversial whether one should pursue extensive biochemical studies for a patient who has passed a single stone, particularly in the absence of

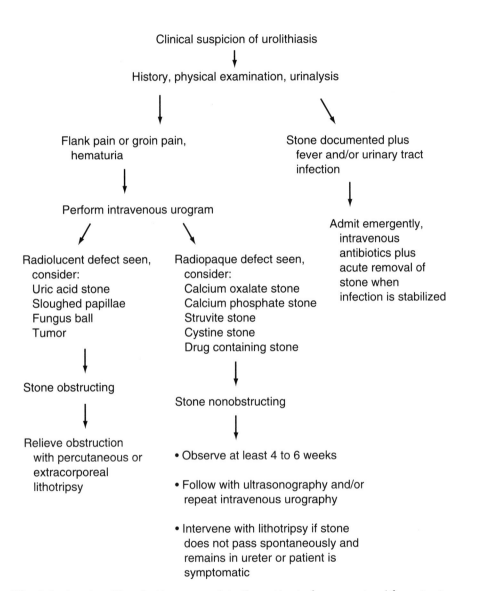

Clinical suspicion of urolithiasis

History, physical examination, urinalysis

Flank pain or groin pain, hematuria

Stone documented plus fever and/or urinary tract infection

Perform intravenous urogram

Radiolucent defect seen, consider:
Uric acid stone
Sloughed papillae
Fungus ball
Tumor

Radiopaque defect seen, consider:
Calcium oxalate stone
Calcium phosphate stone
Struvite stone
Cystine stone
Drug containing stone

Admit emergently, intravenous antibiotics plus acute removal of stone when infection is stabilized

Stone obstructing

Stone nonobstructing

Relieve obstruction with percutaneous or extracorporeal lithotripsy

• Observe at least 4 to 6 weeks

• Follow with ultrasonography and/or repeat intravenous urography

• Intervene with lithotripsy if stone does not pass spontaneously and remains in ureter or patient is symptomatic

Fig. 8-1. An algorithm for the approach to the patient who presents with acute stone passage.

current evidence of continued stone formation. Prospective follow-up of patients with single stones revealed that 11 percent formed a new stone within 3 years, a value similar to that seen for the recurrence rate of individuals who had previously formed multiple stones.[17] Although the decision to proceed with diagnostic studies and laboratory evaluation should be individualized, most physicians delay evaluations until new stones form or in situ stones increase in size.[18] Recurrence of nephrolithiasis is the rule, with a 50 percent chance by 5 years[19] and greater than 60 percent incidence by 9 years.[20] Overall, the natural history of stone disease appears to be one of chronicity with persistence of the tendency to recur well into the seventh decade.[21]

Some patients are particularly prone to recurrent stone disease and should be managed accordingly. This category includes patients with mixed calcium and uric acid stones who have nearly double the rate of recurrence of calcium stone-formers in general[22] and twice that of patients with primary hyperparathyroidism.

Laboratory Evaluation

Once the decision is made to proceed with a more detailed evaluation, which is the case in the majority of patients, one should perform duplicate measurements of 24-hour urine for calcium, phosphate, uric acid, citrate, oxalate, cystine, creatinine, and urea nitrogen and volume while the patient consumes a self-selected diet and fluid intake. Modification of dietary intake before the assessment may obscure any role of diet and fluid in the cause of the patient's stone diathesis. Concomitant plasma determinations of calcium, phosphate, creatinine, uric acid, bicarbonate, and urea nitrogen should be obtained. Fasting urinary pH should be checked in all cases but especially in those with radiologic evidence of nephrocalcinosis, hypokalemia, or hyperchloremic acidosis—all findings of distal RTA. Urinary microscopy, looking for crystals and signs of infection, should be performed, and specimens should be sent for urine culture in all cases.

It is important to emphasize that the complete evaluation should be delayed for at least 6 weeks after an episode of acute nephrolithiasis because the stone passage itself may spawn a number of confounding tubular abnormalities.[23]

Radiologic Studies

Radiologic studies should be performed to localize in situ stones, to document current stone size, and to assess the efficacy of future therapy. Therapy aimed at shrinking stones and preventing new stone formation can be followed in light of these baseline studies. Relative to sonography, IVU has a better sensitivity and specificity for identifying stones and affords the additional benefit of supplying a functional assessment of obstruction. In one study, the overall accuracy rates for identifying stones were 78 percent for sonography and 82 percent for IVU. These rates were 83 percent and 85 percent respectively, in the cases of upper ureteral calculi, and 68 percent and 74 percent, respectively, in lower ureteral stones. When the studies were combined, however, the diagnostic accuracy rate for both modalities increased to 98 percent, 94 percent and 97 percent for upper, lower, and all stones, respectively.[24]

A flat plate with or without tomography should be obtained and contrasted with previous films to identify changes in the size, number, and location of stones.[8]

Computed tomography (CT) scan of the kidney is an excellent modality to identify all radiolucent or radio-opaque calculi.[25,26] Cost, however, limits its routine use.

Diagnostic Approach to Determining Cause

In the Western Hemisphere, 75 percent of stones are calcium-containing (40 percent apatite and 35 percent oxalate), 10 percent are composed of uric acid, 10 percent struvite, and 2 to 3 percent are cystine stones. This distribution varies in other parts of the world, e.g., in Israel, 75 percent of the stones are composed of uric acid.[27]

Crystallographic analysis of the stone serves as the basis for the diagnostic evaluation. This usually means the evaluation of calcium-containing stones, but the exceptions must be carefully pursued as well (vide infra). Factors contributing to stone formation include the quantitative excretion of the stone-forming constituents and the composition of urine, i.e., volume, pH, and the various inhibitors of crystal formation, aggregation, and growth. Unfortunately, at this time, the stone constituents are the major factors that can be routinely assayed, although a few factors that are known to influence the tendency to crystal nucleation, aggregation, and growth have been identified and may be assayed in routine clinical laboratories.

The following summaries will define the approach to the evaluation of a patient with recurrent stone formation after determining the chemical composition of the stone.

Calcium-Containing Stones

The risk factors for calcium-containing stones include (1) increased crystalloid concentration (hypercalciuria, hyperoxaluria, and decreased urine volume); (2) decreased concentration of inhibitors (hypocitraturia, magnesium deficiency, and nephrocalcin deficiency or qualitative abnormalities); and (3) promoters of stone formation (hyperuricosuria and alkaline urinary pH in the case of calcium phosphate stones).

Hypercalciuria

Urinary calcium excretion is normally less than 300 mg/24 hours in males and less than 250 mg/24 hours in females or less than 4 mg/kg body weight per 24 hours.[21] Hypercalciuria may be associated with specific diseases that increased the filtered load of calcium (i.e., hypercalcemia) like primary hyperparathyroidism, sarcoidosis, and other granulomatous diseases, intoxication with either vitamin A or vitamin D, or thyrotoxicosis. It may also be the result of disorders that reduce tubular calcium, reabsorption such as distal renal tubular acidosis and chronic hypophosphatemia.

However, more than 90 percent of the cases of calcium stone formation are idiopathic, and 50 percent of these demonstrate hypercalciuria without hypercalcemia, known tubular disorder, or systemic disorder. Thus, 45 percent of calcium-associated nephrolithiasis results from "idiopathic hypercalciuria." Diet may play a key role in this latter syndrome (vide infra).

Secondary Hypercalciuria

Specific tubular disorders. Distal (type 1) RTA should be suspected when calcium nephrolithiasis is associated with one or more of the following: punctate medullary nephrocalcinosis, a non-anion gap metabolic acidosis, alkaline urine pH, and hypokalemia. These findings, however, can be absent in cases of so-called *incomplete distal RTA*. In this latter instance, a mild form of predominantly intracellular acidosis is manifest by a reduction in the urinary excretion of citrate, the principal chelator of calcium in the urine. Citrate excretion is always reduced in states of acidosis because its proximal reabsorption is stimulated by metabolic acidosis.[28] Fasting urinary pH should be measured in all patients with calcium-containing stones. If fasting urinary pH is greater than 5.5 in the absence of urinary tract infection (a potential cause of increased urinary pH if the infecting organism produces the ectoenzyme urease, vide infra), then one should proceed to an ammonium chloride acid loading test (100 mg/kg body weight, with 500 mg/5 ml solution). If urinary pH does not fall to less than 5.4 at a time when serum bicarbonate falls below 20 mEq/L, classic distal RTA is present. In this condition, hypercalciuria results from the chronic action of acidosis to enhance bone resorption and directly reduce distal nephron reabsorption of calcium.

Hypercalcemic states and hypercalciuria. Primary hyperparathyroidism accounts for 5 percent of calcium stones. Hypercalcemia increases the filtered and therefore the excreted load of calcium despite the opposing action of PTH to enhance calcium reabsorption. The serum calcium level should be measured on at least two separate occasions because intermittent hypercalcemia may be seen in occasional patients with mild hyperparathyroidism.[29,30] One should remember, however, that the normal serum calcium level is lower in women (8.5 to 10.0 mg/dl) than in men (9.0 to 10.5 mg/dl). Therefore, a high "normal" serum calcium level may well represent "hypercalcemia" in a female patient.

The functional state of the parathyroid gland should be analyzed by direct immunoassay of intact immunoreactive PTH (iPTH), but a complete review of the approach to this diagnosis is beyond the scope of this chapter.[31] A hypercalcemic patient with nephrolithiasis, however, likely has primary hyperparathyroidism because patients with tumor-associated hypercalcemia virtually never present with stone disease as the manifestation of the hypercalcemia.[32]

Sarcoidosis and, very rarely, other granulomatous conditions, can cause a particularly severe form of hypercalciuria because the increased filtered load of calcium is combined with secondary suppression of PTH from the hypercalcemia. Urinary calcium excretion rates maybe as high as 600 to 700 mg/day. Circulating levels of 1,2-dihydroxy vitamin D_3 may be increased in these conditions. Vitamin D intoxication may present as hypercalciuria through a similar mechanism. Patients receiving vitamin D supplements to prevent osteoporosis may develop severe hypercalciuria and nephrolithiasis as an unfortunate consequence of this therapy. A careful history for vitamin D intake and measurement of 1,25-hydroxy vitamin D_3 and 25-hydroxy vitamin D_3 will prove the diagnosis of vitamin D intoxication.

Thyroid excess, from inappropriate hormone replacement therapy or from spontaneous disease, may induce hypercalciuria and nephrolithiasis.[33] Characteristic clinical features may be present, but more often, thyroid hormone assays will be required to confirm the diagnosis. Serum calcium is usually normal, but urinary calcium excretion is high in this situation.

Diet-associated hypercalciuria. *Sodium*: The categorization of patients with idiopathic hypercalciuria into diet-dependent or absorptive hypercalciuria, or renal or fasting hypercalciuria has recently been shown to be highly dependent on the dietary sodium intake.[34] *Absorptive hypercalciuria* refers to a condition in which hypercalciuria occurs only with a high dietary intake of calcium or after the oral ingestion of a large calcium load. *Renal hypercalciuria* is defined by an increased urinary calcium excretion (calcium/creatinine, mg/mg greater than 0.12) after an overnight fast.[35-37] In fact, fasting hypercalciuria may be attributable to excess dietary sodium intake in the previous 24 hours in many if not the majority of these patients. Sodium and calcium are handled at similar sites along the nephron, and factors that increase urinary sodium excretion tend to increase urinary calcium excretion as well. For example, increased dietary sodium, hyperaldosteronism in the escape phase, and loop-active diuretics all increase both calcium and sodium excretion.

We reported that "renal" hypercalciurics ingested approximately 50 mEq/d more sodium than the patients designated as "diet-dependent" hypercalciurics (Fig. 8-2). Moreover, restriction of dietary sodium intake can produce a marked and predictable fall in urinary calcium excretion and leads to the recategorization of patients with so-called "renal hypercalciuria" to "diet-dependent hypercalciuria." This apparent dependence of urinary calcium excretion on dietary sodium intake has led to the proposal that specific therapy of hypercalciuria based on such a classification is unwarranted.[34] It logically leads to the proposal that modification of the dietary sodium intake could be a rational form of therapy in these patients.

Dietary protein: The evidence that high dietary protein is an important contributing factor to the risk of recurrent nephrolithiasis derives from the

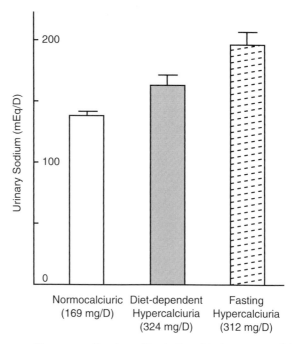

Fig. 8-2. Urinary sodium excretion in patients found to be normocalciuric (open bar), diet-dependent (absorptive) hypercalciuric (shaded bar), and fasting (renal) hypercalciuric (cross-hatched). Initial classifications were based on the measurement of fasting urine calcium/creatinine ratios. This suggests that the level of sodium excretion, and therefore intake, was a determinant of the apparent differences rather than an intrinsic difference in calcium metabolism. (Data from Lau et al.[37])

following findings: (1) population studies that show the clear correlation between the societal consumption of animal protein and the prevalence of upper tract stone disease[8,39]; (2) increased dietary protein ingestion raises urinary calcium, uric acid, and possibly oxalate excretion in normal individuals[40]; (3) the hypocitraturic effect of high dietary protein (which results in the fall in excretion of a principal factor in the chelation of urinary calcium)[41,42]; and (4) the beneficial effect of dietary protein restriction in both studies of vegetarians and in specific therapeutic trials, particularly in individuals who ingest an excessive amount of protein.[43]

In studies from our unit, Wasserstein et al. found that patients with recurrent stone disease tend to be hyper-responsive to the calciuric actions of high dietary protein because they excrete larger amounts of calcium at any level of dietary protein intake than do control subjects.[44]

The underlying mechanism whereby dietary protein leads to hypercalciuria and the reasons for the specific increased sensitivity of patients with recurrent nephrolithiasis to the hypercalciuric action of dietary protein, remain unknown. It is clear, however, that protein effect is expressed at the level of the renal tubule or on an increased glomerular filtration rate rather than any action to raise the level of ionized calcium in the circulation.

The metabolism of dietary protein constituents to strong mineral acids results in increased urinary acid excretion. There is a strong correlation between an increased renal acid excretion and hypercalciuria,[45] probably via a direct inhibition of calcium reabsorption in the distal nephron.[33] The hypercalciuric action of dietary animal protein may thus be a manifestion of increased acidity in the diet and the consequent inhibition of distal nephron calcium reabsorption. However, studies in which the acid load of a high dietary protein was neutralized by exogenous sodium bicarbonate suggested that other, non–acid-related factors may contribute.[46]

Other etiologic factors in recurrent calcium stone formation. *Hyperoxaluria:* Normal 24-hour urinary excretion of oxalate is 55 mg or more in males and 50 mg or less in females, or 0.7 mg/kg/24 h.[47] According to physicochemical considerations, small increments in the urinary oxalate excretion may actually contribute more to calcium oxalate stone formation than a proportional increment in urinary calcium excretion.[48]

Oxalate is an end product of glycine metabolism. The bulk of urinary oxalate is derived from various metabolic pathways, with approximately 40 percent generated from ascorbate while the remainder derives from the metabolism of glycolate, glycine, hydroxyproline, and α-hydroxy-β-ketoadipate.[48] These precursors are primarily found in dietary protein. Under most normal circumstances, the pathways for the metabolism of ascorbate to oxalate are saturated so that any increase in vitamin C intake does not raise the urinary excretion of oxalate.[49] In some individuals, however, marked increases in urinary oxalate excretion occur following the ingestion of 1 to 2 g of ascorbate. Vitamin B_6, pyridoxine, is a cofactor in the interconversion of glycine and glyoxalate. A deficiency of this vitamin results in the increased formation and excretion of oxalate.[49] This fact serves as the basis for recommending pyridoxine therapy for patients with idiopathic hyperoxaluria.

Oxalate itself is a common component of foodstuffs. While ingestion of foods with a very high oxalate content can lead to hyperoxaluria, most foods have a very low oxalate content (less than 0.01 mmol/100 g)[50] so that dietary intake of excessive oxalate is relatively uncommon, even in stone formers. Nonetheless, some studies have found that the urinary oxalate level is higher in patients with recurrent calcium oxalate stones.[48]

The cause of hyperoxaluria in patients with calcium oxalate stones could be multifactorial. Excess dietary oxalate is occasionally seen, but no consistent increase was demonstrated in controlled studies.[51] Evidence for hyperabsorption of oxalate, per se, has been reported in some but not all studies.[52,53] Unabsorbed, unbound calcium in the intestinal lumen can complex with oxalate ions and prevent the anion's absorption. Conversely, a reduction in calcium in the intestinal lumen enhances oxalate absorption. This mechanism has been proposed to explain the hyperoxaluria commonly seen in states of gastrointestinal malabsorption.[48] In these conditions, calcium complexes with unabsorbed fat, rendering dietary oxalate more easily absorbed, and its subsequent excretion leads to hyperoxaluria. Also, alterations in colonic permeability to oxalate (perhaps induced by unabsorbed bile salts) may explain the intestinal hyperabsorption of oxalate in patients with intestinal hyperoxaluria.[48]

Because calcium hyperabsorption is seen in patients with idiopathic hypercalciuria, it has been proposed that the consequent reduction of the calcium content in the more distal portions of the small intestine increases the absorbtion of dietary oxalate.[54] There is no evidence of excess oxalate synthesis in patients with recurrent nephrolithiasis.

The efficacy of reducing dietary oxalate intake in lowering urinary oxalate excretion has been questioned.[48] Several studies, however, have shown that in patients with recurrent idiopathic calcium oxalate stone formation and even in those with primary hyperoxaluria, reducing dietary oxalate intake lowers the renal excretion of oxalate.[55] Moreover, this is particularly effective in patients whose self-selected diet is rich in oxalate. The utility of dietary modification is supported by the observation that no pharmacologic therapy has been consistently successful in reducing urinary oxalate excretion.

Rarely, hyperoxaluria may be due to overproduction (autosomal recessive inheritance in types I and II primary hyperoxaluria). To differentiate between primary and secondary hyperoxaluria, one can measure urinary glycolic acid and L-glyceric acid. Glycolic acid excretion is increased in type I primary hyperoxaluria while L-glyceric acid excretion is increased in type II.[56–58]

Hypocitraturia: Normal urinary excretion of citrate approximates 300 to 900 mg/24 hr with values substantially higher in premenopausal women than in men. Hypocitraturia is usually profound in distal RTA and is perhaps the most important factor for calcium oxalate stone formation in that condition.[28,59] In this condition, as noted, the systemic or, in the case of incomplete RTA, intracellular acidosis is causative. Other causes of hypocitraturia include potassium depletion (presumably because of the intracellular acidosis), bacteriuria (because the organisms may metabolize the urinary citrate), acidifying conditions (e.g., renal failure, chronic diarrhea), and an idiopathic variety that may be associated with recurrent nephrolithiasis.[60]

Hyperuricosuria: In addition to the implications of hyperuricosuria in uric acid stone disease, Coe observed a relationship between hyperuricosuria and a particularly severe form of recurrent calcium oxalate nephrolithiasis.[22] Several groups have studied this phenomenon with a view to unraveling the relationship between uric acid excretion and calcium oxalate stone formation.[61,62] Experimental in vitro studies in highly defined artificial solutions had suggested that urate but not uric acid crystals could act as epitaxial templates and promote calcium oxalate crystal growth.[63] Uric acid crystals, however, are the predominant form in urine; urate crystals are rarely found in urine and are rather poor promoters of crystal growth in highly defined artificial "urines" used in experimental studies defining the nature of crystal growth.[63] Recent studies have suggested an explanation to these inconsistencies. Uric acid crystals can serve to adsorb glutamic acid crystals.[64] This may be the basis for the potency of uric acid as a promoter of crystallization in urine (which contains various organic compounds that act as crystallization inhibitors) but not in defined artificial solutions. In the former, the adsorption of naturally occurring, low molecular weight, organic inhibitors may allow crystal growth and aggregation.

Hyperuricosuria in patients with hypercalciuric, hyperuricosuric stones is a function of excess dietary purine consumption rather than any particular intrinsic abnormality in purine metabolism.[65] Moreover, recent carefully controlled studies have clearly shown the beneficial effects of allopurinol in reducing the frequency of recurrent calcium oxalate stone formation in patients with hyperuricosuria but not hypercalciuria.[66]

Reduced urine volume: Urinary volume is a crucial determinant of the risk of recurrent nephrolithiasis. The risk of calcium stone formation is substantially increased if the urine output is less than 15 ml/kg/d in children[67] and perhaps if less than 2,000 ml/24 h in adults.[8]

Abnormalities in the excretion of inhibitors of stone formation: Those patients who have no identifiable abnormality in any of the previously mentioned urinary constituents and who have recurrent calcium-containing stones probably lack some urinary inhibitors of stone formation or have idiopathic calcium stones. The urine of normal individuals and stone formers is often supersaturated with respect to calcium oxalate; however, inhibitors of crystallization prevent stone formation in most normal individuals. Inhibitors of calcium oxalate crystal growth and aggregation[68,69] in normal urine prevent spontaneous formation of new crystals and inhibit crystal growth at higher concentrations of calcium oxalate than are usually encountered. The growth of crystals in calcium oxalate solutions is markedly decreased in even highly diluted normal urine. Stone formers, on the other hand, produce urine that is deficient in various inhibitors of crystal growth and aggregation.[70–72]

A function relating urine supersaturation and inhibitory activity, the "saturation-inhibition index" was highly correlated with crystalluria and the rate of new stone episodes and is considered the best way to separate normals from stone formers.[70] Additional evidence for the role of inhibitors in preventing calcium oxalate nephrolithiasis comes from the observation that urine from patients with calcium stones, but not from those with uric acid stones, was deficient in inhibitory activity.[71]

Protein macromolecules account for most of the inhibition of crystal growth observed in in vitro assays of normal urine.[72,73] Lower molecular weight urinary substances, including magnesium, pyrophosphate, and citrate, also show inhibitory activity.[74,75] Nakagawa and co-workers[75] have isolated a 14-Kd glycoprotein that has been called *nephrocalcin*, because it contains γ-carboxyglutamic acid (gla), a vitamin K–dependent amino acid that is also found in osteocalcin. Abnormalities in the structure and function of nephrocalcin isolated from the urine and stones of patients with calcium oxalate stones have been detected and include decreased functional activity in crystal growth assays, decreased formation of stable films at the air–water interfaces, decreased affinity of urinary nephrocalcin for calcium oxalate surfaces, and decreased gla content.[75] Taken together, these data suggest that nephrocalcin from stone formers is functionally deficient as a consequence of its decreased gla content. Individuals with this molecular defect would appear to be predisposed to stone formation.

When the assays for urinary crystal inhibitors such as nephrocalcin become widely available, they should increase our understanding of the nature of recurrent kidney stone formation and may suggest exciting new avenues for therapy.

Uric Acid Stones

Although relatively uncommon, uric acid stones may recur frequently and are particularly susceptible to treatment. It must be remembered that uric acid stones are radiolucent; however, it is not uncommon to find them mixed with or coated by calcium crystals so that slight radiopacity my be found in some.

Only 10 to 20 percent of uric acid stones are associated with hyperuricosuria. Typically, serum uric acid and urinary uric acid levels are normal in patients with recurrent uric acid stones. However, excretion of more than 1,000 mg/24 h with an average urinary pH of 5.6 is probably a risk factor for uric acid stone formation.[76] Therefore, 24-h urinary uric acid should be measured particularly in those patients in whom uric acid stone formation has been detected and increased production of uric acid has been suspected.

Urine pH actually has greater impact on stone formation than the urinary uric acid concentration. When the urinary pH decreases from 6 to 5, the undissociated uric acid concentration increases sixfold. Undissociated uric acid solubility is only 90 mg/L. Although the presence of persistently acid urine is an important cause of uric acid stone formation, repeated testing of urine pH to verify this finding generally is unnecessary.

Xanthine and 2,8 dihydroxyadenine (DHA) stones are rare forms of radiolucent stones that may be mistaken for uric acid stones. Both the conditions are inherited as autosomal recessive disorders. The normal urinary xanthine excretory rate is 5.1 to 8.6 mg/24 h. The presence of 2,8 DHA in the urine and gross reduction of adenine phosphoribosyl transferase in erythrocytes allow for the diagnosis of 2,8 DHA stones.[77,78] These two rare forms of radiolucent stone formation are virtually never detected by any means other than actual stone analysis.

Struvite Stones

Infection of the urinary tract with organisms that secrete the ectoenzyme urease can greatly increase the urinary ammonia concentration and pH. The NH_3 formed when urea is deaminated binds protons, thereby alkalinizing the urine. These conditions dramatically increase the risk of forming stones composed of magnesium-calcium-ammonium phosphate (struvite). Characteristically, these stones are very large, extending between minor calyces (i.e., staghorn appearance). The stones are radio-opaque but to a lesser degree than those composed of calcium. The crystals appear "coffin-top" shaped (Table 8-1). Urine and fragments of the stone itself, if available, should be cultured for microorganisms. Many patients with struvite stones also have an underlying metabolic disorder such as hypercalciuria.[79,80] Therefore, a complete metabolic workup should be done to identify the underlying defect once the presence of struvite stones has been detected.

Cystine Stones

Cystinuria is an autosomal recessive condition with an associated disorder of dicarboxylic amino acid (cystine, ornithine, lysine and arginin—COLA) transport involving the intestinal epithelia and renal tubular cells. Cystine stones are moderately radio-opaque as a result of the sulfur atom. Urinalysis may demonstrate characteristic hexagonal crystals in approximately 50 percent of patients, but the cyanide nitroprusside test is more useful for screening. The nitroprusside test is positive at a concentration of greater than 75 mg/g of creatinine.[47] If a qualitative test is positive for cystinuria, a 24-hour quantitative urinary cystine excretion rate should be determined. Some cystinuric patients will not present until the fifth or even sixth decade, so the patient's age should not deter one from pursuing this diagnosis.[81]

PREVENTION AND TREATMENT OF KIDNEY STONES

The long-term treatment goal for patients with recurrent hephrolithiasis is to prevent both new stone formation and the growth of existing stones. Prevention of renal stone formation can be accomplished by (1) reducing the concentration of stone-forming factors in the urine, (2) manipulating the ionic milieu of the urine to favor solubilization of these stone-producing factors, and (3) correcting any mechanical or structural abnormalities that are associated with stasis in the urinary tract.

Therapy of Idiopathic Hypercalciuria

The initial treatment strategy for patients with recurrent calcium-containing stones or for any patient with recurrent stone disease is to treat the underlying disorder. One must be certain, however, that treatment is being recommended for active stone-forming disease. Thus, it is important to know if a patient's stones have been formed recently and to know that a stone that is currently being passed is not one formed months or even years ago. Patients should not receive specific therapy unless radiologic evidence indicates stone growth or new stone formation in the preceding 6 months.

Dietary Modification

In cases of active stone formation, there is a persistent reliance on pharmacologic therapy for the prevention of recurrent kidney stone formation. In fact, the evidence for the efficacy of various pharmacologic treatments for the prevention of recurrent nephrolithiasis is quite weak,[82] and the long-term safety of such drugs as thiazide diuretics has recently been questioned.[83] The reliance on pharmacologic therapies comes in the face of increasing evidence of a marked benefit of mere entry into a nonpharmacologic diet and fluid modification protocol at a clinic specializing in the evaluation and therapy of recurrent nephrolithiasis (the "Stone Clinic Effect"[18]). As noted previously, the epidemic of nephrolithiasis that has occurred in the developed world during the 20th century is in part the result of the diet consumed in these affluent nations.[38] High dietary protein intake is probably the most important factor.[84] The patients who develop nephrolithiasis in the population may also have an increased calciuric response to dietary protein and perhaps to dietary sodium. The benefits of dietary modification include not only a tendency toward a reduction in urinary calcium excretion but also an increase in urinary citrate excretion[85] and reduction in urinary oxalate excretion. The latter two factors also ameliorate the tendency toward stone formation. Prescription of a high fluid intake is also an important component of therapy.[76]

The benefits of dietary therapy in patients with recurrent stone formation have not as yet been rigorously tested in controlled studies, but there are also very few valid clinical studies of various pharmacologic agents such as thiazides, phosphates, allopurinol, or citrate.[82] In the absence of clear-cut advantage of any specific pharmacologic agent, it appears that many patients may benefit from dietary modification before embarking on a lifelong use of medications to prevent stone recurrences. Certain other specific therapies are obviously indicated in certain conditions; for example, patients with primary hyperparathyroidism require surgery, whereas those with distal RTA require alkali therapy.

In some patients, however, dietary modification may fail if patients are persistently hypercalciuric despite dietary modification or if patients persistently form stones; then, pharmacologic therapy should be considered. The agents currently available for the reduction of urinary calcium excretion include thiazide diuretics and dietary phosphate supplementation. Each of these agents has been shown to be effective in the prevention of recurrent kidney stones. However, few long-term controlled studies have been carried out. Therefore, pharmacologic treatment of hypercalciuria should be reserved for patients with active stone formation, evidence of new stones within the prior 6 to 12 months, hypercalciuria, and failure to respond to dietary manipulation.

Pharmacologic Therapy

Hydrochlorothiazide. Hydrochlorothiazide, 50 to 100 mg/d, effectively reduces calcium excretion. Failure of this therapy is usually due to a concomitant and marked increase in sodium intake.[86] Thiazides must reduce ECF volume to effect its full hypocalciuric action.[87] The impact of the diuretic's side effects (e.g., hyperlipidemia, glucose intolerance, and mild hypokalemia) has not been extensively studied in patients with urolithiasis. It has been shown that bone mineralization probably increases in individuals given long-term thiazides.[88,89] To date, however, no clinically detectable abnormalities in bone have resulted from thiazide usage in patients with urolithiasis. Those who have underlying disorders of calcium metabolism, such as primary hyperparathyroidism, or those individuals treated with vitamin D supplements, may be at risk of hypercalcemia when receiving thiazide therapy. Serum calcium levels should be monitored for a 2-month period after initiating thiazide therapy.

Amiloride. Amiloride also has a hypocalciuric action, probably by secondarily stimulating a Gasolateral Na/Ca antiporter and thereby stimulating calcium transport in the distal convoluted tubule.[90] It may be a particularly useful agent, because it tends to retard potassium excretion and prevent typical thiazide-induced hypokalemia. Potassium depletion leads to intracellular acidosis and tends to lower urinary citrate excretion.[60] Therefore, when thiazide therapy is contraindicated or ineffective (as it is in approximately 7 to 15 percent of patients treated[21,86]), amiloride could be used as an adjuct or substitute.

Neutral sodium or potassium phosphate. Neutral sodium or potassium phosphate is an effective therapy for hypercalciuria.[91] Phosphates act by both reducing bone resorption of calcium and promoting renal calcium reabsorption. They have little direct effect on gut calcium absorption, although they may interfere with the activation of vitamin D. Long-term studies of phosphate therapy suggest that it is a safe and effective treatment even though short-term side effects like diarrhea are a frequent problem.[92,93] These agents must be administered four times each day and thus are somewhat inconvenient to take. Acid-containing phosphate salts should not be used because the effects of acidosis on bone and kidney (hypocitraturia and hypercalciuria) may override the beneficial effects of the phosphate salt per se.[94]

Cellullose phosphate. Cellulose phosphate has been advocated as an effective treatment for calcium stone disease, particularly in cases of renal failure induced by sarcoid-associated nephrocalcinosis, hypercalcemia, and hypercalciuria after parathyroidectomy, and in children who have shown inadequate response to thiazide therapy.[95–97] This drug acts as a nonabsorbable ion exchange resin that binds calcium in the gastrointestinal tract.[98,99] This effect, of course, increases the risk of secondary hyperoxaluria and may negate the beneficial action of this agent on urinary calcium excretion.

Potassium citrate. A subpopulation of patients with calcium-containing stones may not be hypercalciuric but rather may demonstrate a marked hypocitraturia. This entity may be the result of an underlying metabolic disorder or be a function of one of the various forms of chronic acidosis. Recent studies suggest that dietary supplementation of a citrate-containing salt (1 mEq/kg body weight) raises the level of urinary citrate excretion. This effect results from the alkali load produced by citrate supplementation rather than from the direct appearance of ingested citrate in the urine. In long-term studies, citrate therapy has been shown to effectively reduce the frequency of new stone formation.[85,100–102]

Therapy of Hyperoxaluria

If urinary oxalate excretion exceeds the normal range in patients with recurrent stone formation, it is often *not* the result of excess dietary oxalate.[58] However, as noted, hyperabsorption of oxalate may result from hyperabsorption of calcium. In certain patients, particularly those with inflammatory bowel disease, additional intake of calcium, as calcium carbonate (500 mg four times a day), may bind intestinal oxalate and reduce its absorption. Oxalate absorption can be reduced by such ionic exchange resins as cholestyramine. This resin binds bile acid, the free form of which is known to increase the colonic absorption of oxalate by increasing its permeability to the intestinal wall.[54]

Pyridoxine (250 to 500 mg/d) has been shown to significantly reduce the urinary excretion of oxalate.[103] Pyridoxine acts by altering the cellular metabolism of glycine, and a trial is indicated in those cases in which the dietary restriction of oxalate and increase of calcium intake are not effective in reducing hyperoxaluria.

Finally, the finding of both hypercalciuria and hyperuricosuria has been proposed as a cause of a particularly virulent form of recurrent urolithiasis. The therapy of hyperuricosuria with dietary purine restriction or with allopurinol may be beneficial in this subpopulation of patients if the usual therapy for hypercalciuria fails to alleviate the disorder.[104]

Therapy of Uric Acid Stones

In those patients with increased excretion of uric acid, the options for treatment include dietary purine restriction, urinary alkalinization, and the administration of allopurinol. Urinary alkalinization can be achieved with sodium bicarbonate (1 to 1.5 mEq/kg/d) or its equivalent. Although such therapy substantially reduces the risk of further uric acid stones, it is also possible that the risk of calcium phosphate stone formation increases because of the alkaline urine pH. Patients must be instructed in the measurement of urinary pH with nitrazine paper and must strive to maintain the value above 7 but under 7.5 pH units.

Allopurinol therapy (200 to 300 mg/24 h) is quite effective in reducing uric acid excretion in patients with hyperuricosuria and is the preferred treatment. The side effects of rash and other hypersensitivity phenomena must be carefully monitored.

In the majority of patients with uric acid stones, uric acid excretion is quantitatively normal. In these patients, alkali therapy is more likely to be effective and should be advocated. Allopurinol may also be useful in such patients if alkalinization and fluid therapy fail.

Therapy of Struvite Stones

Preventing recurrences of struvite stones depends on the success in sterilizing the urine. Because organisms may exist in the interstices of the calculus material itself, it is crucial that all such material be removed from the urinary tract.[105] To achieve this goal, percutaneous or extracorporeal shock wave lithotripsy (ESWL) has almost completely supplanted standard surgical procedures. The combination of nonsurgical stone removal and irrigation of the urinary tract with a solution of strong organic acids (10 percent citric acid compound [Renacidin]) can successfully remove all visible calculus material.[106,107] This approach and organism-specific, prolonged antimicrobial therapy can result in complete cure of struvite stones in over 90 percent of those treated.[105]

In rare cases where such treatment cannot be attempted, the use of medical therapy is indicated as a second-line approach. Acetohydroxamic acid is an orally active urease inhibitor.[108,109] This agent has been shown to be effective in preventing stone growth even when stone fragments and bacterial infection persist. Unfortunately, it has several significant side effects including hemolytic anemia, intractable headache, and possible thrombophlebitis.[109,110]

Therapy of Cystine Stones

Medical treatment consists of (1) reducing the urinary cystine concentration by hydration, (2) increasing cystine solubility by alkalanization, and (3) lowering the urine cystine concentration with agents such as D-penicillamine or thiola.

Cystine solubility limits in urine with a pH less than 7.5 is approximately 300 mg/L. To prevent stone formation or growth in cystinuric patients excreting more than 500 mg/d, continuous fluid therapy over 24 hours is required. Occasionally, patients can achieve this goal, but the majority fail, particularly adolsecents or young adults in whom compliance with high fluid intake may be difficult to achieve. A patient whose 24-hour urinary excretion of cystine is greater than 1,000 mg, a relatively common finding, requires a urine volume of at least 4 L/d spread uniformly over a 24-hour interval to prevent stone growth. This daunting task guarantees that most patients will fail fluid therapy combined with alkalinization.

Alkali therapy is beneficial because the solubility limit of cystine can be doubled (to 600 mg/L of urine) by maintaining urinary pH at 7.5 to 7.8.[111] Such levels are difficult to achieve but may be attempted in highly motivated patients. Unfortunately, a key side effect of this treatment is the increased propensity to calcium phosphate stone formation. Recent studies also suggest that reduction of dietary sodium intake may increase renal cystine reabsorption and thereby reduce the urinary burden.[111]

In some patients, therapy with D-Penicillamine[113] or related drugs (e.g., α-mercaptopropyl glycine (AMPG)[113] and captopril[114] may be required. These compounds form mixed, soluble disulfides with cysteine and thereby prevent cystine stone formation. Unfortunately up to 90 percent of patients treated with D-Penicillamine develop a side effect that causes its discontinuation. However, comparative study with AMPG showed that serious adverse effects requiring cessation of therapy were approximately 50 percent less frequent than with D-Penicillamine administration[113]. Side effects from D-Penicillamine therapy range from insomnia and dysgeusia to a vasculitis syndrome and Goodpasture's syndrome. Insomnia and dysgeusia can be prevented by zinc supplements. Pyridoxine supplements are required to prevent its deficiency. The therapeutic benefit claimed for captopril therapy was based on a study of only two patients.[114] This therapeutic approach requires further study.

Daytime fluid therapy combined with night-time D-Penicillamine administration may be an effective approach in reducing the risk of cystine stone formation while reducing the risk of D-Penicillamine toxicity. A lower, and, therefore, less toxic, dose of the drug is used in this protocol.

Lithotripsy

The treatment of renal and ureteral stones has undergone rapid and major changes since 1980. ESWL has become the most commonly used modality for the treatment of renal and upper ureteral stones. Ureteral stones, however, are more commonly being approached by retrograde techniques. Percutaneous and open surgical nephrolithotomy offer viable alternatives in certain clinical situations.[115] These revolutionary approaches, however, should not supplant a careful prophylactic program of fluid, dietary, and pharmacologic therapy for the amelioration of the various disorders that lead to nephrolithiasis.

FOLLOW-UP OF PATIENTS WITH RECURRENT NEPHROLITHIASIS

The objective of periodic follow-up visits of patients is to detect recurrent stone formation, any complications of urolithiasis and, of course, to monitor the effects of treatment. The physician should monitor the rate of stone growth, the presence of new stone formation, document passage of stones or gravel within the past year and determine whether obstruction and/or infection is present. Yearly abdominal flat plate, sonogram, and/or IVU may be needed to assess the "metabolic activity" of such patients. The choice and frequency of the study should be individualized. The general recommendation is to see the patient at 6- to 12-month intervals, but this interval may be shorter for patients in whom exuberant stone formation has been documented. Follow-up flat plate films may be all that is necessary to assess the activity of radio-opaque stones. For radiolucent stones, sonography or IVU may be required. In addition to radiologic follow-up, routine urinalysis and 24-hour urine collection are needed to measure volume, calcium, sodium, urea nitrogen, citrate, uric acid, and oxalate excretion. For those patients treated with pharmacologic therapy, other follow-up parameters should be mentioned. First, urinary phosphate excretion should be monitored in those patients treated with neutral phosphate salts. Urinary phosphate excretion should exceed 1,500 mg/24 h in such individuals. Also, those patients treated with thiazides should excrete less than 125 mEq/24 h of sodium, should have slightly reduced serum potassium level (greater than 3.5, less than 4.3 mEq/L) and urine potassium excretion equal to the normal intake of 60 mEq/24 h. Review of the diet by a dietician may be necessary to counsel those patients who demonstrate excessive urinary urea nitrogen (indicating excessive dietary protein intake) or who have hypercalciuria that is due to excess sodium intake.

ACKNOWLEDGMENTS

These studies were supported by research grants from the National Institutes of Health, grant no. DK39727, an NIH Training Grant no. T32-AM07006, and grant no. M01-RR0040.

REFERENCES

1. O'Brien W, Rotolo J, Pahira J: New approaches in the treatment of renal calculi. AFP 36:181, 1987
2. Drach C: Urinary lithiasis. p. 1094. In Walsh PC (ed): Campbell's Urology. WB Saunders, Philadelphia, 1986

3. Hadidy S, Shamma M, Kharma A: Some features of pediatric urolithiasis in a group of Syrian children. Int Urol Nephrol 19:3, 1987
4. Borrero E, Queral L: Symptomatic abdominal aortic aneurysm misdiagnosed as nephroureterolithiasis. Ann Vasc Surg 2:145, 1988
5. Stapleton F: Idiopathic hypercalciuria: association with isolated hematuria and risk for urolithiasis in children. The Southwest Pediatric Nephrology study group. Kidney Int 37(2):807, 1990
6. Wilson D: Clinical and laboratory approaches for evaluation of nephrolithiasis. J Urol 141:770, 1989
7. Kapoor R, Saha M, Pandey K: Renal stone presenting as an abdominal lump. J Urol 140:354, 1988
8. Wilson D: Clinical and laboratory evaluation of renal stone patients. Endocr Metab Clin North Am 19:773, 1990
9. Batlle D, Arruda J, Kurtzman N: Hyperkalemic distal renal tubular acidosis associated with obstructive uropathy. N Engl J Med 304:373, 1981
10. Zangerle K, Iserson K, Bjelland J: Usefulness of abdominal flat-plate radiographs in patients with suspected ureteral calculi. Ann Emerg Med 14:316, 1985
11. Roth C, Bowyer B, Berquist T: Utility of the plain abdominal radiograph for diagnosing ureteral calculi. Ann Emerg Med 14:316, 1985
12. Stewart C: Nephrolithiasis. Emerg Med Clin North Am 6:617, 1988
13. Kuuliala I, Niemi L, Ala-Opas M: Ultrasonography for diagnosis of obstructing ureteral calculus. Scand J Urol Nephrol 22:275, 1988
14. Kunz B, Baars H, Heuer H, Pfannenberg C: Diagnostic strategy in urolithiasis. Radiol Diagn 30:429, 1989
15. Bazzocchi M, Stacul F, Cressa C, Dalla-Palma L: Echography in renal colic. Radiol Med 76:78, 1988
16. Urivetzky M, Ravalli R, Weinberg J, Smith A: Biochemical evaluation of calcium stone patients: how soon can it be done after stone surgery/passage? Urology 36(5):410, 1990
17. Strauss A, Coe F, Parks J: Formation of a single calcium stone of renal origin. Arch Intern Med 142:504, 1982
18. Hosking D, Erickson S, Van Den Berg C et al: The stone clinic effect in patients with idiopathic calcium urolithiasis. J Urol 130:1115, 1983
19. Blacklock N: The pattern of urolithiasis in the Royal Navy. p. 235. In Nordin BEC, Hodgkinson A (ed): Proceedings of the Renal Stone Research Symposium. Churchill Livingstone, London, 1969
20. Williams R: Long-term survey of 538 patients with upper urinary tract stones. Br J Urol 35:416, 1963
21. Coe F: Treated and untreated recurrent calcium nephrolithiasis in patients with idiopathic hypercalciuria, hyperuricosuria or no metabolic disorder. Ann Intern Med 87:404, 1977
22. Coe F: Calcium-uric acid nephrolithiasis. Arch Intern Med 138:1090, 1978
23. Jaeger P, Portmann L, Ginalski JM, et al: Tubulopathy in nephrolithiasis: consequence rather than cause. Kidney Int 29:563, 1986
24. Saita H, Matsukawa M, Fukushima H et al: Ultrasound diagnosis of ureteral stone: its usefulness with subsequent excretory urography. J Urol 140:28, 1988
25. Segal A, Spataro R, Linke C, Frank IN et al: Diagnosis of nonopaque calculi by computed tomography. Radiology 129:447, 1978

26. Federle M, McAninch JW Kaiser JA et al: Computed tomography of urinary calculi. Am J Roentgenol 136:255, 1981
27. Atsman A, Devries A, Frank M: Uric Acid Lithiasis. Elsevier, Amsterdam, 1963
28. Simpson D: Citrate excretion: A window on renal metabolism. Am J Physiol 244:F223, 1983
29. Ladenson J, Lewis J, McDonald J et al: Relationship of free and total calcium in hypercalcemic conditions. J Clin Endocrinol Metab 48:393, 1978
30. Muldowney F, Freaney R, McMullin J et al: Serum ionized calcium and parathyroid hormone in renal stone disease. Q J Med 45:75, 1976
31. Blind E, Schmidt-Gayk H, Scharla S, et al: Two-site assay of intact parathyroid hormone in the investigation of primary hyperparathyroidism and other disorders of calcium metabolism compared with midregion assay. J Clin Endocrinol Metab 67:353, 1988
32. Blomqvist CP: Malignant hypercalcemia—a hospital survey. Acta Med Scand 220:455, 1986
33. Agus Z, Goldfarb S, Wasserstein A: Calcium transport in the nephron. Rev Physiol Biochem Pharmacol 90:155, 1981
34. Wasserstein A, Agus Z: How extensive should the workup be for hypercalciuric patients with nephrolithiasis? The case for a limited evaluation. p. 303. In Narins RG (ed): Controversies in Nephrology and Hypertension. Churchill Livingstone, New York, 1984
35. Reusz G, Tulassay T, Szabo A et al: Studies on the urinary calcium excretion in children with hematuria of postglomerular origin: effect of the variation of dietary calcium and sodium intake. Int J Pediatr Nephrol 7(4):221, 1986
36. Pak C: Pathogenesis of idiopathic hypercalciuria. p. 205. In Hypercalciuric States, Pathogenesis, Consequences, and Treatment. Grune & Stratton, Orlando, FL, 1984
37. Lau Y, Wasserstein A, Westby G et al: Proximal tubular defects in idiopathic hypercalciuria: resistance to phosphate administration. Miner Electrolyte Metab 7:237, 1982
38. Andersen D: Environmental factors in the etiology of urolithiasis. p. 130. In Civuentes-Delatte RA, Hodgkinson A (eds): Urinary calculi. Karger, Basel, 1973
39. Robertson W, Peacock M, Heyburn P: Risk factors in calcium stone disease of the urinary tract. Br J Urol 50:449, 1981
40. Lemann J Jr, Gray W, Maierhofer W et al: The importance of renal net acid excretion as a determinant of fasting urinary calcium excretion. Kidney Int 29:743, 1986
41. Nicar M, Skurla C, Sakhaee K et al: Low urinary citrate excretion in nephrolithiasis. Urology 21:8, 1983
42. Schwille P, Scholz D, Schwille K et al: Citrate in urine and serum and associated variables in subgroups of urolithiasis. Nephron 31:194, 1982
43. Robertson W, Peacock M, Heyburn P: Should recurrent calcium oxalate stone formers eat less animal protein? p. 359. In Urolithiasis: Clinical and Basic Research. Plenum, New York, 1981
44. Wasserstein A, Stolley P, Goldfarb S, Agus Z: Case control study of risk factors for calcium nephrolithiasis. Miner Electrolyte Metab 13:85, 1987
45. Lemann J Jr, Adams N, Gray R: Urinary calcium excretion in human beings. N Engl J Med 301:535, 1979
46. Lutz J: Calcium balance and acid-base status of women as affected by increased

protein intake and by sodium bicarbonate ingestion. Am J Clin Nutr 39:281, 1984

47. Smith L: Urolithiasis. p. 785. In Schrier R, Gottschalk CW (eds.): Diseases of the Kidney. Little, Brown, Boston, 1989

48. Larsson L, Tiselius H-G: Hyperoxaluria. Miner Electrolyte Metab 13:242, 1987

49. Tiselius H-G, Almgard L: The diurnal excretion of oxalate and effect of pyridoxine and ascorbate on the oxalate excretion. Eur Urol 3:41, 1977

50. Kasidas G, Rose G: Oxalate content of common foodstuffs: determination by an enzymatic method. J Hum Nutr 34:2555, 1980

51. Menon M, Mahle C: Oxalate metabolism and renal calculi. J Urol 137:148, 1982

52. Tiselius H-G, Ahlstrand C, Lundstrom B: [^{14}C]-oxalate absorption by normal persons, calcium oxalate stone formers, and patients with surgically disturbed intestinal function. Clin Chem 27:1682, 1981

53. Hodgkinson A: Evidence of increased oxalate absorption in patients with calcium containing renal stones. Clin Sci Mol Med 54:291, 1978

54. Dobbins J, Binder H: Effect of bile salts and fatty acids on the colonic absorption of oxalate. Gastroenterology 70:1096, 1976

55. Tiselius H-G: Oxalate and renal stone formation. Scand J Urol Nephrol 53(suppl):135, 1980

56. Danpure C, Jennings P: Peroxisomal alanine: glyoxylate aminotransferase deficiency in primary hyperoxaluria type I. Publication of Federation of European Biochemical Societies 201:20, 1986

57. Danpure C, Purkiss P, Jennings P, Watts R: Mitochondrial damage and the subcellular distribution of 2-oxoglutarate: glyoxylate carboligase in normal human and rat liver and in the liver of patient with primary hyperoxaluria type I. Clin Sci 70:417, 1986

58. Williams H, Smith L Jr: Primary hyperoxaluria. p. 204. In Stanbury JB, Wyngaarden JB, Fredrickson DS et al (eds): The Metabolic Basis of Inherited Disease. 5th Ed. McGraw-Hill, New York, 1983

59. Cohen J, Kamm D: Renal metabolism relation to renal function. p. 126. In Brenner B Rector FC Jr (eds): The Kidney. vol. 1. WB Saunders, Philadelphia, 1976

60. Pak C, Fuller C: Idiopathic hypocitraturic calcium-oxalate nephrolithiasis successfully treated with potassium citrate. Ann Intern Med 104:33, 1986

61. Sarig S, Hirsch D, Garti N: An extension of the concept of epitaxial growth. Crystalline Growth 69:92, 1984

62. Pak C, Waters O, Arnold L: Mechanisms for calcium urolithiasis among patients with hyperuricosuria. J Clin Invest 59:426, 1977

63. Coe F, Lawton R, Goldstein R: Sodium urate accelerates precipitation of calcium oxalate in vitro. Proc Soc Exp Biol Med 149:926, 1975

64. Sarig S: The hyperuricosuric calcium oxalate stone former. Miner Electrolyte Metab 13:251, 1987

65. Coe F, Moran E, Lavalich A: The contribution of dietary purine over consumption to hyperuricosuria in calcium oxalate in vitro. Proc Soc Exp Biol Med 149:926, 1975

66. Ettinger B, Citron J, Tang A et al: Prophylaxis of calcium oxalate stones: clinical trials of allopurinol, magnesium hydroxide, and chlorthalidone. p. 549. In Urolithiasis and Related Clinical Research. Plenum, New York, 1985

67. Miller L, Stapleton F: Urine volume in children with urolithiasis. J Urol 141:918, 1989

68. Rose MB: Renal stone formation The inhibitory effect of urine on calcium oxalate precipitation. Invest Urol 12:428, 1975
69. Meyer JL, Smith LH: Growth of calcium oxalate crystals II. Inhibition by natural urinary crystal growth inhibitors. Invest Urol 13:36, 1975
70. Robertson WG, Peacock M, Marshall RW et al: Saturation-inhibition index as a measure of the risk of calcium oxalate stone formation in the urinary tract. N Engl J Med 294:249, 1976
71. Coe FL, Margolis HC, Deutsch LH, Strauss AL: Urinary macromolecular crystal growth inhibitors in calcium nephrolithiasis. Mineral Electrolyte Metab 3:268, 1980
72. Fleisch H: Inhibitors and promoters of stone formation. Kidney Int 13:361, 1978
73. Fleisch H, Bisaz S: Isolation from urine of pyrophosphate: a calcification inhibitor. Am J Physiol 203:671, 1962
74. Ito H, Coe FL: Acidic peptide and polyribonucleotide crystal growth inhibitors in human urine. Am J Physiol 233:F455, 1977
75. Nakagawa Y, Abram V, Parks JH et al: Urine glycoprotein crystal growth inhibitors: evidence for a molecular abnormality in calcium oxalate nephrolithiasis. J Clin Invest 76:1455, 1985
76. Members of the Consensus Development Panel NIH: Prevention and treatment of kidney stones. JAMA 260(7):977, 1988
77. Gault M, Simmonds H, Snedden W et al: Urolithiasis due to 2,8-dihydroxyadenine in an adult. N Engl J Med 305:1570, 1981
78. Witten F, Morgan J, Foster J et al: 2,8-Dihydroxyadenine urolithiasis: review of the literature and report of a case in the United States. J Urol 130:938, 1983
79. Resnick M: Evaluation and management of infection stones. Urol Clin North Am 8:265, 1981
80. Segura J, Erickson S, Wilson D et al: Infected renal lithiasis: result of long-term surgical and medical management. p. 195. In Smith LH, Robertson WG, Finlayson B (eds): Urolithiasis: Clinical and Basis Research, Plenum, New York, 1981
81. Dahlberg P, Van Den Berg C, Kurtz S et al: Clinical features and management of cystinuria. Mayo Clin Proc 52:533, 1977
82. Churchill D: Medical treatment to prevent recurrent calcium urolithiasis: a guide to critical appraisal. Miner Electrolyte Metab 13:294, 1987
83. Churchill D, Taylor D: Thiazides for patients with recurrent calcium stones: still an open question. J Urol 133:749, 1985
84. Allen L, Oddoye E, Margen S: Protein-induced hypercalciuria: a longer term study. Am J Clin Nutr 32:741, 1979
85. Pak C, Fuller C, Sakhaee K et al: Long-term treatment of calcium nephrolithiasis with potassium citrate. J Urol 134:11, 1985
86. Yendt E: Renal calculi. Can Med Assoc J 102:479, 1970
87. Suki WN: Calcium and the kidney—from stones to molecules. Verh K Acad Geneeskd Belg 52:203, 1990
88. Steiniche T, Mosekilde L, Chistensen M, Melsen F: Histomorphometric analysis of bone in idiopathic hypercalciuria before and after treatment with thiazide. APMIS 97:302, 1989
89. Ray W, Griffin M, Downey W, Melton L: Long-term use of thiazide diuretics and risk of hip fracture. Lancet 1:687, 1989
90. Scoble J, Goligorsky M, Westbrook S et al: Role of Na/Ca exchange in calcium

transport by canine proximal tubular (PT) cell monolayer. Fed Proc 44:1899, 1985

91. Insogna K, Ellison A, Burtis W et al: Trichlormethiazide and oral phosphate therapy in patients with absorptive hypercaciuria. J Urol 141:269, 1989

92. Smith L, Thomas W, Arnaud CD: Orthophosphate therapy in calcium renal lithiaais. Urinary Calculi 188, 1973

93. Thomas WJ: Use of phosphates in patients with calcareous renal calculi. Kidney Int 13:390, 1978

94. Lau K, Wolf C, Nussbaum P et al: Differing effects of acid versus neutral phosphate therapy of hypercalciuria. Kidney Int 16:736, 1979

95. Burke J, Cowley D, Mottrem B, Buckner P: Cellulose phosphate and chlorothiazide in childhood idiopathic hypercalciuria. Aust NZ J Med 16:43, 1986

96. Evans R: Hypercalcaemia: what does it signify? Drugs 31:64, 1986

97. Waron M, Weissgarten J, Gil I et al: Sarcoid nephrocalcinotic renal failure reversed by sodium cellulose phosphate. Am J Nephrol 6:220, 1986

98. Pak C: Clinical pharmacology of sodium cellulose phosphate. Clin Pharmacol 19:451, 1979

99. Blacklock N, MacLeod M: The effect of cellulose phosphate on intestinal absorption and urinary excretion of calcium. Br J Urol 46:385, 1974

100. Pak C, Fuller C, Sakhaee K et al: J Urol 13:1003, 1986

101. Pak C, Peterson R: Successful treatment of hyperuricosuric calcium oxalate nephrolithiasis with potassium citrate. Arch Intern Med 246(5): 863, 1986

102. Pak C, Peterson R, Sakhaee K et al: Correction of hypocitraturia and prevention of stone formation by combined thiazide and potassium citrate therapy in thiazide-unresponsive hypercalciuric nephrolithiasis. Am J Med 79:284, 1985

103. Mitwalli A, Ayiomamitis A, Grass L, Oreopoulos D: Control of hyperoxaluria with large doses of pyridoxine in patients with kidney stones. Int Urol Nephrol 20:353, 1988

104. Coe F: Uric acid and calcium oxaiate nephrolithiasis. Kidney Int 24:392, 1983

105. Griffith D, Osborne C: Infection (urease) stones. Miner Electrolyte Metab 13:278, 1987

106. Stegmayr B, Anneroth G, Bergman B, Tomic R: Urinary tract calculi dissolved by means of renacidin. an experimental study. Scand J Urol Nephrol 24:215, 1990

107. Spirnak J, DeBaz B, Green H, Resnick M: Complex struvite calculi treated by primary extracorporeal shock wave lithotripsy and chemolysis with hemiacidrin irrigation. J Urol 140:1356, 1988

108. Williams J, Rodman J, Peterson C: A randomized double-blind study of acetohydroxamic acid in struvite nephrolithiasis. N Engl J Med 311:760, 1984

109. Griffith D, Khonsari F, Skurnick J, James K: A randomized trial of acetohydroxamic acid for the treatment and prevention of infection-induced urinary stones in spinal cord injury patients. J Urol 140:318, 1988

110. Rodman J, Williams J, Jones R: Hypercoagulability produced by treatment with acetohydroxamic acid. Clin Pharmacol Ther 42:346, 1987

111. Singer A, Das S: Cystinuria: a review of the pathopaphysiology and management. J Urol 142:669, 1989

112. Jaeger P, Portmann L, Saunders A et al: Anticystinuric effects of glutamine and of dietary sodium reatriction. N Engl J Med 315:1120, 1986

113. Pak C, Fuller C, Sakhaee K et al: Management of cystine nephrolithiasis with alpha-mercaptopropionylglycine. J Urol 136:1003, 1986

114. Sloand J, Izzo J: Captopril reduces urinary cystine excretion in cystinuria. Arch Intern Med 147:1409, 1987

115. Kishimoto T, Yamamoto K, Sugimoto T et al: Two years' clinical experiences with extracorporeal shock-wave lithotripsy and transurethral ureterolithotripsy for ureteral stones. Eur Urol 16:343, 1989

9

The Value of the Renal Biopsy

Melvin M. Schwartz
Stephen M. Korbet
Edmund J. Lewis

INTRODUCTION

The renal biopsy has defined the advancement of knowledge of kidney disease in the modern era of clinical nephrology. Performed at the onset and throughout the course of the disease, renal biopsy has given us current diagnostic terminology, demonstrated involvement of the immune system in the pathogenesis of renal disease, defined new diseases, and provided insights into the pathogenesis of others. It is undeniable that renal biopsy has contributed to our understanding of renal disease and has a role as a research tool. In addition, the renal biopsy continues to play a central role in patient management.

The "renal biopsy-guided" approach makes certain assumptions about the management of renal disease. It assumes that there is a "best" treatment for each patient and that the renal biopsy is the only way to be certain of the diagnosis. This approach may also assume that prognosis, which is a function of the disease, is important information for the patient. The renal biopsy provides a great deal of unique information, which is obtained at a relatively low risk.[1] Although treatment of a given "syndrome" plays a role in management, the enhanced information provided by biopsy expands the ability of a physician to diagnose and treat a specific patient. Despite limitations in the current therapeutic armamentarium, this approach is not merely intellectually more satisfying but becomes more efficacious as more disease-specific treatment becomes available.

An alternative point of view suggests that the management of certain renal diseases does not require a tissue diagnosis. Its proponents point out that results of renal biopsy rarely enable the physician to make a specific diagnosis without clinical support. Because the clinical presentation of renal disease leads to a limited differential diagnosis, the experienced clinician is required to integrate noninvasive laboratory tests and clinical information not to reach an accurate diagnosis but rather to decide whether to treat a patient. We contend that this approach will lead to many missed diagnoses. When the question is the application of expensive and potentially dangerous therapy, good medical care requires a diagnosis that is more than a probability statement. Finally, to the clinician faced with an emergent situation, the renal biopsy leads to the correct therapeutic approach in the quickest and most efficient manner.

A variant of the "no biopsy" approach is suggested by those who maintain that a diagnosis is not as important as response to therapy and a satisfactory cost/risk/benefit ratio. The only formal presentation of this position is in the treatment of the idiopathic nephrotic syndrome in adults.[2] Even if one accepts the many assumptions in that analysis, including the putative steroid responsiveness of membranous glomerulonephritis, the implication that renal biopsy is not necessary in any clinical situation does not follow.

Our approach in this chapter will be to prioritize the clinical situations in which a biopsy provides important and unique information (Table 9-1). We will begin with situations in which a renal biopsy provides such key informa-

Table 9-1. Priorities for Renal Biopsy

1. Biopsy always indicated for optimal patient management
2. Biopsy indicated under exceptional circumstances
3. Biopsy indicated in a "morbid" condition
4. Discovery of new diseases

tion that therapy should not be begun without morphologic support. In these instances, a biopsy is always indicated for optimal patient management. We will then consider the indications for biopsy in the management of diseases that often do not require a renal biopsy. In this group, the anatomic diagnosis and the course of the renal disease have been established by previous biopsy studies, and we will only concern ourselves with the deviations from the expected clinical course. There are diseases in which the overall clinical course is so discouraging that renal biopsy is deferred in the belief that a morphologic diagnosis of the renal problem is will not contribute to the patient's well-being. However, we will examine this assumption and suggest that even patients who are allegedly "terminal" may benefit from disease-specific therapy. We will conclude by indicating that truly new diseases begin with morphologic characterization. At each level, we will discuss the necessity of a biopsy, provide illustrative examples, and explain how the biopsy helped in patient management. We wish to emphasize that the cases serve as examples of the value of renal biopsy in the management of various clinical situations. These are not examples of rare or unusual occurrences of the "case report" type. Our point of view is that biopsy is a diagnostic tool of immeasurable value in common presentations of renal disease.

BIOPSY INDICATED FOR OPTIMAL PATIENT MANAGEMENT

Nephrotic Syndrome in the Adult

The principal problem for the clinician confronted by an adult with the nephrotic syndrome is that only a small proportion has a renal lesion that is completely responsive to any of the currently known therapeutic modalities. In addition, unlike the pediatric nephrologist, the adult nephrologist is confronted by patients in their third through ninth decades. Obviously, treatment is effected not simply to corroborate a diagnosis but is critical in managing the patient's disease. The causes of the nephrotic syndrome are legion, but they may be broadly classified into primary glomerulopathies, glomerular involvement in certain systemic diseases, drugs, infections, malignancies, circulatory disturbances, infantile or congenital forms, and rare miscellaneous diseases. When the secondary forms of nephrotic syndrome are excluded, there remains a group of patients with idiopathic nephrotic syndrome who can only be differentiated with certainty by renal biopsy. This latter category includes minimal change glomerulopathy and its histologic variants[3] focal segmental glomerular sclerosis[4] and membranous glomerulonephritis.[5] Heptinstall collected 11 series comprising mainly adults with nephrotic syndrome.[6] In 845 adult nephrotic patients in whom diabetes mellitus, amyloidosis, and systemic lupus erythematosus (SLE) were excluded, 23 percent had minimal change glomerulopathy, 29 percent had membranous glomerulonephritis (GN), and 46 percent had some other form of GN. Although segmental glomerular sclerosis was not separately classified, it contributed 15 percent of the cases in our personal series.[7] In contrast, four series of children with the nephrotic syndrome exclusive of systemic disease totaling 1,253 cases had 66 percent minimal change glomerulopathy, 8 percent focal glomerular sclerosis, 4 percent membranous GN, and 8 percent membranoproliferative glomerulonephritis. The remaining cases were other forms of proliferative GN, chronic GN, and unclassified lesions.[6]

The different prevalence of the various lesions in children and adults seems to imply a different approach if specific therapeutic intervention is being considered. The situation is more complex in adults than in children because the cause of the nephrotic syndrome is much wider and because only minimal change glomerulopathy, comprising approximately 25 percent of the patients, has a proven benefit from steroids. Also, adults appear to require a longer course of therapy before they respond, as compared to children.[8] Although the other lesions may respond to different therapies such as chlorambucil for membranous glomerulonephritis and platelet inhibitors for membranoproliferative glomerulonephritis, the potential side effects make it imperative to only expose patients with potentially responsive diseases to these drugs.[7] Thus, our approach to adults is to recommend renal biopsy to patients with the idiopathic nephrotic syndrome and to treat the underlying glomerular pathology with the most beneficial and proven drug regimen that is consistent with the patient's clinical condition.

The decision to determine treatment of adults with the nephrotic syndrome on the demonstration of specific renal pathology by renal biopsy is based on the goal of treating specific diseases rather than symptoms and signs. The goal of therapy is not always the same in different diseases. Increased life expectancy[2] is just one of several outcomes that may be important to the individual patient. In fact, in younger patients, the quality of life and the ability to work and support a family may actually be overriding concerns. Even when the same therapeutic agent is being considered, the goals of therapy may vary between diseases. The goal of steroid therapy in minimal change glomerulopathy is remission. In membranous GN, a decreased level of proteinuria or diminished progression to renal failure may be considered as satisfactory outcomes. Finally, therapeutic protocols, tailored to specific diseases, have emerged from controlled clinical trials for minimal change glomerulopathy, membranous GN, and membranoproliferative GN. To assert that all patients with proteinuria should be treated blindly and in a similar fashion ignores the major thrust of clinical research in this area since 1970.

Clinical Presentation

A 20-year-old white woman presented with a 6-month history of fatigue and the nephrotic syndrome. Her serum creatinine was 0.5 mg/dl, albumin 3.0 g/dl, and cholesterol 208 mg/dl. The urine sediment was benign, and a 24-hour urine protein was 6 g. There was no obvious secondary cause for her proteinuria based on history. Her blood pressure was 124/70 mmHg, and she had 2^+ pretibial edema. The serologic workup was completely negative including negative antinuclear antibody (ANA) and normal serum complements. Her nephrologist, who felt she had an idiopathic nephrotic syndrome, opted not to do a renal biopsy but to give her a trial of daily high-dose steroids for 9 weeks. After completing the treatment, a follow-up urine protein continued to be elevated at 1.9 g/24 h. As a result of the persistent proteinuria, the patient and her family sought a second opinion.

Pathology Findings

The glomeruli showed mild mesangial hypercellularity and increased mesangial matrix by periodic acid-Schiff (PAS) and silver staining. One glomerulus had a segmental scar, but there were no other segmental lesions. The basement membranes showed widespread abnormalities best seen with the silver stain and consisting of irregular lucent areas in the en face sections and focal discrete spikes on the epithelial side of the glomerular basement membrane (GBM). Immunofluorescence microscopy showed diffuse granular deposits of immunoglobulins and complement components (C3 and C1q) along the GBM (Fig. 9-1) with negative staining of the mesangium and extraglomerular structures. Electron microscopy confirmed the presence of electron-dense deposits in a subepithelial and intramembranous location. No mesangial electron-dense deposits or tubuloreticular structures were observed.

This patient presented with the nephrotic syndrome and was treated empirically with steroids. Although her proteinuria decreased, she continued to excrete 1.9 g/d after 9 weeks of prednisone. She sought a second opinion, and before she embarked on further therapy, a renal biopsy demonstrated membranous GN. The renal biopsy findings clearly impacted on the long-term management and therapeutic expectations in this patient.

Membranous GN is a chronic disease with a 10-year survival of approximately 50 percent,[9] but a significant number of the survivors will either be in remission or will have persistent proteinuria with preservation of renal function. Because many of the patients on whom the survival data are based were treated in an uncontrolled manner, we need to examine the survival of untreated patients to arrive at the true natural history of membranous GN. Donadio et al.[10] retrospectively studied 140 patients with biopsy-proven membranous GN, 89 of whom were not treated with steroids or immunosuppressive agents and 50 of whom received a short course of prednisone as the primary treatment. No significant difference was noted between nontreatment and treatment groups, and survival without renal failure was 71 per-

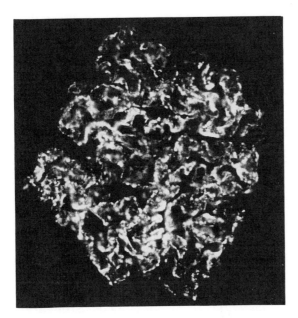

Fig. 9-1. Membranous glomerulonephritis. Immunofluorescence microscopy of a glomerulus staining in a granular pattern along the peripheral capillary basement membrane. (lgG, × 550.)

cent at 5 years, and 58 percent at 10 years. The outcome of proteinuria was quite variable, but no differences were observed between the treated and untreated groups. The majority, or 41 of 72 (57 percent), of untreated patients and 17 of 42 (40 percent) treated patients had achieved either partial or complete remission from the nephrotic syndrome at final assessment. However, the authors found considerable variability in the degree of proteinuria when it was examined over the long-term course of membranous GN. In a prospective, randomized trial of 6 months using alternate-day prednisone as compared with a placebo, Cattran et al.[11] found no differences in survival or preservation of renal function between 81 prednisone-treated and 77 control patients. After 3 years, the authors observed no differences in the outcome of proteinuria. Twenty-five percent of the control and 20 percent of the treated patients had achieved a complete remission, and a comparable proportion were in a partial remission. These data suggest that our patient's decrease in protein excretion may reflect the natural history of membranous GN rather than a specific effect of therapy.

Several features in the patient's history suggest that the diagnosis of SLE could become evident in the future. She is a young woman; she gave a vague history of fatigue that preceded the onset of the nephrotic syndrome; and she developed membranous GN at a young age. The diagnosis of SLE is based on a clinical constellation of signs and symptoms, and in this case they are certainly not adequate to make the diagnosis. It is well known that lupus may present with membranous GN, but it may be years before the patient develops either systemic disease or positive serology to support a diagnosis of SLE. The renal biopsy in the present case had several unusual features, and we should consider how strongly they support the diagnosis of SLE. A segmental scar was noted in one glomerulus. Although this finding is nonspecific, it raises the possibility of an antecedent proliferative lesion that would be highly suggestive of a systemic disease with renal involvement such as SLE. However, we have found isolated segmental scars in up to 10 percent of our cases of idiopathic membranous GN with prolonged follow-up, and although it is possible that they too represent occult cases of SLE, the finding of a segmental scar is too nonspecific to make the diagnosis of SLE.[5] The biopsy showed significant mesangial hypercellularity. Although increased mesangial matrix and cellularity are general features of membranous GN, it is usually mild and requires morphometric techniques to demonstrate. Jennette et al.[12] studied a number of pathologic features in lupus and nonlupus membranous GN including mesangial hypercellularity. Diffuse mesangial hypercellularity had a low sensitivity for lupus membranous GN (27 percent) and a specificity of 85 percent. Thus, its presence was of less value in making the diagnosis than its absence was in excluding the diagnosis of SLE.

In the present case, the renal biopsy demonstrated membranous GN. Given the natural history of this lesion, it is unlikely that the patient will respond to further treatment. Thus, the renal biopsy provided information that directly effects the clinician's attitude toward further therapy, and it gives the patient a prognosis based on the behavior of a specific disease.

Systemic Lupus Erythematosus

SLE with renal involvement confronts the clinician with a unique problem. The diagnosis is usually established on the basis of the clinical criteria, and although the biopsy may suggest the diagnosis of SLE, the histopathology is diagnostic in only a minority of the cases. Because the biopsy is not required for the diagnosis of SLE, some have questioned the utility and the indications for a renal biopsy in this clinical situation.[13,14] Despite this sanguine attitude, SLE is a complex disease, and the kidney may be affected by the disease itself or by its therapy. One major problem for the clinician is the lack of correlation between clinical and laboratory data and the severity of the renal lesion. It has been said that serious renal disease can occur in patients with SLE who have no evident abnormality of urinalysis or renal function. Although this is true in occasional patients, the yield of renal biopsy in this patient population is low, and the information obtained that would impact on therapy, is relatively small. Thus, we will limit our discussion to patients with SLE who have clinical abnormalities that are indicative of renal involvement.

The degree to which the kidneys are involved in SLE correlates with overall prognosis. It would appear that the kidney mirrors the severity of systemic disease. Classifications of a patient's glomerular lesion therefore become important. The relationship between renal function, serology, and physical findings and the renal pathology of SLE has been the subject of repeated investigations. The principal glomerular lesion is cellular proliferation, and variations in the amount and distribution of hypercellularity have formed the basis for most classification schemes.[15-17] However, when the clinical data are used to predict the morphologic classification of the glomerular pathology, the results have been disappointing.[16,18-21] Despite the considerable clinical overlap among patients with different categories of SLE GN, renal biopsy studies have demonstrated that the histologic category predicts outcome.[15,17,18]

Renal biopsy studies have shown that diffuse proliferative GN has a worse prognosis than any of the other histologic variants of lupus.[15,18,22] In addition, high doses of prednisone increased survival in patients with diffuse GN by decreasing systemic activity of the disease process and delaying the onset of renal failure.[17,22] These results were so definitive that no controlled clinical trials of the efficacy of steriods were ever attempted, and the success of subsequent therapeutic agents has been measured against the proven benefits of steroids. Although current therapy has improved survival, patients with diffuse lupus GN still suffer more lupus-related deaths and loss of renal function than do all the other histologic categories combined.[23] The poor prognosis of lupus GN requires a precise definition of this histologic category. The information that is obtained is of value in several ways. First, the prednisone dose and treatment may be determined by the severity of the lesion. Second, the addition of other agents, particularly cytotoxic drugs, may be determined by the type and severity of the pathology. Last, the biopsy provides information regarding nonresolvable damage, which may be of considerable importance in deciding how actively a patient should be treated.

There is a spectrum of glomerular pathology in patients with diffuse SLE GN that includes (1) severe segmental GN (50 percent or more involvement)[15-17]; (2) diffuse proliferative GN; and (3) membranous GN with superimposed severe segmental or diffuse GN.[16,20] When the effect of these morphologic variants on outcome was examined, we found that clinical or serologic criteria did not predict the morphology. All three variants had sufficient morbidity and mortality to warrant inclusion in the category of diffuse GN, and patients with membranous GN and superimposed proliferative lesions had the worst prognosis.[19] As our ability to treat the acute inflammatory lesions that form the basis of the morphologic classification has improved, several attempts have been made to define morphologic features that are better predictors of outcome.[9] However, the reproducibility and therapeutic guidance afforded by the World Health Organization (WHO) histologic classification have made it the standard approach to evaluating the renal biopsy in SLE.

Clinical Presentation

A 26-year-old black woman presented with fever, myalgias, and swelling of the face and ankles. She had previously been healthy, but 7 months prior, she had presented with preeclampsia requiring delivery by caesarian section. Following delivery, she was normotensive; her serum creatinine was 0.9 mg/dl; and her urine was negative for protein. On physical examination, however, her blood pressure was 160/110 mmHg with a temperature of 102°F, and she had periorbital edema with bibasilar rales and 1+ pretibial edema. Her serum creatinine was 0.9 mg/dl with an albumin 3.0 g/dl, and she was anemic. Her urinalysis had 4+ protein with a benign sediment. Urine protein excretion was 5.4 g/24 h. The ANA titer was 1:500 in a speckled pattern; anti-ds DNA antibody was positive at 100 percent; and the C3 and C4 titers were both low at 22 and less than 6 mg/dl, respectively.

Pathology Findings

Diffuse proliferative GN was observed with widespread hyaline thrombi in glomerular capillaries and arterioles (Fig. 9-2). The glomeruli were diffusely hypercellular, and the capillary lumens were restricted by mesangial expansion and endocapillary proliferation. In addition, patchy, intense areas of interstitial inflammation and focal tubular atrophy were noted. Immuno-

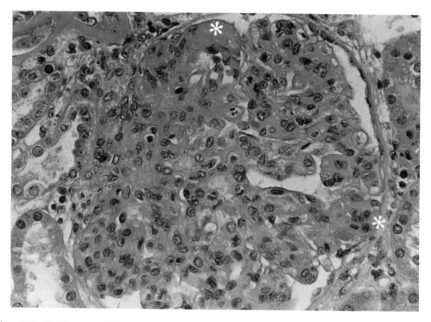

Fig. 9-2. Diffuse proliferative systemic lupus erythematosus glomerulonephritis. There is diffuse mesangial expansion and hypercellularity with lobulation of the glomerular tuft. In addition, there are large eosinophilic deposits in the glomerular capillary walls (asterisks). (H&E, × 550.)

fluorescence microscopy showed mesangial, discontinuous granular, and capillary and arteriolar thrombotic deposits of immunoglobulins and complement. Granular deposits of IgG were observed on 25 percent of the tubular basement membranes. Electron microscopy demonstrated mesangial and massive subendothelial electron-dense deposits and capillary thrombi.

The patient developed the clinical and serologic stigmata of SLE postpartum. Despite the active serology with hypocomplementemia, elevated anti-native DNA, and positive ANA, the principal renal manifestation was the nephrotic syndrome. Based on her otherwise normal renal function and bland urinary sediment, the clinical diagnosis was SLE membranous GN. Treatment of SLE membranous GN is the subject of controversy, but few would be as active in the pharmacologic approach to that lesion as would be the case with diffuse GN. However, the biopsy demonstrated a lesion that clearly required active therapeutic intervention. Thus, this is an example in which the clinical presentation was misleading, and the renal biopsy provided the rationale for the approach to drug therapy.

Clinical Presentation

A 35-year-old black women with a history of SLE presented to an outside hospital with a fever of 105°F, disorientation, and an elevated white blood cell (WBC) count with a left shift in the differential count. She had oliguria with a serum creatinine of 7.7 mg/dl, and her urinalysis had 4+ protein with microscopic hematuria and waxy casts. Neurologic evaluation demonstrated a diffusely abnormal electroencephalogram (EEG). It was felt that she was septic and had oliguric lupus GN and cerebritis. She was transferred to our hospital for aggressive immunosuppressive therapy and plasmapheresis. On transfer, her serum creatinine was 8.4 mg/dl, and she continued to have oliguria, ultimately requiring hemodialysis. Her ANA was 1:500 in a homogeneous pattern with the anti-ds DNA antibody positive at approximately 100 percent. The C3 was 49 mg/dl and C4 less than 5 mg/dl. The creatine phosphokinase was 14,000 IU/L, aldolase 35.7 mU/ml (normal, less than 8.1) and myoglobin level elevated at 1,250 mg/ml.

Pathology Findings

The patient had membranous GN with mild mesangial proliferation (Fig. 9-3), and immunofluorescence and electron microscopy confirmed the histologic diagnosis by demonstrating diffuse granular deposits of immunoglobulin and complement and subepithelial and intramembranous electron-dense deposits, respectively. In addition, widespread tubulointerstitial nephritis was noted, with acute tubular necrosis and regeneration (Fig. 9-4).

In this case, the patient presented with acute renal failure thought to be secondary to lupus GN and was considered for immunosuppression and plasmapheresis. Although her history of SLE and very active serology led to a clinical diagnosis of severe lupus GN, the renal biopsy demonstrated that her acute renal failure was not of glomerular origin. The use of aggressive

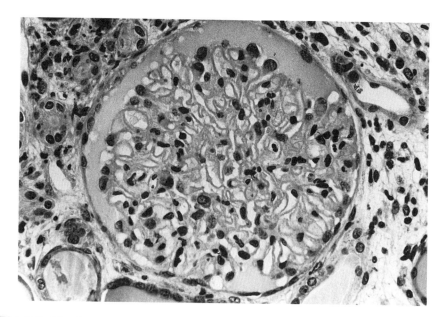

Fig. 9-3. Membranous systemic lupus erythematosus glomerulonephritis. There is diffuse thickening of the glomerular basement membranes with only mild increase in the mesangial matrix and cellularity. (H&E, × 550.)

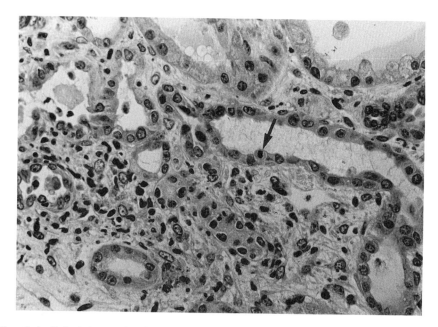

Fig. 9-4. Tubulointerstitial nephritis in a case of membranous systemic lupus erythematosus glomerulonephritis. There is tubular atropy with thinned epithelium, hyperchromatic regenerative nuclei, and tubular mitosis (arrow). The interstitium contains numerous lymphocytes, histiocytes, and occasional plasma cells. (H&E, × 550.)

immunosuppression and plasmapheresis is controversial in a septic patient, and the renal biopsy obviated the decision to treat the glomerular lesion. She eventually recovered renal function with supportive therapy only.

These two cases demonstrate the lack of correlation between clinical presentation and glomerular pathology that is a frequent problem in the management of SLE GN. In the first case, the bland presentation of severe glomerular inflammation would have led to undertreatment, and in the second case, the severity of the renal failure and assumptions about the glomerular pathology would have led to unnecessary treatment. In both, the renal biopsy diagnosis led to appropriate therapy.

Crescentic Glomerulonephritis

After Ellis noted the relationship between a "rapidly progressive course" to renal failure and the glomerular crescent, the biopsy finding of crescentic GN assumed its current value as an adverse prognostic sign.[29] The glomerular crescent is a sign of severe injury, and the involved glomerulus almost always shows histologic evidence of necrosis.[30] However, the proportion of glomeruli with crescents is variable, and an adverse outcome correlates with increasing levels of glomerular involvement. Thus, the literature reports a poor prognosis for patients with crescents in more than 50 percent of their glomeruli.[31,32] Conversely, isolated glomerular necrosis, occurring in the absence of crescent formation, implies qualitatively less severe glomerular damage and a less dismal prognosis.[30]

The glomerular cresent is an impressive sign of glomerular injury, but with few exceptions it is etiologically nonspecific. Cresents have been reported in virtually every type of GN[30] and have also been associated with membranous GN. The pathogenesis of crescentic GN is diverse, for they are associated with three types of immunologic injury: anti-GBM antibody, immune complex disease, and nonantibody mediated GN (pauci-immune). When systemic diseases are excluded, the pauci-immune form of crescentic GN is the most frequent.[33,34]

Pauci-immune GN is seen in three quarters of patients with idiopathic crescentic GN,[33,34] but the proportion drops in patients with fewer cresents.[34] In both anti-GBM and immune complex GN, the crescents are explained by antibody activation of the inflammatory process via the complement system, but the pathogenesis of pauci-immune GN is less clear. The presence of lymphocytes and macrophages in the crescents and examples of destructive granulomatous inflammation in the periglomerular interstitium have suggested the possibility that pauci-immune GN is mediated by cellular immunity. This hypothesis receives some support from clinical studies in anti-GBM and poststreptococcal GN[35] and experimental models.[36,37] Once severe injury has damaged the glomerular capillary wall, the crescent may follow as a consequence of the initiating event, but the nature of this initial injury is not known. Because many of the diseases associated with crescent formation affect blood vessels throughout the body, necrotizing GN with crescent formation may be considered a localized form of vasculitis. This is specifically true in pauci-immune GN, and the recent recognition of a serologic test that correlates with pauci-immune GN may provide the link between localized manifestations of non-immunoglobulin-mediated GN in the kidney and systemic vasculitis.

Antineutrophil cytoplasmic antibodies (ANCA) are circulating antibodies directed against the contents of neutrophil and monocyte granules. When ANCA-positive sera are tested against alcohol-fixed human neutrophils, two patterns are demonstrable by indirect immunofluorescence microscopy. The cytoplasmic ANCA (C-ANCA) is directed against a serine proteinase in neutrophil primary granules (proteinase 3), and the perinuclear ANCA (P-ANCA) is usually reactive with myeloperoxidase.[38] A positive ANCA was initially thought to be specific for Wegener's granulomatosis with the titer related to disease activity, but subsequent studies have demonstrated ANCA in a variety of systemic vasculitic syndromes with pauci-immune necrotizing and crescentic glomerular involvement.[34] Despite this improvement in diagnostic serologic parameters, the treatment of crescentic GN still demands a knowledge of the extent of glomerular damage. Hence, the ANCA test has enhanced our ability to predict the immunopathology that will be found at biopsy and is some indicator of therapeutic choices that must be considered.[39] The most accurate decision regarding management of the patient, in our view, still requires evaluation of degree of severity of glomerular disease. Hence, the renal biopsy remains an important feature of the workup of these patients.

Clinical Presentation

A 41-year old white woman who was previously well presented with a 1-week history of an upper respiratory tract infection consisting of sinus congestion and fever of 102°F and swelling in her feet. Over the past year, she had several upper respiratory infections that were treated with antibiotics. In addition, she had a recent history of arthritis and tendonitis involving the hands. Her blood pressure was 136/90 mmHg. She had 1+ edema of the lower extremities, and joints appeared normal. Her serum creatinine was 4.3 mg/dl, and the urine had 3+ protein with microscopic hematuria and red blood cell (RBC) casts. Sinus radiographs were negative. The ANA and complement levels were normal, but ANCA was significantly positive with a cytoplasmic pattern.

Pathology Findings

Severe crescentic GN was demonstrated with involvement of more than 80 percent of glomeruli. The glomerular pathology ranged from segmental areas of necrosis with fibrinoid exudation, epithelial cell proliferation, and karyorrhexis to diffuse cresent formation (Fig. 9-5). There was collapse of the capillary tuft, complete destruction of the glomerulus with only a fibrous remnant, and periglomerular inflammatory cells that broke through Bow-

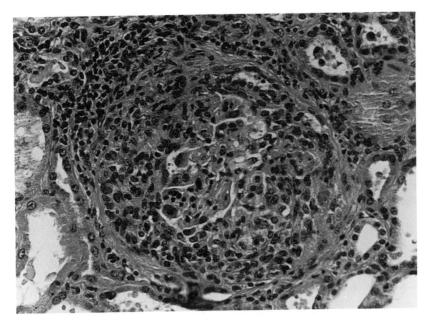

Fig. 9-5. Crescentic glomerulonephritis. The glomerulus is compressed by the cellular crescent in Bowman's space, but it shows only mild reactive proliferation. There is an associated intense interstitial cellular infiltrate. (H&E, × 550.)

man's capsule into the crescent. The glomeruli contained no significant deposits of immunoglobulin or complement components by immunofluorescence microscopy, but there were segmental deposits of fibrin. Ultrastructural examination showed no electron-dense deposits.

This was a typical example of pauci-immune crescentic GN. There was no evidence of extrarenal vasculitis, and inflammatory lesions were limited to the glomeruli. The C-ANCA is frequently positive in Wegener's granulomatosis, but in the absence of pulmonary or upper respiratory involvement, the patient's disease is best classified as microscopic polyarteritis. Immunosuppression with cyclophosphamide has been effective in treating some types of pauci-immune crescentic GN,[39] but once the glomeruli are destroyed and scarred, treatment aimed at controlling the inflammatory lesion becomes ineffective. Despite the high proportion of glomeruli with crescents, indicating a poor prognosis for survival of renal function, she was given a course of cyclophosphamide. Although further treatment with plasmapheresis or high-dose prednisone might have been considered, the advanced state of her glomerular lesion, as seen on renal biopsy, led her physicians to abandon further therapy when she failed to respond. Thus, a precise knowledge of the extent of the glomerular damage helped the physician in his determination to terminate therapy and spared the patient a more aggressive approach to which her scarred glomeruli could not possibly have responded.

Pulmonary-Renal Syndrome

The pulmonary-renal syndrome is a broad category of diseases that affects both the lungs and the kidneys with disease processes as diverse as Goodpasture's syndrome, vasculitis, SLE, and nephrotic syndrome with pulmonary embolism. However, when renal involvement is limited to necrotizing glomerulonephritis and crescents, there is considerable overlap between patients presenting with a pulmonary-renal syndrome and rapidly progressive glomerulonephritis (RPGN). Not only do many diseases presenting as RPGN have pulmonary involvement, but many of the same pathogenetic and therapeutic considerations apply to both situations.

Clinical Presentation

A 44-year-old white man presented to an outside hospital with a 6-week history of fatigue and fever and progressive dyspnea over the previous week. His temperature was 103° F, and a systolic ejection murmur was noted. He was treated for pneumonia with 600,000 U of intramuscular penicillin G and cephradine to be taken as an outpatient. When his condition did not improve, he received a course of erythromycin. His serum creatinine was 3.8 mg/dl, and the hemoglobin concentration was 5.9 g/dl. Urinalysis demonstrated 4+ protein with pyuria, microscopic hematuria, and RBC and WBC casts. A urine protein was 14.5 g/24 h. The patient's pulmonary status deteriorated, and chest radiographs showed extensive reticulonodular infiltrates, bilaterally. A transbronchial biopsy had numerous hemosiderin-laden macrophages. A presumptive diagnosis of Goodpasture's syndrome was made, and he was given pulse doses of methylprednisolone. He was then transferred to our medical center for immunosuppressive therapy and plasmapheresis. The serum creatinine was 4.1 mg/dl with an albumin of 2.5 g/dl, and the serologic work up was remarkable for severely depressed C3 and C4 levels, an elevated rheumatoid factor, and an elevated cryoglobulin level. The ANA was negative, as was the antistreptolysin O titer. An indirect assay for antiglomerular basement membrane antibody was negative. Echocardiogram demonstrated a 5 × 45-mm vegetation on the anterior mitral valve leaflet, but repeated blood cultures were negative. A renal biopsy was performed to obtain information rapidly regarding the cause of this man's pulmonary-renal syndrome and the appropriate management approach.

Pathology Findings

The biopsy demonstrated a diffuse proliferative and exudative GN. In addition to endocapillary proliferation and neutrophilic exudates, we observed large subendothelial deposits and segmental reduplication of the glomerular capillary walls. Immunofluorescence microscopy showed focal segmental discontinuous linear deposits and focal capillary thrombi of immunoglobulins, complement components, and fibrin; and electron-dense deposits were seen between the basal lamina and the endothelial cell in segmental areas (Fig. 9-6). Thus, this was an immune complex-mediated acute GN with focal membranoproliferative features.

The patient initially presented with a febrile illness and was treated empirically with several different antibiotics. When renal involvement was manifested, the diagnosis shifted to Goodpasture's syndrome, and he was given intravenous methylprednisolone. Although the clinical suspicion of bacterial endocarditis was reinforced by the ultrasound demonstration of a mitral valve vegetation, the nature of the renal lesion was uncertain in the presence of negative blood cultures. The renal biopsy identified an acute, immune complex-mediated GN. Plasmapheresis was, therefore, not carried out. Switching the patient from pulse methylprednisolone to broad-spectrum antibiotics reversed his deteriorating renal function, normalized his serum complements and cryoglobulins, and achieved a gratifying diminution of protein excretion. As the case presented, the correct diagnosis was obscure, but continuing therapy with steroids could have been catastrophic. The renal biopsy results indicated that antibiotics were specific therapy for this particular pulmonary-renal syndrome, and treatment led to a resolution of the patient's renal disease.

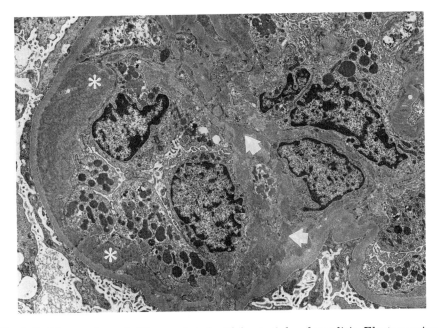

Fig. 9-6. Glomerulonephritis associated with bacterial endocarditis. Electron micrograph shows mesangial infiltration by macrophages containing electron-dense lysosomes and similar lysosomes in proliferating endothelial cells. Electron-dense deposits are in the subendothelial space (asterisks) and mesangium (arrows). All electron micrographs stained with uranyl acetate and lead citrate. ($\times$ 8,400.)

Paraproteinemia With Renal Involvement

Paraproteinemias are diseases characterized by the elaboration of immunoglobulin fragments that are abnormal in quantity or quality. Their renal effects may manifest as albuminuria, light chain proteinuria (Bence-Jones proteinuria), or renal failure. Plasma cell dyscrasia with the proliferation of a single clone of immunoglobulin-producing plasma cells is the classic example, and multiple myeloma, Waldenstrom's macroglobulinemia, and heavy chain disease are included in this group. Other paraproteinemias are characterized by systemic deposition of immunoglobulin fragments: light chain deposition disease and its variants and some cases of amyloidosis are examples. For completeness, essential monoclonal gammopathy and cryoglobulinemia are included with the paraproteinemias. The diseases are related because of the elaboration of related proteins, but we discuss them here because of the various ways in which they all may effect the kidney.

The diseases listed here are diagnosed by the nature of the circulating protein and the extent of systemic involvement, and renal biopsy is not usually required to make a diagnosis. Even when the clinical diagnosis is obvious, however, one disease may be associated with renal lesions of very different prognosis and therapeutic responsiveness. For example, multiple myeloma is diagnosed by the presence of monoclonal serum protein, evidence of bone marrow infiltration by malignant plasma cells and Bence-Jones proteinuria. Three different forms of renal disease are seen with multiple myeloma: amyloidosis, nonamyloid paraprotein deposition, and myeloma cast nephropathy. The majority of myelomas may be typed immunologically as IgG, but the frequency of renal involvement roughly parallels the frequency of light chain proteinurias.[40] Hill[41] provided evidence that variability in the isoelectric point (pI) and/or the degree of polymerization of the free light chains underlies the different morphologic manifestations of myeloma. When the pI is low, the light chains are negatively charged and do not appear to pass the glomerular filter in any quantity. A high degree of polymerization of the light chains has the same effect. In either instance, the light chains are deposited in the glomerulus as amyloid or nonamyloid paraprotein deposits. Proteinuria is due to the glomerular lesion, and free light chains are present in the urine. When the light chains are less negatively charged or are present as low molecular weight dimers or trimers, they are freely filtered and give rise to myeloma cast nephropathy. In these cases, the urine contains free light chains. The specific renal diagnosis in paraproteinemia is not only of morophologic interest because these lesions have different prognostic and therapeutic implications.

Clinical Presentation

A 70-year-old white man presented with a serum creatinine of 5.5 mg/dl and proteinuria (2.4 g/24 h). His blood pressure was 160/80 mmHg, and he had 2+ pretibial edema. A monoclonal IgA-κ was found in the serum, and free κ-light chains were detected in the urine. The bone marrow was not diagnostic of multiple myeloma with less than 20 percent plasma cells, and a bone survey was negative for lytic lesions. In addition, a fat aspirate was negative for the presence of amyloid.

Pathology Findings

The glomeruli were diffusely and strikingly abnormal with diffuse mesangial expansion and mild to moderate increase in mesangial cellularity. In several glomeruli, there was a marked increase in the mesangial matrix with the formation of multiple acellular nodules. The nodules were PAS positive and methenamine silver stain negative, and even in the most severely involved glomeruli, the capillary lumens appeared open (Fig. 9-7). The biopsy showed diffuse interstitial expansion and fibrosis with focal tubular atrophy associated with the most severely sclerotic glomeruli. Interstitial cellular infiltrates are sparse. Congo red stain for amyloid was negative. Immunofluorescence microscopy showed staining of the mesangium in general and the mesangial nodules in particular with IgG and most strongly with κ. We also noted diffuse staining of the tubular basement membranes for κ-light chains (Fig. 9-8). Electron microscopy confirmed the mesangial expansion seen by light microscopy, but we observed no evidence of microfibrils or organization of the deposits.

The patient had paraproteinemia with an immunoglobulin A (IgA)

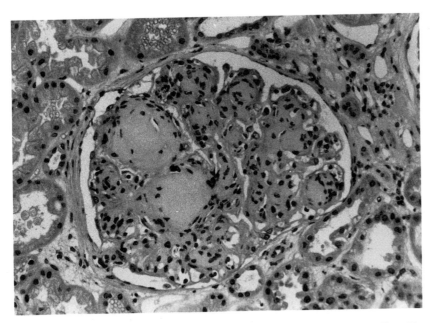

Fig. 9-7. Light chain deposition disease. Glomerulus with multiple small and large acellular mesangial nodules. The capillary loops are generally patent, and mesangial cellularity is only slightly increased. (H&E, $\times$ 550.)

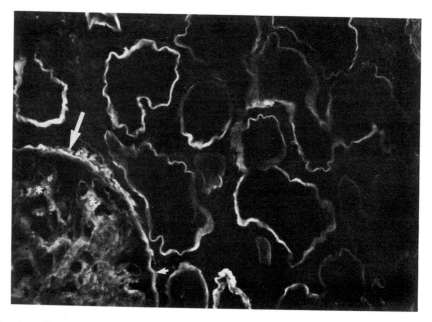

Fig. 9-8. Light chain deposition disease. The glomerular mesangium (asterisks), Bowman's capsule (arrows), and the tubular basement membranes stain for κ-light chain.(× 550.)

κ-monoclonal protein, and he fit the criteria for myeloma with low plasma cell volume.[42] The biopsy demonstrated the combined glomerular and tubular lesion of light chain deposition disease (LCDD). The presence of heavy chain determinants in cases such as this suggests that a more appropriate name is light and heavy chain deposition disease. The clinical findings and light microscopy suggest LCDD, but the diagnosis is usually based on the demonstration of glomerular and tubular basement membrane deposits of immunoglobulin light chains.

Ganeval et al.[43] reviewed the topic and their experience at the Necker Hospital in Paris. They contrast LCDD with amyloidosis and emphasize the importance of making this distinction, because amyloidosis resulting from plasma cell dyscrasias has a very short course to death, whereas LCDD may be responsive to therapy. The frequency of LCDD may be underestimated unless the biopsy is examined with antisera to light chain determinants. This is especially true in the myeloma patient with the nephrotic syndrome, who, until the description of LCDD, was assumed to have developed amyloidosis. The nodular form of the glomerular lesion seen in our patient may be confused with diabetic glomerular sclerosis, and some of the reported cases of nodular nondiabetic glomerular sclerosis may represent misdiagnosed LCDD. Finally, it must be emphasized that LCDD occurs in the absence of overt myeloma in approximately one-third of the cases. When LCDD occurs in the absence of myeloma, nothing separates it clinically from the other causes of the nephrotic syndrome in adults. LCDD is a systemic disease, and like amyloidosis, tissue deposits are found in multiple organs. Although renal and cardiac disease have been the dominant problems in a few cases, renal involvement with proteinuria and early, frequent renal failure are the main problems in most.

When LCDD occurs in a patient with multiple myeloma, the patient is usually treated for the myeloma. Uncontrolled evidence, however, indicates that treatment will also benefit those in whom renal LCDD occurs in the absence of lymphoplasmacytic malignancy. Ganeval et al.[43] state that treatment of LCDD without myeloma can be rationalized in the hope of improving or stabilizing the renal failure and preventing extrarenal depositon of light chains. In six patients treated early in their courses, before the onset of advanced renal failure, only one required hemodialysis, and the others were either stable or improved after 4 years of follow-up. In contrast, five patients, treated either late in their courses or not at all, developed end stage renal disease 2, 3, 4, 18, and 22 months after diagnosis.

In our patient, the renal biopsy diagnosis has important prognostic and therapeutic implications. Because the patient developed the nephrotic syndrome as a complication of multiple myeloma, LCDD must be distinguished from amyloidosis and its grim prognosis. In addition, the biopsy demonstration of LCDD raises the possibility of disease-specific therapy. In LCDD, with or without associated multiple myeloma, the patient may profit from therapy directed at the benign or malignant clone of plasma cells that are producing the light chain responsible for the tissue deposits.

BIOPSY INDICATED UNDER EXCEPTIONAL CIRCUMSTANCES

Nonresponsive Nephrotic Syndrome in a Child

Nephrotic syndrome in childhood is due to minimal change glomerulonephropathy in at least 70 percent of the reported cases. Because this lesion is usually responsive to prednisone therapy, current medical practice is to give the patient a trial of steroid therapy and not perform a renal biopsy at this point in the course. If the child does not respond to the standard 8-week course of prednisone,[44] the prediction that he has a lesion other than minimal change nephrotic syndrome would be incorrect in about 25 percent of the cases and in as many as one half of the patients 6 years of age or younger. Thus, a renal biopsy becomes indicated after failure of the initial course of therapy and during relapse, especially if the relapses are frequent. The information gained from a specific biopsy-derived diagnosis (1) would encourage further steroid therapy or a course of steroid-sparing immunosuppressive drugs in the patient with minimal change glomerulonephropathy, (2) would spare the child with unresponsive focal segmental glomerular sclerosis further therapy, and (3) would suggest a different specific therapy for the patient with membranoproliferative glomerulonephritis.

Clinical Presentation

A 3-year-old Hispanic boy presented with abdominal pain and was found to have the nephrotic syndrome. His blood pressure was 104/58 mmHg, and he had periorbital and pretibial edema with ascites. The serum creatinine was 0.7 mg/dl, and the serum albumin was 1.5 g/dl. The urinalysis had 4+ protein and 4+ blood. Protein excretion was 124 mg/m^2/hour. He was placed on prednisone 60 mg/m^2/d but failed to respond over the next month. Serologic evaluation was negative for ANA, antistrepotolysin O antibodies, and hepatitis, and the C3 and C4 titers were normal.

Pathology Findings

The biopsy showed focal segmental glomerular sclerosis with collapsed segments and adhesions in 7/30 glomeruli (Fig. 9-9). The uninvolved glomeruli and the uninvolved portions of the glomeruli with segmental scars were unremarkable. Immunofluorescence microscopy showed no significant deposits, and the glomerular epithelial cells showed diffuse foot process effacement.

The patient was biopsied after he failed to respond to prednisone therapy. Although he was a primary treatment failure, he remained quite symptomatic from the nephrotic syndrome, and the clinicians were considering another course of therapy. Despite his therapeutic history, the clinical diagno-

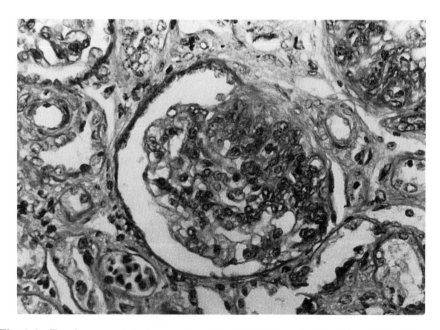

Fig. 9-9. Focal segmental glomerular sclerosis. The involved portion of the glomerulus is collapsed with obliteration of the architecture and adhesion to Bowman's capsule. The remainder of the glomerulus has patent capillaries and only a mild increase in mesangial cellularity. (H&E, × 550.)

sis remained mimimal change glomerulonephropathy. Because the clinicians were contemplating another course of therapy because of the profound nephrotic syndrome, they performed a biopsy. The diagnosis of focal segmental sclerosis suggested that this patient would remain unresponsive even to cyclophosphamide and that the prognosis was very poor.

Acute Renal Failure That Does Not Resolve

Elevation of blood urea nitrogen (BUN) and creatinine in a patient with previously normal renal function is a common clinical problem. When these parameters increase daily with or without oliguria, the diagnosis of acute renal failure (ARF) is made and the etiology is sought. About half of the cases of ARF are related to surgery or trauma, 25 percent occur in a medical setting, 13 percent are related to pregnancy and 9 percent are caused by nephrotoxins.[45] A variety of parenchymal lesions underlie ARF as a result of intrinsic renal diseases, but 75 percent of the cases are due to acute tubular necrosis (ATN). ATN occurs in the context of renal ischemia; exposure to nephrotoxins; radiocontrast studies in patients with multiple myeloma, diabetes mellitus, and preexistent renal disease; and massive myoglobinuria or hemoglobinuria. Although the cause of ARF is usually apparent from the history and the clinical setting, some cases may require the full range of the nephrologist's diagnostic tools including renal biopsy.

ARF that is due to ATN often has an oliguric phase that begins shortly after the initiating event and persists for 1 to 2 weeks, but when oliguria continues for more than 4 weeks, the diagnosis should be reconsidered. This is an important point because a delay in resolution of ATN may be the most important clue that the lesion is not ATN. It is well-known that the prognosis of ARF is related to the nature of the precipitating condition. The first principle of management is to rule out the reversible causes of ARF. Thus, any suggestion that the renal parenchymal cause of ARF is not ATN should lead the clinician to renal biopsy.

Clinical Presentation

A 20-year-old black woman presented during her 18th gestational week with normotensive acute renal insufficiency. Her only medication was prenatal vitamins. During her first trimester, the serum creatinine was 1.0 mg/dl, and at presentation, it was 4.6 mg/dl. The serum calcium was mildly elevated, 10.9 mg/dl, with a serum albumin of 3.6 g/dl. The urine demonstrated 2+ protein with pyuria and WBC casts but a negative culture for bacteria. Urinary protein excretion was 1.2 g/24 h. The workup was negative for SLE, hepatitis, and paraproteinemia. The cryoglobulin level was normal. She was not thought to be preeclamptic. The kidneys were normal by ultrasound and were not obstructed. Following renal biopsy, the patient was started on prednisone. Her ARF resolved and she delivered a normal-term infant.

Pathology Findings

The biopsy showed widespread granulomatous interstitial nephritis with glomerular and vascular sparing. The granulomas were noncaseating, and they contained many giant cells (Figure 9-10). Special stains for microorganisms were negative.

The incidence of ARF during the course of pregnancy has two periods of high risk. The early cases relate to septic abortions. A later peak, which was also not relevant to our patient, occurs as a result of preeclampsia and obstetric bleeding.[46] Thus, our patient had an atypical presentation which led to a renal biopsy and to a specific diagnosis. Sarcoidosis is a multisystem disease and granulomas within the kidney are a common autopsy finding. Clinically evident renal involvement is only rarely a consequence of granulomatous interstitial nephritis. The present case[47] had a number of important features: It occured in the absence of systemic evidence of sarcoidosis; ARF that is due to sarcoid interstitial nephritis is a rare event, and this was the first case reported during pregnancy; and the patient had a gratifying response to therapy without a negative effect on the fetus. She was biopsied because she had no apparent cause for her ARF, and the biopsy demonstrated a lesion that was responsive to specific therapy with prednisone.

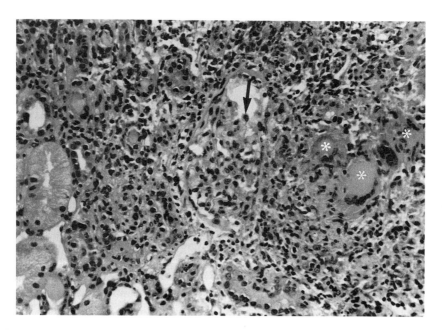

Fig. 9-10. Sarcoidosis. The kidney shows a granulomatous interstitial nephritis with numerous giant cells (asterisks). Surviving glomeruli (arrow) and tubules are widely separated by the intense infiltrate. (H&E, × 550.)

Hypertension During Preganancy With Atypical Features

Hypertension developing during pregnancy is a critical clinical sign, because it may be a harbinger of a true medical emergency. The syndrome of hypertension developing during the last trimester of pregnancy, associated with proteinuria, is called preeclampsia. The diagnosis of preeclampsia on clinical grounds is somewhat problematic because other diseases may present with hypertension and proteinuria, but once seizures occur, the clinical diagnosis is unfortunately secure. Autopsies and renal biopsies, performed in large numbers of pregnant patients and during the puerperium have demonstrated that the kidney of the hypertensive proteinuric patient may show the lesions of preeclampsia, nephrosclerosis, primary or secondary renal (and glomerular) disease, or normal histology. If a hypertensive patient is assumed to be preeclamptic, the clinical diagnosis will be incorrect in fully one third of the cases.[48] Although protein excretion is usually modest in preeclampsia, this lesion is still the most common cause of the nephrotic syndrome during pregnancy. Case reports have documented the occurrence of numerous other causes of the nephrotic syndrome during pregnancy, and because many of these conditions do not respond to corticosteroids or may even be worsened by them, the importance of establishing a diagnosis before initating therapy is apparent. Despite this caveat, all too frequently, the practice is to follow the patient and treat symptomatically without performing a renal biopsy.[49]

Preeclampsia and eclampsia occur most commonly in primiparas during the first pregnancy carried into the third trimester. Although it occurs in some multiparas, the frequency is six to eight times greater in primiparas. Preeclampsia usually occurs late in pregnancy with the onset after the 30th week in 95 percent of cases. Hypertensive symptoms may be prominent, but the level of hypertension is variable, as is the level of protein excretion. The GFR is usually reduced, although the decrease may be masked by the physiologic increase that accompanies pregnancy. Reflecting the decreased GFR associated with preeclampsia, it has been emphasized that a serum creatinine greater than 0.8 mg/dl and uric acid level greater than 6.0 mg/dl may be abnormal in a pregnant patient. Although the clinical presentation has been correlated with the severity of the glomerular lesion, the long-term prognosis for preeclampsia is excellent. When a pregnant patient deviates from the usual clinical course or when the hypertension and proteinuria persist into the puerperium for more than 4 weeks, a renal biopsy becomes necessary to distinguish among the underlying diseases and to guide therapy.

Clinical Presentation

A 29-year-old white woman presented at 28 weeks' gestation with hypertension and the nephrotic syndrome. She was first found to be mildly hypertensive at 9 weeks' gestation. Her urine protein remained normal until 25 weeks' gestation, when it was 3.0 g/24 h, and the serum albumin was 3.0 g/dl with a serum creatinine of 0.8 mg/dl. Her blood pressure was 150/104 mmHg while taking medication, and she had 3+ edema. She continued to have a normal serum creatinine with hypoalbuminemia, and urine protein excretion rose to 6.0 g/24 h. Her uric acid concentration was elevated. No serologic evidence of SLE was noted in the past, she had three spontaneous abortions, all between the fourth and seventh weeks of gestation. During the present admission, she was thought to have preeclampsia, and 18 hours after admission, she underwent an emergent delivery by caesarian section and had an open renal biopsy.

Pathology Findings

The glomeruli were "bloodless" with swollen endothelial cells and diminished capillary lumens. Some large PAS-positive deposits protruded into the capillary lumens (Fig. 9-11). The tubules and blood vessels showed no evidence of chronic disease or hypertensive injury. Mesangial and finely granular capillary deposits of IgM and C3 were noted. Electron microscopy confirmed the presence of swollen endothelial cells, lipid inclusions in subendothelial macrophages and endothelial cells, and subendothelial finely granular electron-dense deposits. These findings are all consistent with the glomerular lesion of preeclampsia.

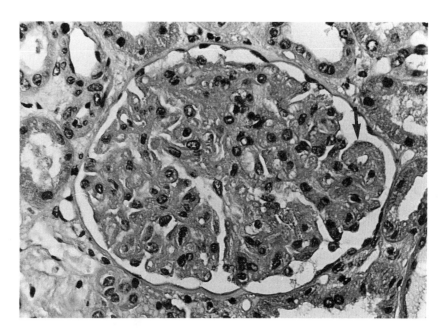

Fig. 9-11. Preeclampsia. The glomerulus has marked reduction of the capillary lumens, prominent, swollen endothelial cells, and thickening of the glomerular capillary wall (arrow). (H&E, × 550.)

As mentioned, the patient had three prior pregnancies that all ended in spontaneous abortions between weeks 4 and 7. She had no prior history of hypertension but was first noted to have an elevated blood pressure by the ninth week which rose to 130/108 by 17 weeks of gestation. She did not initially have proteinuria, but it appeared at 25 weeks and progressed to frank nephrotic syndrome by week 30. She had an elevated serum uric acid and creatinine, but she was biopsied at the time of caesarian section with the plan of treating the nephrotic syndrome if she had a responsive glomerular lesion.

The biopsy demonstrated the typical lesion of preeclampsia, and thus, despite the atypical presentation, the patient was not treated and would be expected to resolve the nephrotic syndrome without residual deficits of renal function shortly after terminating the pregnancy.

Chesley[50] presented the follow-up of 270 women who survived eclampsia and were followed for a mean of 33 years. He found an increased mortality among women who had eclampsia as multiparas, and the increase in late mortality was the consequence of an increased incidence of cardiovascular diseases. Black primiparas and multiparas both had an increase in the incidence of cardiovascular disease compared to the white primiparas, which the author attributed to the increased incidence of hypertension in blacks. When the eclamptic patients were compared to age-matched controls, the white primiparas suffered no increase in the incidence of death, but the white mutiparas and the black primiparas and multiparas all had an increased ratio of actual/expected deaths. Furthermore, those who had eclampsia as primiparas did not have an increased level of hypertension at follow-up, whereas hypertensive multiparas did. The author concluded that eclampsia is not a sign of latent hypertension or renal disease and that it does not cause chronic hypertension. Despite the dramatic nature of our patient's atypical clinical presentation, the renal biopsy findings suggested that her long-term prognosis for normal renal function and resolution of the nephrotic syndrome were excellent. She was not expected to develop hypertension or its cardiovascular sequela at a greater rate than women of her age who have not experienced preeclampsia.

BIOPSY INDICATED IN A "MORBID" SITUATION
Human Immunodeficiency Virus Infection and Glomerulopathy

The patient with human immunodeficiency virus (HIV) infection may develop a variety of renal complications that occur not only in the fully developed acquired immunodeficiency syndrome (AIDS) and AIDS-related complex (ARC) but that, also occur with asymptomatic HIV infections.[51] Glomerular disease or HIV nephropathy is manifested by proteinuria, frequently with the nephrotic syndrome, and varying degrees of renal failure. Preoteinuria is common in patients with HIV infection, but nephrotic range proteinuria is seen in fewer than 10 percent.[52,53] The renal failure progresses rapidly to end stage in most, and this feature, plus 3- to 6-month reported survival[54] have supported the contention that HIV nephropathy is a clinicopathologic syndrome with a particularly poor prognosis. Various glomerular pathologies have been described in patients with HIV infections including mesangial hyperplasia, minimal change glomerulopathy, and other histologic categories of glomerulonephritis, but focal segmental glomerular sclerosis is the most common lesion associated with HIV nephropathy.[51]

The poor prognosis of idiopathic focal glomerular sclerosis and an understandable reluctance to use immunosuppressive drugs in patients with compromised immunity have discouraged the aggressive evaluation and treatment of patients with HIV nephropathy. There is a tendency to assume that proteinuria and the nephrotic syndrome in patients with HIV infections are signs of untreatable glomerular lesions that identify a group of terminally ill patients. There is evidence, however, that not all proteinuric HIV-positive patients have a progressive renal disease, and if identified, some of them may profit from disease specific therapy.

Clinical Presentation

A 31-year-old HIV positive homosexual black man with a past history of intravenous drug abuse was found to have 4+ protein by dipstix and microscopic hematuria. His blood pressure was 132/96 mmHg; there were small hard posterior cervical glands; and he had 2+ pretibial edema, bilaterally. His serum creatinine was 1.0 mg/dl with a serum albumin of 2.1 g/dl. A 24-hour urine had 12 g of protein. The T-cell helper/suppressor ratio (CD4/CD8) was 0.2 (normal 0.8 to 2.9). The ANA test was negative, and the C4 titer was normal. The rheumatoid factor (latex) was 1:320, and the C3 titer was low at 59 mg/dl (normal 80 to 180). The cryoprecipitate was 0.7 percent (normal, less than 0.1 percent), and the Lowry protein 504 μg/ml (normal, less than 2μg/ml). Immunofixation of serum and urine were negative for paraproteins. Serum was negative for hepatitis B surface antigen. The antistreptolysin O antibody was less than or equal to 2,400 lU/ml. Numerous blood cultures were negative. An echocardiogram did not demonstrate any vegetations. The patients renal function began to deteriorate (serum creatinine (1.7 mg/dl). However, a renal ultrasound revealed normal-sized kidneys with no increase in echogenicity or obstruction.

Pathology Findings

The principal renal lesion was diffuse proliferative and exudative glomerulonephritis. Segmental areas of endocapillary proliferation were observed, but no signs of segmental scars were noted. Immunofluorescence microscopy demonstrated mesangial and discontinuous linear and granular deposits of IgG and C3. Electron microscopy showed large subepithelial electron-dense deposits (humps) (Fig. 9-12). The glomerular capillary endothelial cells con-

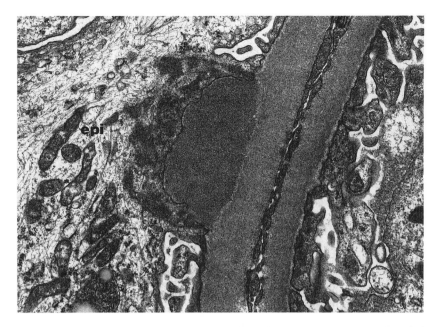

Fig. 9-12. Acute post-streptococcal glomerulonephritis. There is an isolated, large subepithelial electron-dense deposit with condensation of the overlying glomerular epithelial cell (epi) cytoplasm. (× 42,000.)

tained tubular reticular structures, but none of the other ultrastructural features of HIV nephropathy were seen.[55]

The biopsy showed a diffuse proliferative GN with immunohistologic and ultrastructural features of a postinfectious GN. Postinfectious GN runs an acute self-limited course. By 6 months, most patients have completely resolved their glomerular lesions or have only isolated abnormalities of the urinary sediment. In our patient, the nephrotic syndrome and hematuria persisted for 6 months, suggesting that the complex immunologic abnormalities of HIV infection prolonged the usual benign course of postinfectious GN, which placed the prognosis of this patient in doubt. This case raises several important points concerning the evaluation of the patient with HIV nephropathy.

This renal biopsy emphatically demonstrated that proteinuria and renal failure in an HIV-positive patient are not synonymous with HIV nephropathy. Although HIV nephropathy has a poor prognosis, not all HIV-positive patients with renal failure share the same dismal outlook. If the glomerular diagnosis is not determined, significant prognostic differences will be missed. Our patient had a number of clinical features that were atypical for HIV nephropathy including hypertension, hematuria, edema, and hypocomplementemia. Certainly, in this case with its atypical presentation, the need for a renal biopsy was supported, but existing evidence suggests that even a broader application of renal biopsy is indicated in the HIV-positive patient with glomerular disease.

The stage of the AIDS infection appears to be a more important prognostic indicator than the development of renal failure. Thus, survival in hemodialyzed HIV-positive patients depends on how advanced their underlying disease is rather than the presence of renal failure.[56] In addition, the possibility of specific therapy depends on a biopsy-proven diagnosis. If HIV nephropathy proves responsive to zidovudine as some case reports suggest, the value of early histologic diagnosis and treatment may become critical in the care of these patients. Because the HIV-positive patient may also have steroid-responsive lesions such as minimal change glomerulonephropathy,[57] the need to aggressively diagnose the glomerular disease will increase as further lesion-specific therapy becomes available.

DISCOVERY AND DESCRIPTION OF NEW DISEASES
Immunotactoid Glomerulopathy

All patients presenting for the evaluation of renal disease cannot be assigned a specific diagnosis after even a complete clinical and laboratory examination. When renal involvement occurs in the context of a systemic disease such as SLE, diabetes mellitus, and amyloidosis, a renal biopsy may not be required for diagnosis, but as discussed previously, morphologic information may still be required for patient management. In broad clinical classes such as nephrotic syndrome and rapidly progressive glomerulonephritis, the biopsy is required because of the prognostic and therapeutic implications of the different diseases responsible for the syndrome. There is a further justification for renal biopsy in patients whose renal symptoms are unexplained. If we wait until autopsy, the diagnostic specificity may no longer be apparent in the end stage kidney. It is usually from carefully studied biopsies, obtained early in the course of the disease, that new diseases are recognized. Examples include IgA nephropathy as a major cause of hematuria, "thin basement membrane disease" as a nonprogressive form of hereditary nephritis separate from Alport's syndrome, and LCDD as a nonamyloid paraprotein deposit.

Clinical Presentation

A 66-year-old white woman presented with hypertension and 3+ proteinuria and microscopic hematuria. Her blood pressure was 140/80 mmHg, and she had no edema. Her serum creatinine serum creatinine was 1.8 mg/dl, and the serum albumin 2.8 g/dl. The urine protein was 1.06 g/24 h. The serologic workup was negative for a paraproteinemia, SLE, and cryoglobulinemia. A renal biopsy demonstrated organized microtubular deposits of IgG. Even though the congo red stain was negative, she was given the diagnosis of amyloidosis. Seven years later, her serum creatinine was 6.7 mg/dl, and urinary protein excretion was 10 g/24 h. She progressed to end stage renal disease over the next year and was placed on hemodialysis. Three years later she was otherwise in excellent health and received a cadaveric renal transplant, which functioned well for more than 5 years with no evidence of recurrent disease or the development of another systemic disease. Because of her favorable course, which was unusual for amyloidosis, her original biopsy was reevaluated.

Pathology Findings

The glomeruli showed diffuse mesangial expansion by PAS-positive congo red negative material without a significant increase in cellularity. The mesangium stained for IgG and C3 by immunofluorescence microscopy (Fig. 9-13). Electron microscopy showed mesangial expansion by randomly arranged fibrils (mean diameter 20 nm) (Fig. 9-14). Fibrils were also focally present in the basal lamina, mainly in the subepithelial region but also transmembranous. The ultrastructural, immunochemical, and histochemical features defined immunotactoid glomerulopathy.[58]

This patient illustrates the diagnostic confusion that frequently surrounds this disease, because she carried the diagnosis of congo red-negative amyloidosis through renal failure and successful transplantation until her course, which was prolonged for amyloidosis, prompted reevaluation of the renal biopsy. There are now enough patients with immunotactoid glomerulopathy reported to define the clincal features of this condition. The patients all present with proteinuria, and over half are nephrotic. Renal failure is evident at presentation in half, and after 4 years, approximately half have progressed to end stage renal failure. Immunotactoid glomerulopathy appears to represent a primary GN, because there is no evidence of a systemic disease. This disease must be distinguished from other diseases that may have organized immune deposits in the glomeruli. In addition to amyloidosis, these include mixed essential cryoglobulinemia, SLE, multiple myeloma, and light chain disease. The pathology of immunotactoid disease suggests that there is either an abnormal production of a monoclonal protein or of immune complexes. It is clinically important to distinguish this entity from the other disorders in the differential diagnosis because immunotactoid glomerulopathy has a more favorable prognosis, especially in comparison to amyloidosis.[59]

CONCLUSION

In many clinical situations a renal biopsy provides unique information that is important in patient management, and the ones we have chosen to discuss reflect our experience. The prognosis of the diseases that bring the renal patient to the attention of a physician are quite different. For example, hematuria may result from a benign condition such as thin basement membrane disease, chronic slowly progressive conditions such as IgA nephropa-

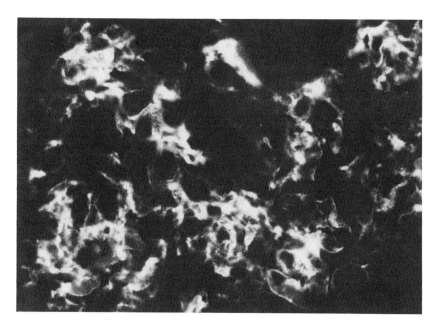

Fig. 9-13. Immunotactoid glomerulopathy. Immunofluorescence microscopy demonstrates diffuse mesangial deposits of IgG (γ-chain determinant). (× 550.)

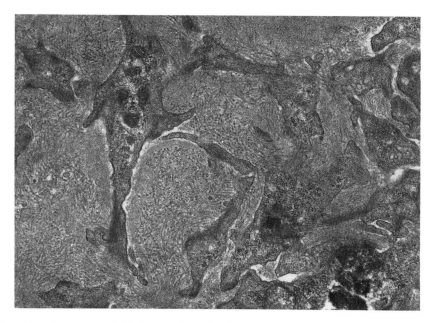

Fig. 9-14. Immunotactoid glomerulopathy. Electron microscopy demonstrates mesangial deposits of randomly arranged fibrils with a mean diameter of approximately 20 nm. (× 34,000.)

thy and membranoproliferative GN, and emergent conditions such as crescentic GN. The same prognostic considerations apply to the other clinical presentations of renal disease including proteinuria, nephritis, nephrotic syndrome, rapidly progressive glomerulonephritis, acute renal failure, and chronic renal failure.

The histologic diagnosis obtained by renal biopsy is important to the physician because it is appropriate medical practice to treat a patient rather than a symptom or syndrome. By establishing the anatomic diagnosis with a renal biopsy, clinicians can apply a therapeutic regimen that has been developed specifically for a disease. They can remain alert for known complications of therapy and for further expressions and evolutions of the underlying disease. Not only is this therapeutic approach more efficient for the patient with a known disease, but it avoids treating patients with potentially toxic and dangerous drugs to which their disease may not be responsive.

The limitations of the current therapeutic armamentarium should not be taken as a lack of justification for making an anatomic diagnosis by renal biopsy. Biopsy may demonstrate subgroups in histologic categories of some glomerular diseases that are responsive to available modalities of therapy. For example, recent studies suggest that early stages of membranous GN will respond to corticosteroids.[60] In addition, biopsy studies continue to demonstrate new diseases and to identify the mechanisms of known diseases. As new specific therapies become available, these morphologic classifications will become the basis for assigning therapy.

REFERENCES

1. Burstein DM, Schwartz MM, Korbet SM: Percutaneous renal biopsy with the use of real time ultrasound. Am J Nephrol 11:195, 1991
2. Kassirer JP: Is renal biopsy necessary for optimal management of the idiopathic nephrotic syndrome? Kidney Int 24:561, 1983
3. International Study of Kidney Disease in Children: Primary nephrotic syndrome in children: Clinical significance of histopathologic variants of minimal change and of diffuse mesangial hypercellularity. Kidney Int 20:765, 1981
4. White RHR, Glasgow EF, Mills RJ: Clinicopathological study of nephrotic syndrome in childhood. Lancet 1:1353, 1970
5. Schwartz MM: Membranous glomerulonephritis. p. 559. In Heptinstall RH (ed): The Pathology of the Kidney. 4th Ed. Little, Brown, Boston, 1991
6. Heptinstall RH: The nephrotic syndrome. p. 637. In Heptinstall RH (ed): The Pathology of the Kidney. 3rd Ed. Little, Brown, Boston, 1983
7. Lewis EJ: Management of the nephrotic syndrome in adults. p. 461. In Cameron JS, Glassock RJ (eds): The Nephrotic Syndrome. Marcel Dekker, New York, 1988
8. Korbet SM, Schwartz MM, Lewis EJ: The prognosis of focal segmental glomerular sclerosis of adulthood. Medicine 65:304, 1986
9. Cameron JS: The Natural History of Glomerulonephritis In Black D, Jones NF (eds): Renal Disease. 4th Ed. Blackwell Scientific, Oxford, England, 1979
10. Donadio JV Jr, Torres VE, Velosa JA et al: Idiopathic membranous nephropathy: The natural history of untreated patients. Kidney Int 33:705, 1988

11. Cattran DC, Delmore T, Roscoe J et al: A randomized controlled trial of prednisone in patients with idiopathic membranous nephropathy. N Engl J Med 320:215, 1989
12. Jennette JC, Iskandar SS, Dalldorf FG: Pathologic differentiation between lupus and nonlupus membranous glomerulopathy. Kidney Int 24:377, 1983
13. Fries JF, Porta J, Liang MH: Marginal benefit of renal biopsy in systemic lupus erythematosus. Arch Intern Med 138:1386, 1978
14. Whiting-O'Keefe Q, Riccardi PJ, Henke JE et al: Recognition of information in renal biopsies of patients with lupus nephritis. Ann Intern Med 96:723, 1982
15. Muehrcke, RC, Kark RM, Pirani CL, Pollak VE: Lupus nephritis: a clinical and pathologic study based on renal biopsies. Medicine 36:1, 1957
16. Baldwin DS, Lowenstein, J, Rothfield NF et al: The clinical course of the proliferative and membranous forms of lupus nephritis. Ann Intern Med 73:929, 1970
17. Baldwin DS, Gluck MC, Lowenstein J, Gallo GR: Lupus nephritis. Clinical course as related to morphologic forms and their transitions. Am J Med 62:12, 1977
18. Pollak V, Pirani CL, Schwartz F: The natural history of the renal manifestations of systemic lupus erythematosus. J Lab Clin Med 63:537, 1964
19. Schwartz MM, Lan S, Bonsib SM et al: The Lupus Nephritis Collaborative Study Group: Clinical outcome of three discrete histologic patterns of injury in severe lupus glomerulonephritis. Am J Kidney Dis 13:273, 1989
20. Mahajan SK, Ordonez NG, Feitelson PJ et al: Lupus nephropathy without clinical renal involvement. Medicine 56:493, 1977
21. Pollak VE, Pirani CL, Kark RM: Effect of large doses of prednisone on the renal lesions and life span of patients with lupus glomerulonephritis. J Lab Clin Med 57:495, 1961
22. Hill GS, Hinglais N, Tron F, Bach J-F: Systemic lupus erythematosus. Morphologic correlations with immunologic and clinical data at the time of biopsy. AM J Med 64:61, 1978
23. Esdaile JM, Levinton C, Federgreen W et al: The clinical and renal biopsy predictors of long-term outcome in lupus nephritis: a study of 87 patients and review of the literature. Q J Med 72:779, 1989
24. Churg J, Sobin LH: Lupus nephritis. p. 127. In: Renal Disease. Classification and Atlas of Glomerular Diseases. Igaku-Shoin, New York, 1982
25. Schwartz MM, Kawala KS, Corwin HL, Lewis EJ: The prognosis of segmental glomerulonephritis in systemic lupus erythematosus. Kidney Int 32:274, 1987
26. Austin HA III, Klippel JH, Balow JE et al: Therapy of lupus nephritis. Controlled trial of prednisone and cytotoxic drugs. N Engl J Med 314:614, 1986
27. Austin HA III, Muenz LR, Joyce KM et al: Diffuse proliferative lupus nephritis: identification of specific pathologic features affecting renal outcome. Kidney Int 25:689, 1984
28. Schwartz MM, Bernstein J, Hill GS et al: The Lupus Nephritis Collaborative Study Group: Predictive value of renal pathology in diffuse proliferative lupus glomerulonephritis. Kidney Int 36:891, 1989
29. Ellis A: Natural history of Bright's disease: clinical and experimental observations. Lancet 1:1, 1942
30. Schwartz MM, Korbet SM: Crescentic glomerulonephritis. Progress in Reproductive and Urinary Tract Pathology. 1:163, 1989
31. Morrin PAF, Hinglais N, Nabarra B, Kreis H: Rapidly progressive glomerulonephritis: a clinical and pathologic study. Am J Med 65:446, 1978
32. Whitworth JA, Morel-Maroger L, Mignon F, Richet G: The significance of extra-

capillary proliferation. Clinicopathological review of 60 patients. Nephron 16:1, 1976

33. Stilmant MM, Bolton WK, Sturgill BC et al: Crescentic glomerulonephritis without immune deposits: Clinicopathologic features. Kidney Int 15:184, 1979

34. Jennette JC, Wilkman AS, Falk RJ: Anti-neutrophil cytoplasmic autoantibody-associated glomerulonephritis and vasculitis. Am J Pathol 135:921, 1989

35. Fillit HM, Zabriskie JB: Cellular immunity in glomerulonephritis. Am J Pathol 109:227, 1982

36. Bhan AK, Collins AB, Schneeberger EE, McCluskey RT: A cell-mediated reaction against glomerular bound immune complexes. J Exp Med 150:1410, 1979

37. Bolton WK, Tucker FL, Sturgill BC: New avian model of experimental glomerulonephritis consistent with mediation by cellular immunity. J Clin Invest 73:1263, 1984

38. Falk RJ: ANCA-associated renal disease. Kidney Int 38:998, 1990

39. Salant DJ: Immunopathogenesis of crescentic glomerulonephritis and lung purpura. Kidney Int 32:408, 1987

40. Pruzanki W: Clinical manifestations of multiple myeloma: Relation to class and type of M component. Can Med Assoc J 114:896, 1976

41. Hill GS: Multiple myeloma, amyloidosis, Waldenstrom's macroglobulinemia, and benign monoclonal gammopathies. p. 995. In Heptinstall RH (ed): Pathology of the Kidney. 3rd Ed. Little, Brown, Boston, 1983

42. Durie BG, Salmon SE: A clinical staging system for multiple myeloma: Correlation of measured myeloma cell mass with clinical features, response to treatment and survival. Cancer 36:842, 1975

43. Ganeval D, Noel L-H, Preud'homme J-L et al: Light-chain deposition disease: its relation with AL-type amyloidosis. Kidney Int 26:1, 1984

44. The International Study of Kidney Disease in Children: The primary nephrotic syndrome in children. Identification of patients with minimal change nephrotic syndrome from initial response to prednisone. J Pediatr 98:561, 1981

45. Levinsky NG, Alexander EA, Venkatachalam MA: Acute renal failure. p. 1181. In Brenner BM, Rector FC, Jr (eds): The Kidney. 2nd Ed. WB Saunders, Philadelphia, 1981

46. Smith K, Browne JCM, Shackman R, Wrong OM: Renal failure of obstetric origin. Br Med Bull 24:49, 1968

47. Warren GV, Spraque SM, Corwin HL: Sarcoidosis presenting as acute renal failure during pregnancy. Am J Kidney Dis 12:161, 1988

48. Fisher KA, Luger A, Spargo BH, Lindheimer MD: Hypertension in pregnancy: clinical-pathological correlations and late prognosis. Medicine 60:267, 1981

49. Lindheimer MD, Katz Al: Hypertension in pregnancy: Current concepts. N Engl J Med 313:675, 1985

50. Chesley LC: Remote prognosis after eclampsia. p. 31. In Lindheimer MD, Katz Al, Zuspan FP (eds): Hypertension in Pregnancy. John Wiley & Sons, New York, 1976

51. Bourgoignie JJ: Renal complications of human immunodeficiency virus type 1. Kidney Int 37:1571, 1990

52. Rao TK, Filippone EJ, Nicastri AD et al: Associated focal and segmental glomerulosclerosis in the acquired immunodeficiency syndrome. N Engl J Med 310:669, 1984

53. Pardo V, Aldana M, Colton RM et al: Glomerular lesions in the acquired immunodeficiency syndrome. Ann Intern Med 101:429, 1984

54. Rao TK, Friedman E, Nicastri A: The types of renal disease in the acquired immunodeficiency syndrome. N Engl J Med 316:1062, 1987

55. Chander P, Soni A, Suri A et al: Renal ultrastructural markers in AIDS-associated nephropathy. Am J Pathol 126:513, 1987

56. Ortiz C, Meneses R, Jaffe D et al: Outcome of patients with human immunodeficiency virus on maintenance hemodialysis. Kidney Int 34:248, 1988

57. Appel RG, Neill J: A steroid-responsive nephrotic syndrome in a patient with human immunodeficiency virus (HIV) infection. Ann Intern Med 113:892, 1990

58. Korbet SM, Schwartz MM, Rosenberg BF, Lewis EJ: Immunotactoid glomerulopathy. Medicine 64:228, 1985

59. Korbet SM, Schwartz MM, Lewis EJ: Immunotactoid glomerulopathy (review). Am J Kidney Dis 17:247, 1991

60. Schulze M, Baker PJ, Johnson RJ et al: Urinary complement C5b-9 excretion in membranous nephropathy (MN). Kidney Int 33:331, 1988

10

Radionuclide Techniques for the Diagnosis of Urinary Tract Disease

M. Donald Blaufox

INTRODUCTION

Conventional chemical assessment of renal function has many shortcomings. The clinical evaluation of renal function is relatively simple but also relatively crude; blood concentrations of compounds excreted by the kidney may fall within the broad range of normal values despite significant loss of renal function. More accurate chemical techniques require urine sampling, which is notoriously unreliable under routine clinical conditions.

Despite problems with routine clinical evaluation of renal function, radionuclide studies of the kidney remain underutilized. This underutilization is due largely to a lack of familiarity or understanding on the part of both consumers (urologists and nephrologists) and providers (nuclear medicine physicians). Study of the kidneys in many medical centers is restricted to the traditional tools of chemical analyses of blood and urine for assessment of overall kidney function and to traditional urography (roentgenography) to obtain anatomic information.

Measurement of effective renal plasma flow with radionuclide agents excreted primarily by tubular secretion, combined with imaging, can greatly enhance the physician's ability to diagnose and evaluate urinary tract abnormalities. This review outlines some of the opportunities afforded by such radionuclide studies, including the ability to measure renal function indirectly with relatively simple methodology and to determine the function of individual kidneys, an otherwise difficult task.

The functional nature of nuclear medicine studies offers tremendous advantages over conventional roentgenography for use in studies of the kidney, where problems frequently involve functional difficulties and not simply anatomic abnormalities. Nuclear medicine studies also offer advantages over traditional methods of determining renal function. They allow more accurate quantitation of various parameters of renal function as well as the power to generate sequential images of kidney activity over time.

Before discussing specific nuclear medicine techniques, it will be useful to outline some basic principles of renal function and physiology as they relate to the techniques I will discuss.

THE CLEARANCE CONCEPT

Clearance of a given substance is defined as the amount of that substance appearing in the urine in a given time period (in ml/min) divided by the plasma concentration during the same time period, when plasma concentration is held constant. Clearance $= UV/P$ where U is urine concentration, V is urine volume, and P is plasma concentration. When radioactive materials are used, concentrations are expressed in cpm/ml instead of mg/ml.

Normal blood constituents, like creatinine, are excreted by the kidney, and their circulating concentration is maintained at stable, steady-state levels, which can be used to measure renal clearance. In the case of creatinine, the clearance approximates the glomerular filtration rate (GFR). No substance normally is present in the blood that can be used to estimate the renal plasma flow.

KIDNEY STRUCTURE

The kidneys, located posteriorly in the retroperitoneal space, are encased in fatty tissue and surrounded by a connective tissue capsule. The ureters, blood vessels, lymph vessels, and nerves converge and enter the kidney at the hilum (Fig. 10-1). The renal pelvis is a cavity in the central portion of the kidney that connects to the ureter at the ureteropelvic junction. The parenchyma of the kidney may be divided anatomically into the cortex and the medulla. The medulla consists of the cone-shaped renal pyramids, the apexes of which converge and empty into the calyces. The calyces in turn empty into the pelvis.

The cortex surrounds the medulla, and portions of it enter the medulla and support the vascular supply. The cortex is composed of the glomerulus and the proximal and distal convoluted tubules of the nephrons. The portion of the nephron that connects the proximal and distal tubule, the loop of Henle, extends down into the medulla between the pyramids.

KIDNEY FUNCTION

A large portion of each nephron lies in the central portion of the kidney (Fig. 10-2).[1] The distal tubule leads into the collecting duct, and these collecting tubules converge in the pyramidal projections, which are each covered by a lesser calyx.

If a substance is filtered freely at the glomerulus and is neither secreted nor reabsorbed by the tubules, it may be used to measure the GFR. The GFR is a quantitative expression of the amount of plasma filtered by the glomerulus per unit time and approximates 20 percent of incoming blood. Compounds that are totally, or almost totally, removed from the blood perfusing the kidney by tubular secretion may be used to estimate the renal plasma flow (RPF), which is approximated by the blood clearance of these compounds. Even very highly extracted substances are not completely removed from the blood, so the term *effective renal plasma flow (ERPF)* is used to describe the measurement obtained from their clearance.

Glomerular Filtration

As blood flows through the glomerular capillaries, water and solutes are filtered out into Bowman's capsule, which surrounds the glomerulus and is the proximal end of the renal tubule. The GFR is autoregulated as perfusion

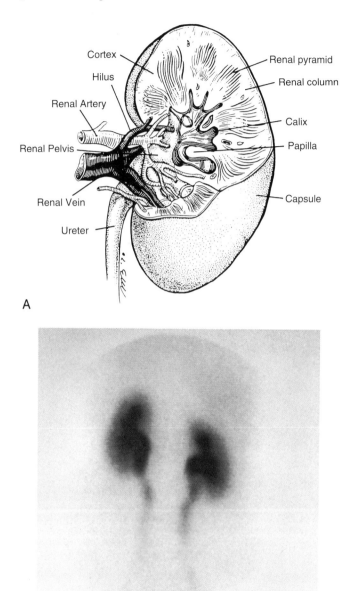

Fig. 10-1. (A & B) Intrarenal anatomy. Renal scintigram illustrates imaging capability of modern agents. The renal parenchyma, pelvis, and upper ureter can be readily identified by inspecting the image of this normal patient. (Scintigram produced with TechneScan MAG3, courtesy of Mallinckrodt Medical, Inc. From Austrin and Austrin,[69] with permission.)

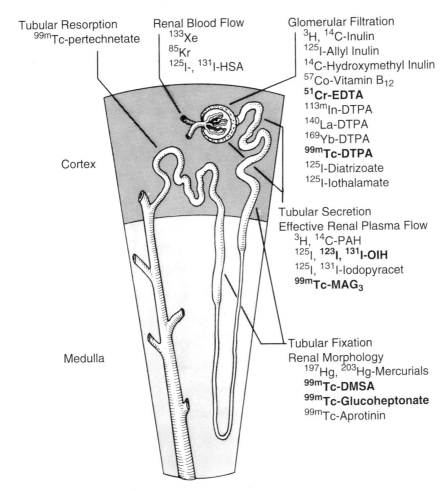

Tubular Resorption
^{99m}Tc-pertechnetate

Renal Blood Flow
^{133}Xe
^{85}Kr
^{125}I-, ^{131}I-HSA

Glomerular Filtration
^{3}H, ^{14}C-Inulin
^{125}I-Allyl Inulin
^{14}C-Hydroxymethyl Inulin
^{57}Co-Vitamin B$_{12}$
^{51}Cr-EDTA
^{113m}In-DTPA
^{140}La-DTPA
^{169}Yb-DTPA
^{99m}Tc-DTPA
^{125}I-Diatrizoate
^{125}I-Iothalamate

Cortex

Tubular Secretion
Effective Renal Plasma Flow
^{3}H, ^{14}C-PAH
^{125}I, **^{123}I, ^{131}I-OIH**
^{125}I, ^{131}I-Iodopyracet
^{99m}Tc-MAG$_{3}$

Tubular Fixation
Renal Morphology
^{197}Hg, ^{203}Hg-Mercurials
^{99m}Tc-DMSA
^{99m}Tc-Glucoheptonate
^{99m}Tc-Aprotinin

Medulla

Fig. 10-2. Some agents that have been used for the measurement of renal function. In boldface type are those with the most extensive clinical use or greatest clinical potential. (Figure prepared by L.R. Chervu. From Blaufox,[1] with permission.)

pressure is varied and remains relatively constant between approximately 80 and 160 mmHg; beyond this range of perfusion pressures, the GFR is directly related to systemic blood pressure. As blood pressure decreases below the level of autoregulation, there is a decrease in glomerular pressure and in the GFR.

Tubular Reabsorption

Resorption of water, electrolytes, and nutrients occurs in the proximal convoluted tubules by active and passive transport mechanisms. Transfer of sodium (also ascorbic acid, acetoacetic acids, basic amino acids, and many other substances) out of the tubular lumen, across the cell membrane, and into the interstitial fluid is primarily an active process.

Tubular Secretion

Movement of material from the peritubular circulation into the tubular lumen is known as tubular secretion. This occurs by an active secretory process and affects many substances including penicillins, hippuric acid, and several iodinated contrast media.

MEASURED PARAMETERS

Radionuclide studies can measure several parameters of renal function. Chief among these are *ERPF* and *GFR*. Functioning *renal mass* also may be estimated with nuclear medicine techniques, although the clinical role of renal mass determination is not yet clear.

Effective Renal Plasma Flow

ERPF, until recently, has been used primarily as a research tool, with limited use in direct clinical practice. Recognition of the diagnostic information that can be acquired by renal imaging, and the development of procedures such as captopril renography, is expanding interest in the use of ERPF measurements. The availability of clinically useful, cost-effective ERPF imaging agents is likely to increase the application of this measurement.

In theory, complete extraction from the blood of a substance during a single pass through the kidney would allow measurement of true RPF. However, this is not achieved in practice. A small portion of the blood that passes through the kidney is not presented to secretory tissue but instead perfuses such nonsecretory tissues as perirenal fat, pelvis, and capsule.[2] That portion presented to secretory tissue also may be incompletely removed as a result of limited transport efficiency. The term *ERPF* was coined to refer to the portion of the renal plasma flow presented to renal secretory tissue. The fraction of an agent removed from the blood in a single pass through the kidney is known as the *extraction ratio*. It is unclear how much of the reduction of extraction ratio is due to limited transport efficiency. This may vary with the compound used as a tracer and with the physiologic state of the kidney.

The ERPF may be estimated with an agent that has a high extraction ratio. An ideal ERPF agent would meet the following criteria. It would not be metabolized by the kidneys; be readily dissociated from any plasma protein complex in its transit through the kidney; have nearly total renal extraction; and be possible to quantitate in plasma or urine by a simple analytic method.

In addition, for a single injection clearance, it is desirable that the agent have no extrarenal site of excretion.

The diagnosis of obstructive and renovascular disorders can be facilitated also through measurement of *transit times* through the renal parenchyma and pelvis.

Glomerular Filtration Rate

The GFR is a widely used parameter for following the clinical course of renal disease and the effects of various therapies on renal function. Determination of the GFR based on plasma creatinine[3] does not yield a very precise value. The GFR may be determined with an approximate 5 percent error with continuous infusion of inulin to maintain a steady plasma level, combined with urine collection for measurement of the amount that has been cleared in a given time. This method, however, is cumbersome and impractical in most clinical situations.

The GFR may be estimated by measurement of the blood clearance of substances that satisfy specific criteria. Such substances must be freely filtered through the glomerular capillary membrane; must be physiologically inert and not metabolized in the body; must be excreted only by the kidneys (which becomes unnecessary if urine collections are carried out); must not be secreted or absorbed by the renal tubules; must have not toxic effect and no effect on renal function when infused in large amounts; must be accurately quantifiable in body fluids; must have clearances that are equal to accepted standard tracers that have been shown to measure GFR; and must have a constant clearance at any urine flow rate in order to exclude the influence of tubular reabsorption or secretion.

Radionuclide studies require the substance to be labeled with a radioactive material, and the combination must be radiochemically stable; that is, the radioactive labeling material must be an integral part of the compound.

AVAILABLE RENAL IMAGING AGENTS

A great many agents have been evaluated and used for renal imaging and the evaluation of renal function, but only a few have broad clinical importance. They generally are categorized as ERPF agents or GFR agents, depending on whether they are excreted largely by tubular secretion or glomerular filtration. Their advantages and disadvantages are summarized in Table 10-1.[4]

Other radionuclides are suitable as purely anatomic imaging agents. They allow measurement of functioning renal mass but not of GFR or ERPF. Use of these agents usually is secondary to information previously gathered with urography or ultrasonography. These procedures and agents will not be considered here.

Table 10-1. Advantages and Disadvantages of Renal Agents

Renal Agents	Advantages	Disadvantages
^{99m}Tc DTPA	Measures GFR Low radiation dose Can be used for static and flow images Availability, ease of use Inexpensive	Lower extraction efficiency than tubule-secreted agents Poor uptake in renal failure Poor image quality in renal failure Higher tissue and blood background Approximately 5% aberrant behavior
^{131}I OIH	Measures ERPF High target/background ratio Greater renal uptake than DTPA High extraction efficiency Acceptable images down to 2% renal function	Higher radiation dose Free iodide Poor radiolabel for γ-camera
^{123}I OIH	Measures ERPF High target/background ratio Lower radiation burden Excellent imaging agent Greater renal uptake than DTPA High extraction efficiency Acceptable images down to 2% renal function	Possible radiocontamination Expense Availability
^{99m}Tc MAG3	Measures ERPF High target/background ratio Greater renal uptake than DTPA Excellent imaging agent High extraction efficiency Good images down to 2% renal function Low radiation dose	Variable liver uptake[a] More expensive than DTPA

Abbreviations: DTPA, diethylenetriaminepenta-acetic acid; ERPF, effective renal plasma flow; GFR, glomerular filtration rate; I, iodine; MAG3, mercaptoacetylglycylglycylglycine; OIH, orthoiodohippurate; Tc, technetium.

[a] Not a serious impediment to use as an imaging agent.

ERPF Agents

Radionuclides excreted by tubular secretion may be used to estimate ERPF. Most of the agents in widespread clinical use have been *hippurate-containing compounds*. Renal transport mechanisms such as those involved in tubular secretion have not been well described. However, experience has identified several factors that affect handling of hippurate-containing compounds. These factors include lipophilicity and conjugation to amino acids and lactic acids. Glycine conjugates such as para-aminohippuric acid (PAHA) are vigorously secreted by the renal tubule.[5] PAHA is not a clinically useful substrate because its concentration in the blood can be determined only by time-consuming chemical methods or it can be radiolabeled with a β-emitter. It is used as a reference compound for ERPF determination.

Orthoiodohippurate (OIH) may be labeled with various iodine isotopes by a simple iodine exchange reaction.[6] The clinically important compounds are those labeled with iodine 131 (^{131}I OIH) and iodine 123 (^{123}I OIH). It is possible to prepare compounds with high specific activity[7-12]; however, this may result in significant radiolytic decomposition, releasing free inorganic iodide.[13,14] Quantitative ERPF determinations require quality control of OIH preparations to determine that free iodide content is 2 percent or less.

[131]I OIH is useful clinically for the determination of ERPF.[15,16] Its urinary clearance in humans has been estimated to be only about 80 to 85 percent that of para-aminohippurate (PAH). These differences may be due to the presence of free ^{131}I in the preparation, plasma protein binding, and/or differences in tubular transport.[16-19] This lower extraction ratio results in a slight systematic underestimate of ERPF (Fig. 10-3). The clearance, however, is reproducible and is useful clinically.

Because of its avid uptake by the kidney, ^{131}I OIH often is useful when other agents provide inconclusive results and for patients with major impairment of renal function.[4] It is relatively inexpensive, widely available, and has a high extraction efficiency, providing a low level of background blood and tissue activity in imaging procedures. A major drawback to this agent is the ^{131}I radiolabel. It is imaged poorly with the γ-cameras currently in use[20]

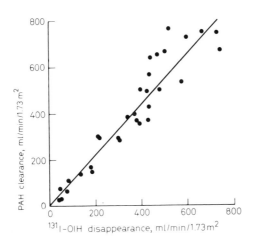

Fig. 10-3. The continuous infusion clearance of para-aminohippuric acid (PAH) against a single-injection clearance of ^{131}I-labeled OIH. The extraction ratio of OIH is slightly lower than that of PAH, resulting in a systematic underestimate. However, the extraction is high enough to provide a useful estimate of the ERPF. (From Chervu and Blaufox,[27] with permission.)

and can be administered only in relatively small doses as a result its long half-life and associated β-emission. This results in poor data quality when kidney function is low. Retention of radioactivity in the kidney in the presence of outflow obstruction results in a significantly increased radiation dose.[21] A low radiation-dose equivalent of ^{131}I OIH has been searched for in renal nuclear medicine for some time.[4] Such an agent would safely provide high-quality images in patients with poor renal function. OIH labeled with different isotopes of iodine has been proposed but may pose problems because of its expense and associated radiation exposure. An analog of OIH labeled with technetium holds more promise.

[123]I OIH is very similar to ^{131}I OIH and is much better suited to the modern γ-camera. It provides excellent images even when renal function is poor, and it is excreted more rapidly than the ^{131}I-labeled substrate. [123]I OIH can be used in adults and children in larger doses than ^{131}I OIH while still imparting a lower radiation burden to the patient.[22–26] However, the low-energy methods of its preparation can result in contamination with [124]I and [126]I. Iodine 126 can contribute a high radiation burden to the patient.

[123]I OIH currently is available commercially but is not in widespread use because of its great expense and short physical half-life. Higher energy methods of producing ^{123}I OIH may result in higher radionuclidic purity and increasing availability at lower cost.

A number of centers have abandoned the use of OIH[4] and directed their efforts at the use of technetium-99m *diethylenetriamine-pentacetic acid* [99m]*Tc (DTPA)*. However, a recently introduced technetium-labeled OIH analog is likely to become a useful agent for renal imaging and ERPF determination. This agent already has achieved widespread use in Europe, where it has been available for several years. *Technetium-99m mercaptoacetylglycylgly-cylglycine* (^{99m}Tc MAG3) is reasonably similar to ^{131}I OIH in renal excretion properties.[27,28] In normal human volunteers, MAG3 and ^{123}I OIH show comparable image quality, renal excretion, blood clearance, and time to peak height of the renogram curve.[29,30] Images obtained with MAG3 are significantly better than images obtained with ^{131}I OIH. Blood and plasma clearances indicate more rapid renal clearance for ^{131}I OIH than for ^{99m}Tc MAG3, although quantitative urinary excretion is similar for the two agents. The two agents also behave similarly in animal models of renovascular hypertension (Fig. 10-4).[31]

Overall, the clearance of ^{99m}Tc MAG3/^{131}I OIH is approximately 80 percent in humans. This proportion, however, appears to be stable across a wide range of renal function, allowing use of ^{99m}Tc MAG3 for the estimation of ERPF. This difference apparently is due to the greater protein binding and the absence of a filtered component for MAG3. So, MAG3 appears to be a "pure" tubular agent.

Taylor and colleagues[32] determined the radiochemical purity of the MAG3 kit using high-performance liquid chromatography (HPLC) and thin-layer chromatography. The preparation was 97.3 percent pure, with 0.7 percent insoluble forms and 2.0 percent non-MAG3-labeled soluble material.[32] They

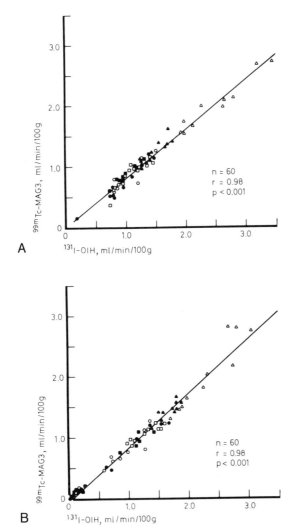

Fig. 10-4. (A) Excellent correlation has been shown between the clearances of MAG3 and OIH in rats with renovascular hypertension. **(B)** This correlation is maintained after captopril adminstration despite the significant change in clearances. (From Chervu and Blaufox,[27] with permission.)

reported that the kit was stable for up to 6 hours after formulation and that it had physiologic and biologic properties similar to those of ^{131}I OIH in patients with suspected renal dysfunction while producing consistently better images. This group also has found the kit formulation to compare favorably with formulations of MAG3 purified by HPLC.[33]

Some precautions may be required in interpretation of MAG3 studies in patients with very low renal function. Taylor and colleagues[33] have reported approximately 1 percent of the injected dose in the gallbladder and approximately 5 percent in the liver 30 to 60 minutes after injection in three patients with renal failure.[33] Our group also has seen liver and biliary uptake in patients with varied levels of renal function. This raises the possibility that the gallbladder may be mistaken for the right kidney. An anterior or lateral view can eliminate this possibility. Liver extraction also could result in an overestimate of renal function when a single injection clearance technique is used to estimate renal function. These features must be considered when using MAG3, but they are not serious impediments to its great potential as an imaging agent.

Technetium labeling of a substance that behaves similarly to OIH can be expected to result in better image quality and clinical utility, even in patients with very low renal function. This has been the case with MAG3.[34,35]

GFR Agents

Ethylenediaminetetra-acetic acid (EDTA) and its analog *DTPA* are chelating agents that have been used for the treatment of toxic metal poisoning. They are eliminated via glomerular filtration without any metabolic alteration and with very little, if any, tubular secretion. They form strong complexes with several radionuclides. The most widely used agent of this group is DTPA in complex with ^{99m}Tc (^{99m}Tc DTPA).

^{99m}Tc DTPA has been tested extensively for nephrologic and urologic applications. The mode of renal elimination may vary, depending on the the exact manufacture and packaging of the agent and the time interval between preparation and use.[36,37] Quality control before GFR determination has been stressed.[38–41]

^{99m}Tc DTPA shows little diffusion of radioactivity into blood cells, but up to 5 percent of the compound may be protein bound,[42,43] and 4 to 5 percent of the administered dose may be detected in various tissues at 24 hours after administration.[44]

Compared with agents transported by tubular secretion, those transported by glomerular filtration alone have a relatively low extraction efficiency. The result is a higher proportion of background activity or "noise" in imaging procedures.

AVAILABLE PROCEDURES AND TECHNIQUES

Many procedures are available to estimate renal function with the aid of radionuclides (Table 10-2).[1] They include renal perfusion studies, renal imaging studies performed to acquire anatomic information only, and renal imaging studies combined with an estimate of renal function. The Department of Nuclear Medicine at the Albert Einstein College of Medicine/Montefiore Medical Center has virtually abandoned nonimaging techniques for the measurement of renal function except for research purposes. In most

Table 10-2. Evaluation of Renal
Function With
Radionuclides

Clearance methods
  Continuous infusion
  Single injection
  Simplified single injection

Radioimmunoassay
  Angiotensin
  Renin activity
  Aldosterone

Radiorenogram
  ^{99m}Tc DTPA
  ^{131}I, ^{123}I OIH
  ^{99m}Tc MAG3
  Miscellaneous

Body spaces

Radionuclide cystogram
  Residual urine
  Ureterovesical reflux

Scintiphotography
  Individual renal function
    ^{99m}Tc DTPA
    ^{99m}Tc MAG3
    ^{131}I, ^{123}I OIH
  Individual renal mass
    ^{99m}Tc-DMSA
    ^{99m}Tc-glucoheptonate
  Perfusion imaging
    Any low-dose ^{99m}Tc agent
  Morphology
    Renal mass agents

Renal blood flow

Abbreviations: DMSA, dimercaptosuccinic acid; DTPA, diethylenetriaminepenta-acetic acid; MAG3, mercaptoacetylglycylglycylglycine; OIH, orthoiodohippurate.

clinical situations, the small additional radiation burden of a renal scintigram is more than warranted by the additional information acquired.

Single-Injection Clearance Methods

The practical clinical use of the single-injection clearance is one of the most
important contributions of radionuclides to nephrology. The dose required
for the accurate chemical quantification of PAH in the performance of a
single-injection clearance would achieve concentrations in the blood above
the maximum secretory ability of the kidney. Therefore, radionuclides are

essential for effective single-injection determinations of ERPF. These agents also provide great convenience in the single-injection determination of GFR, although inulin can be substituted easily, thus avoiding exposure of the patient to radiation.

Single-injection clearances may be determined by several different methods. All of them require that the body be in a steady state, that the material used by excreted only by the kidney, that it not be metabolized, that no chemical or radioactive impurities are present, and that the plasma can be readily sampled and represents the central compartment.[1]

The most accurate of the single-injection techniques uses a two-compartment model.[45] Simplified methods using a one-compartment model and one to three blood samples also can provide clinically acceptable approximations of renal function.[1,45,46] The simplified one-compartment model described by Blaufox and Merrill[47] estimates ERPF with two blood samples taken usually 20 minutes and 30 minutes after administration of ^{131}I OIH. The method described by Tauxe et al. (also with ^{131}I OIH) uses a single timed sample and yields similar results.[48,49] Similar methods of determining GFR usually sample plasma beginning 2 hours after injection because of the slower kinetics of glomerular filtration.

Albert Einstein College of Medicine routinely relies on single-injection clearances for determination of total renal function. Clinical indications for such evaluation include chronic renal disease and renal transplantation. In patients with low levels of renal function, urine sampling may be necessary to achieve optimum accuracy.

External Counting Methods and Scintigraphy

Kidney function also may be estimated with external counting methods.[50,51] After injection of a radionuclide, the kidneys are imaged with a γ-camera interfaced to a computer. The renogram generated during 1 to 2 minutes, corrected for background radioactivity and depth, may be used to determine the ERPF of the individual kidneys or the total ERPF when compared with the injected dose (Fig. 10-5).[52]

The ERPF values for the right and left kidneys derived from external counting methods may be compared to yield relative renal function. Some investigators have advocated using this left/right ratio in combination with a measurement of total renal function derived from plasma clearance measurements to arrive at more precise values for individual renal function.[53] The absolute values of GFR and ERPF determined with camera imaging methods are not as accurate as those obtained with other techniques. However, the techniques are very good; the reproducibility in a given patient is very precise, with correlations greater than 0.98. Better methods of depth correction using sonography or lateral views appear to improve the accuracy of the camera methods.[54–56] In the absence of accurate quantitation of depth, it may be preferable to omit depth correction.

Clinical indications for determination of individual renal function include

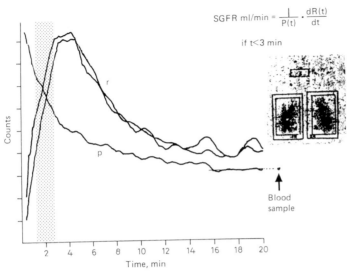

$$SGFR \; ml/min = \frac{1}{P(t)} \cdot \frac{dR(t)}{dt}$$

if $t < 3$ min

Blood
sample

Fig. 10-5. External counting method using the cardiac blood pool and the early portion of the second slope of the renogram, as shown in the shaded portion of the figure. The best portion of the slope in terms of avoiding excretion and minimizing background appears to be between 1 and 2 minutes. Use of the total integral count between 1 and 2 minutes, instead of the slope, will reduce the margin of error. SGFR, single-nephron glomerular filtration rate. (From Piepsz et al.,[52] with permission.)

renovascular hypertension, unilateral renal parenchymal disease, bilateral renal disease with planned surgical intervention, and evaluation of renal function after intervention or during growth. Table 10-3 illustrates the range of clinical utility of nuclear medicine tests.

The scintigram is the mainstay of the radionuclide study in urology and nephrology.[4] This procedure provides both anatomic and functional information. No other technique can provide both the individual renal functional information and the information on urinary flow that this noninvasive radionuclide test can provide (Figs. 10-6, 10-7).

The renal scintigram with OIH has shown prognostic value in acute renal failure, allowing the recognition of residual renal function in patients with severely compromised renal function resulting from obstruction. MAG3 has not yet been adequately studied for this use. Its value will depend on the extent of its uptake by the liver. The same is true in chronic renal failure. In both cases, a technetium-labeled ERPF agent is desired.

A renal scintigram can provide valuable information regarding the upper urinary tract sequelae of bladder neck obstruction or neurogenic bladder.

A major contribution of nuclear medicine to the evaluation of *pyelonephritis* is information regarding relative renal function and functional impairment caused by this disease. Functional agents are less helpful in this situation than agents such as gallium, which can help identify the affected area, or dimercaptosuccinic acid (DMSA), which is very sensitive in diagnosing pyelonephritis and differentiating it from *cystitis*.

Table 10-3. Clinical Conditions Evaluated by Nuclear Medicine

Disease/ Condition	Test	Agent	Value
Acute renal failure	Scintigram	ERPF agent	Prognosis, diagnosis
Bladder-neck obstruction	Scintigram	ERPF or GFR agent	Diagnosis, serial changes
Chronic renal failure	Scintigram	ERPF agent	Location, relative function, serial changes
Neurogenic bladder	Scintigram	ERPF or GFR agent	Diagnosis, serial changes
Obstructive uropathy	Scintigram, renogram	ERPF, GFR agent	Relative function, prognosis, diagnosis, serial changes
Pyelonephritis	Scintigram, renogram	ERPF, GFR, renal parenchymal agent	Diagnosis, relative function, serial changes
Renal arterial embolism	Flow scintigram	ERPF, GFR agent, renal parenchymal agent	Diagnosis, relative function, serial changes
Renal transplantation	Flow scintigram	ERPF, GFR agent	Diagnosis, function, serial changes
Renal trauma	Flow scintigram	ERPF, GFR agent, renal parenchymal agent	Diagnosis, relative function, serial changes
Renovascular hypertension	Scintigram, renogram	ERPF, GFR agent	Diagnosis, relative function, serial changes

Abbreviations: ERPF, effective renal plasma flow; GFR, glomerular filtration rate. (Adapted from Blaufox et al.,[4] with permission.)

The flow scintigram is particularly useful in several situations. *Renal arterial embolism* is a relatively rare but potentially serious condition. Both ERPF and GFR agents are appropriate for diagnosis and evaluation of this condition. However, the greater perfusion and higher uptake and excretion rates of ERPF agents may offer an advantage in patients who are severely compromised.

Until recently, only ^{99m}Tc DTPA was available for initial flow studies in most centers; ^{131}I OIH placed too great a radiation burden on the patient, and ^{123}I OIH was prohibitively expensive. With MAG3, both the flow study and static imaging studies can be performed at a reasonable cost with an ERPF

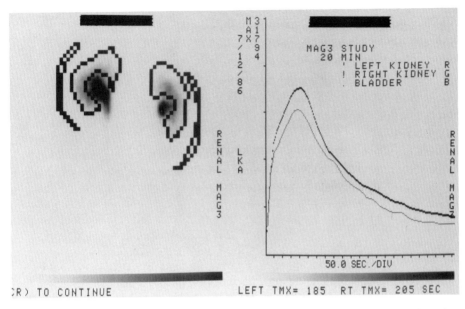

Fig. 10-6. MAG3 scintigram and renogram in a patient with normal renal function, showing the renal and background regions of interest.

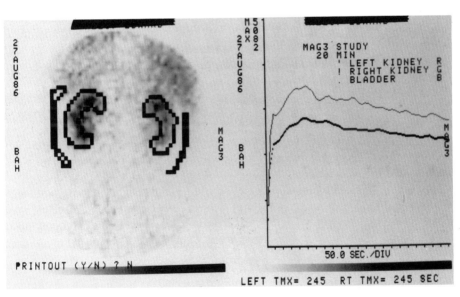

Fig. 10-7. MAG3 scintigram and renogram in a patient with bilateral renal damage. The patient is a 64-year-old man with diabetes and hypertension. Contrast the significantly reduced uptake seen in the renogram with the normal uptake in Figure 10-6. The renal impairment is only slightly asymmetric.

agent. This should be quite helpful in evaluating patients who have undergone *renal transplantation* as well as those with *renal trauma*.

Diuretic Renography

One of the most important applications of radionuclides to the study of the urinary tract is diuretic renography in the differential diagnosis of *obstructive uropathy*. Dilatation of the urinary collecting system may not be diagnostic of clinically significant obstruction in adults or children.[57] It often is necessary to differentiate between nonobstructive dilatation of the collecting system and dilatation associated with obstruction that may require surgical correction to prevent progressive loss of renal function.[58] This problem is made particularly difficult by the complex and variable relationship between hydrostatic pressure, urine flow, and peristalsis in the ureter.[59,60]

Whittaker[61] devised a test to evaluate nonobstructive dilatation that has achieved wide urologic acceptance. It involves placing a tube proximal to the site of the presumed obstruction and infusing saline solution at a predetermined rate. (Usually, the infusion is made into the renal pelvis via a nephrostomy tube or percutaneous needle.) Theoretically, this makes it possible to determine whether or not an abnormal pressure–flow relationship, and therefore obstruction, exists. An intermediate group, however, falls between those patients who show clear obstruction and those who are clearly not obstructed. Ureteral pressure rises to a finite, higher-than-normal point in this group but does not continue to rise as the infusion continues. The clinical significance of Whittaker test results in this middle group is difficult to determine, and the problem remains unresolved.

Radionuclide study of obstructive uropathy is noninvasive and does not affect urine flow rate or urine composition. Thus, it allows the use of a variety of interventions that change urine flow rate and so challenge the collecting system in a manner analogous to the Whittaker test. Diuretic challenge is the logical and most common approach. Water or osmotic diuretics such as mannitol are potent and safe, and thiazide diuretics can be administered intravenously. The great potency of furosemide, however, makes it the most attractive option. It is effective over a wide range of renal function, even in relatively severe renal insufficiency. A wide variety of diuretic agents are available. Their different courses of action allow many possible ways of altering the urinary composition, but little work has been done to determine the differing effects (if any) of different types of diuretic agents on the renogram.[59]

The two radionuclides most commonly used to test the urinary tract are ^{99m}Tc DTPA and ^{131}I OIH. MAG3 apparently yields results that are quite similar to ^{131}I OIH. The GFR agent results in a relatively low radiation dose to the patient, allowing repeated administration of larger amounts. This results in good images and very reliable data. ^{131}I OIH is concentrated more

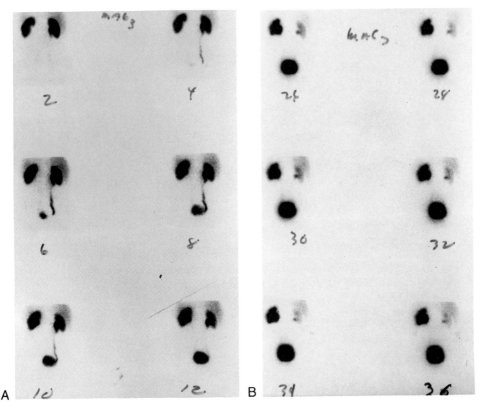

Fig. 10-8. Sequential images from a MAG3 study using 2-minute frames. The images from 4, 8, 12, 26, 28, 30, 32, 34, and 36 minutes are shown. Furosemide was administered at 20 minutes. Note the significant impairment of emptying on the left with increasing pelvic activity.

rapidly, giving it an advantage in imaging severely damaged kidneys. Its more rapid excretion makes it possible to appreciate smaller changes in renal function. This procedure is, of course, most helpful when it allows classification of a patient as obstructed or unobstructed (Figs. 10-8 and 10-9).

A significant proportion of these studies, however, yields only indeterminate results. This is not a failure of the test, but a reflection of the wide spectrum of disease and the inability to control factors such as the patient's state of hydration. Even when results are not definitive, the great sensitivity of this test to changes in renal function can make follow-up studies extremely valuable. Nuclear medicine techniques allow safe, noninvasive study of the kidney serially, rather than at a single point in time. This intermediate group should have adequate follow-up in order to facilitate surgical intervention before irreversible renal damage occurs and to avoid unnecessary surgery in patients with stable function.

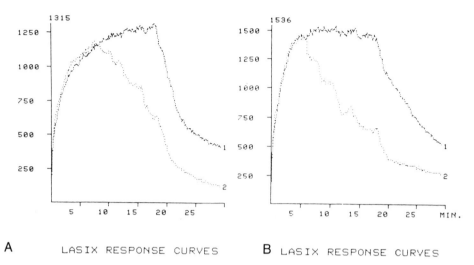

Fig. 10-9. Time–activity curves in a case of left nonobstructive hydronephrosis with **(A)** ^{99m}Tc MAG3 and **(B)** ^{123}I OIH. The vertical scale shows counts per second, the horizontal time in minutes. Furosemide was administered at 18 minutes. Note the comparability of the response in this case between ^{123}I OIH and ^{99m}Tc MAG3. (From Jaffri et al.,[62] with permission.)

Captopril Renography

An increasingly important role for renal radionuclide studies is in the evaluation of hypertensive disease.[63,64] The role of nuclear medicine in the diagnosis of renovascular disease has been controversial, largely because of the lack of specificity of renography in making the diagnosis. Renography is highly sensitive in detecting unilateral renal disease, but it produces an unacceptable number of false-positive results. In the diagnosis of renovascular hypertension (RVH), the intravenous urogram and the scintirenogram have generally been reported to have sensitivities and specificities of approximately 85 percent.[63,64] That is, each test correctly identifies 85 percent of the true-positives tested and correctly identifies 85 percent of the true-negatives tested. In a population with a low prevalence of disease (less than 5 percent of hypertension is due to a correctable lesion), this is not adequate for general screening. The costs involved cannot be supported, to say nothing of the discomfort and small but significant patient risks associated with the urogram.

In the hospital setting, however, it may be possible to select out a population of patients with hypertension in whom the prevalence of RVH is approximately 20 to 30 percent.[64] The definitive diagnosis of RVH requires an angiographic procedure, but routine renography interposed between angiographic procedures can significantly reduce the cost of each case of RVH found.[64]

The recent introduction of captopril renography has spurred new interest in the use of nuclear medicine to diagnose RVH.[65] The rationale for the use of angiotensin-converting enzyme (ACE) inhibition in the renographic diagnosis of RVH is based on the observation that short-term administration of the captopril alters kidney function on the side affected by renal arterial constriction, but has little or no effect on kidneys with a normal blood supply.[66,67] The specificity of these changes offers the potential to greatly increase the accuracy of radionuclide tests in RVH, achieving even greater cost reductions in the diagnosis of RVH. Improvements in imaging properties of tubule-secreted radionuclide preparations also may contribute to the more effective diagnosis of RVH.[68]

CONCLUSION

Continuing refinement of nuclear medicine techniques can serve both patients and the nuclear medicine community. Diuretic renography and captopril renography have captured considerable current interest and can serve to demonstrate the value of renal scintigraphy. Improvements in imaging techniques and materials are forthcoming and should help ensure the diagnostic utility of renal nuclear medicine.

One such improvement lies in the development of improved radionuclide imaging agents. Technetium-labeled imaging agents transported by tubular secretion, such as MAG3, have combined the advantages of diverse earlier agents. The low radiation dose allows repeated administration of large amounts, resulting in good counting statistics and excellent images. Tubular secretion results in greater perfusion and quicker concentration, allowing appreciation of even small changes in renal function.

ACKNOWLEDGMENTS

I thank Mr. Manel Valdez-Cruz for his valuable editorial assistance in the preparation of this manuscript. This work was supported by an educational grant from Mallinckrodt Medical, Inc.

REFERENCES

1. Blaufox MD: Measurement of renal function with radioactive materials. p. 12. In Blaufox MD (ed): Evaluation of Renal Function and Disease with Radionuclides: The Upper Urinary Tract. Karger, Basel, 1989
2. Goldring W, Clarke RW, Smith HW: The phenol red clearance in normal man. J Clin Invest 15:221, 1936
3. Bianchi C: Measurement of the glomerular filtration rate. p. 21. In Blaufox MD (ed): Evaluation of Renal Function and Disease With Radionuclides: The Upper Urinary Tract. Karger, Basel, 1972

4. Blaufox MD, Fine E, Lee H-B, Scharf S: The role of nuclear medicine in clinical urology and nephrology. J Nucl Med 25:619, 1984

5. Despopoulos A: A definition of substrate specificity in renal transport of organic anions. J Theor Biol 8:163, 1965

6. Tubis M, Posnick E, Nordyke RA: Preparation and use of I131 labeled sodium iodohippurate in kidney function tests. Proc Soc Exp Biol Med 103:497, 1960

7. Scheer KE, Meier-Borst W: Die Darstellung von ^{131}I-Orthoiodohippursäure durch Austauschmarkierung. Nucl Med Stuttg 2:193, 1961

8. Mitta AEA, Fraga A, Veall N: A simplified method for preparing ^{131}I-labeled hippuran. Int J Appl Radiat Isot 12:146, 1961

9. Elias H, Arnold CH, Koss G: Preparation of ^{131}I labeled m-iodohippuric acid and its behavior in kidney function studies compared to o-iodohippuric acid. Int J Appl Radiat Isot 24:463, 1973

10. Gillet R, Cogneau M, Mathy G: The preparation of ^{123}I labeled sodium iodohippurate for medical research. Int J Appl Radiat Isot 27:61, 1976

11. Thakur ML, Chauser BM, Hudson FR: The preparation of ^{123}I labeled sodium orthoiodohippurate and its clearance by the rat kidneys. Int J Appl Radiat Isot 26:319, 1975

12. Sinn H, Maier-Borst W, Elias H: An efficient method for routine production of orthoiodohippuric acid labeled with ^{131}I, ^{125}I or [123]I. Int J Appl Radiat Isot 28:809, 1977

13. Hotte CE, Ice RD: The in vitro stability of ^{131}I-O-iodohippurate. J Nucl Med 20:441, 1979

14. Hammermaier A, Reich E, Bogl W: Radiochemical purity and in vitro stability of commercial hippurans. J Nucl Med 27:850, 1986

15. Schwartz FD, Madeloff MS: Simultaneous renal clearances of radiohippuran and PAH in man. Clin Res 9:208, 1961

16. Burbank MK, Tauxe WN, Maher F et al: Evaluation of radioiodinated hippuran for the estimation of renal plasma flow. Proc Staff Meet Mayo Clin 36:372, 1961

17. Mailloux L, Gagnon JA: Measurement of effective renal plasma flow. p. 54. In Blaufox MD (ed): Evaluation of Renal Function and Disease With Radionuclides: The Upper Urinary Tract. Karger, Basel, 1972

18. Haas JP, Prellwitz W: Die Bestimmung der renalen und totalen Clearance mit Jod-131-markiertem Chlorjodpropyl-Inulin, radioaktive Isotope in Klinik und Forschung. Vol. 7. p. 462. Urban & Schwartzenberg, Munich, 1967

19. Maher FT, Tauxe WN: Renal clearance in man of pharmaceuticals containing radioactive iodine. Influence of plasma binding. JAMA 207:97, 1969

20. Zucker LS, Axelrod MS, Wexler JP et al: The implications of decreased performance of new generation gamma cameras on the interpretation of 131-I Hippuran renal images. Nucl Med Commun 8:49, 1987

21. Elliott AT, Britton KE: A review of the physiological parameters on the dosimetry of 123-I and 131-I labelled Hippuran. Int J Appl Radiat Isot 29:571, 1978

22. Zielinski FW, Holly FE, Robinson GD Jr et al: Total and individual kidney function assessment with I123-orthoiodohippurate. Radiology 125:753, 1977

23. Wellman HN, Berke RA, Robbins PJ: Dynamic quantitative renal imaging with I123 Hippuran. A possible salvation of the renogram. J Nucl Med 12:405, 1971

24. Chisolm GL, Short MD, Glass HI: The measurement of individual renal plasma flows using I131 hippuran and the gamma camera. Br J Urol 46:591, 1974

25. Heindenreich P, Lauer O, Fendel H et al: Determination of total and individual kidney function in children by means of I123-hippuran whole body clearance and scintillation camera. Pediatr Radiol 11:17, 1981

26. Carlsen O, Kvinesdal B, Nathan E: Quantitative evaluation of ^{123}I-hippuran gamma camera renography in normal children. J Nucl Med 27:117, 1986

27. Chervu LR, Blaufox MD: Radiopharmaceuticals for the measurement of glomerular filtration rate and renal plasma flow. p. 28. In Blaufox MD (ed): Evaluation of Renal Function and Disease With Radionuclides: The Upper Urinary Tract. Karger, Basel, 1989

28. Fritzberg AR, Kasina S, Eshima D et al: Synthesis and biological evaluation of Tc99m MAG3 as a hippuran replacement. J Nucl Med 27:111, 1986

29. Taylor A, Eshima D, Fritzberg AT er al: Comparison of ^{131}I-OIH and Tc99m-MAG3 renal imaging in volunteers. J Nucl Med 27:795, 1986

30. Taylor A Jr, Eshima D, Alazraki N: Tc 99m MAG3, a new renal imaging agent: preliminary results in patients. Eur J Nucl Med 12:510, 1987

31. Lee HB, Blaufox MD: Tc 99m MAG3 clearances after captopril in renovascular hypertension (RVH), abstract. J Nucl Med 29:849, 1988

32. Taylor A Jr, Ziffer JA, Steves A et al: Clinical comparison of I 131 orthoiodohippurate and the kit formulation of Tc 99m mercaptoacetyltriglycine. Radiology 170:721, 1989

33. Taylor A Jr, Eshima D, Christian PE et al: Technetium-99m MAG3 kit formulation: preliminary results in normal volunteers and patients with renal failure. J Nucl Med 29:616, 1988

34. Taylor A Jr, Ziffer JA, Eshima D: Comparison of Tc 99m MAG3 and Tc 99m DTPA in renal transplant patients with impaired renal function. Clin Nucl Med 15:371, 1990

35. Taylor A Jr, Eshima D, Christian PE, Milton W: Evaluation of Tc 99m mercaptoacetyltriglycine in patients with impaired renal function. Radiology 162:365, 1987

36. Srivastava SC, Meinken G, Smith TD et al: Problems associated with stannous Tc99m radiopharmaceuticals. Int J Radiat Isot 28:83, 1977

37. Carlsen JE, Moller ML, Lund JO et al: Comparison of four commercial Tc99m (Sn) DTPA preparations used for the measurement of glomerular filtration rate. J Nucl Med 21:126, 1980

38. Hosain F: Quality control of Tc99m-DTPA by double tracer clearance technique. J Nucl Med 15:442, 1974

39. Kempi V, Persson RB: Tc99m-DTPA (Sn) dry-kit preparation. Quality control and clearance studies. Nucl Med Stuttg 13:389, 1975

40. Russell CD, Bischoff PD, Rowell KL et al: Quality control of Tc99m-DTPA for measurement of glomerular filtration. Concise communication. J Nucl Med 24:722, 1983

41. Russell CD, Rowell K, Scott JW: Quality control of Tc99m-DTPA. Correlation of analytic tests with in vivo protein binding in man. J Nucl Med 27:560, 1986

42. Chervu LR, Lee HB, Goyal Q et al: Use of Tc99m-Cu-DTPA complex as a renal function agent. J Nucl Med 18:62, 1977

43. Klopper JF, Hauser W, Atkins HL et al: Evaluation of Tc99m DTPA for the measurement of glomerular filtration rate. J Nucl Med 13:107, 1972

44. McAfee JG, Gagne G, Atkins HL et al: Biological distribution and excretion of DTPA labeled with Tc99m and In111. J Nucl Med 20:1273, 1979

45. Rabinowitz A, Wexler JP, Blaufox MD: Quantification of the radionuclide image: theoretical concepts and the role of the computer. p. 261. In Freeman L, Johnson P (eds): Clinical Radionuclide Imaging. Grune & Stratton, Orlando, FL, 1984

46. Russsell CD, Bischoff PG, Kontzen FN et al: Measurement of glomerular filtration rate. Single injection plasma clearance method without urine collection. J Nucl Med 26:1243, 1985

47. Blaufox MD, Merrill JP: Simplified hippuran clearance. Measurement of renal function in man with simplified hippuran clearances. Nephron 3:274, 1966

48. Tauxe WH, Dubovsky EV, Kidd T Jr et al: New formulas for the calculation of effective renal plasma flow. Eur J Nucl Med 7:51, 1982

49. Tauxe WN, Maher FT, Taylor WF: Effective renal plasma flow. Estimation from theoretical volumes of distribution of intravenously injected 131-I orthoiodohippurate. Mayo Clin Proc 46:524, 1971

50. Schlegel JU, Hamway SA: Individual renal plasma flow determination in 2 minutes. J Urol 116:282, 1976

51. Gates GF: Glomerular filtration rate. Estimation from fractional renal accumulation of ^{99m}Tc DTPA (stannous). Am J Radiol 138:565, 1982

52. Piepsz A, Denis R, Ham HR et al: A simple method for measuring separate glomerular filtration rate using a single injection of ^{99m}TC DTPA and the scintillation camera. J Pediatr 93:769, 1978

53. Russell C: A comparison of methods for GFR measurement using TC-99m-DTPA and the gamma camera. p. 173. In Tauxe W, Dubovsky E (eds): Nuclear Medicine in Clinical Urology and Nephrology. Appleton-Century-Crofts, East Norwalk, CT, 1985

54. Fine EF, Axelrod M, Gorkin J et al: Measurement of effective renal plasma flow. A comparison of methods. J Nucl Med 28:1393, 1987

55. Grünewald SM, Collins LT, Fawdry RM: Kidney depth measurement and its influence on quantitation of function from gamma camera renography. Clin Nucl Med 10:398, 1985

56. Nimmon CC, McAlister JM, Cattell WR: Kidney position and the measurement of relative uptake of 131-I hippuran in renography. Estimation from theoretical volumes of distribution of intravenously injected 131-I orthoiodohippurate. Mayo Clin Proc 46:524, 1971

57. O'Reilly PH, Lawson RS, Shields RS et al: Wide ureters: a dilemma in diagnosis. Br J Radiol 51:223, 1978

58. Blaufox MD: Diuretic renography and other interventions in urinary tract disease. p. 519. In Spencer RP (ed): Interventional Nuclear Medicine. Grune & Stratton, Orlando, FL, 1984

59. Ross JA, Edmond P, Kirkland IS: Behavior of the human ureter in health and disease. Williams & Wilkins, Baltimore, 1972

60. Boyarcky S, Tanagho EA, Gottschalk CW et al: Urodynamics: Hydrodynamics of the Ureter and Renal Pelvis. Academic Press, Orlando, FL, 1971

61. Whittaker RH: Methods of assessing obstruction in dilated ureters. Br J Urol 45:15, 1973

62. Jafri RA, Britton KE, Nimmon CC et al: Technetium-99m MAG3, a comparison with iodine-123 and iodine-131 orthoiodohipourate, in patients with renal disorders. J Nucl Med 29:147, 1988

63. Blaufox MD, Fine EJ: Role of nuclear medicine techniques for evaluating hyper-

tensive disease. p. 1509. In Laragh JH, Brenner BM (eds): Hypertension: Pathophysiology, Diagnosis, and Management. Raven Press, New York, 1990

64. Blaufox MD: Cost-effectiveness of nuclear medicine procedures in renovascular hypertension. Semin Nucl Med 19:116, 1989

65. Working group on renovascular hypertension: detection, evaluation and treatment of renovascular hypertension, fifth report. Arch Intern Med 147:820, 1987

66. Lee HB, Blaufox MD: Regional functional changes after angiotensin converting enzyme inhibition or nitroprusside in hypertensive rats. J Hypertension 4 (suppl 5):S266, 1986

67. Oei HY, Geyskes GG, Dorhout Mees EJ, Puylaert CBAJ: The significance of captopril renography in renovascular hypertension. p. 95. In Bischof-Delaloye A, Blaufox MD (eds): Radionuclides in Nephrourology. Vol. 56. Karger, Basel, 1987

68. Lee HB, Blaufox MD: Technetium-99m MAG-3 clearances after captopril in experimental renovascular hypertension. J Nucl Med 30:666, 1989

69. Austrin MG, Austrin HR: Learning Medical Terminology: A Worktext. 6th Ed. CV Mosby, St. Louis, 1987

11

Urinary Tract Infections
Important Diagnostic Procedures

Byungse Suh
Robert G. Narins
Calvin M. Kunin

Differential Culture Methods
    Ureteral Catheterization and Bladder Washout
    Segmented Cultures of the Lower Urinary Tract in the Male (Method of Meares and Stamey)
    Cystoscopic Differentiation Between Bladder Bacteriuria and Renal Bacteriuria (Method of Stamey, Govan, and Palmer)
    Bladder Washout Method in Differentiating the Site of Urinary Tract Infection (Method of Fairley)
Serologic Methods
    Tamm-Horsfall and Cross-Reactive Antigens in Kidney
    Antibody-Coated Bacteria in Urine
Diagnostic Imaging and Radionuclide Methods
Enzymuria
Tests of Renal Function in Urinary Tract Infection
Maximum Urinary Concentrating Test

INTRODUCTION

The clinical syndromes associated with urinary tract infections (UTIs) are all characterized by microbial colonization of the urine and the potential for infecting any portion(s) of the urinary tract, extending from the kidney to the urethral meatus. Infection may be present predominantly at a single site such as the kidney (pyelonephritis), the bladder (cystitis), the prostate (prostatitis), the urethra (urethritis), or it may be restricted to the urine (bacteriuria). The entire system, however, is always at risk of invasion by the causative organism once one of its parts is infected. UTIs can also be divided into two broad categories by host factors; *simple or uncomplicated infections* occur in patients with otherwise normal tracts, while *complicated infections* occur when the integrity of the voiding mechanism is impaired or a foreign body (e.g., nephrolithiasis) is present. The infection may also be classified on the basis of its location into *lower* (bladder) and *upper* (kidney) tract infections. This classification is useful in studies of the natural history of UTIs and in evaluation of chemotherapeutic agents; however, it bears little prognostic value on the final outcome.

Infections of the urinary tract represent one of the most common types of human infections encountered in medical practice today, affecting women far more than men. Approximately 20 percent of women experience symptoms of UTIs at some time during their lives,[1] and over 5 million visits to physicians' offices per year in the United States are accounted for by UTIs.[2] Furthermore, UTI is the leading cause of nosocomial infections and of gram-negative bacteremia and death resulting from sepsis in hospitals.[3] UTI is also the most common type of bacterial infection in renal transplant recipients,[4,5] and approximately 60 percent of the bacteremias seen in this setting originate in the urinary tract.[6]

It is well established that the morbidity caused by UTIs is a significant health problem and that failure to correctly diagnose and treat UTIs may lead to even more serious complications including septicemia[7–9] and death.[10,11]

This chapter discusses the practical aspects of detecting "significant" bacteriuria by microscopic, culture, and chemical methods as well as microscopic and biochemical methods for detecting pyuria. A description of the methods used to localize the site of infection to the upper and lower tract, will also be included. Nephrologists frequently consult on patients with UTIs and are often asked about the various tests for screening for and localizing infections. We have synthesized, updated, and consolidated this information. This discussion updates and extends a previous review by one of the authors.[12]

METHODS FOR DETECTING
SIGNIFICANT BACTERIURIA

Urine is an ultrafiltrate of blood and is normally sterile. The presence of any bacteria in urine obtained by aseptic means (e.g., direct-needle bladder aspiration or bladder catheterization) should be considered abnormal.[13,14]

Conversely, voided urine specimens, regardless of the care taken to avoid contamination, contain 10^2 colony-forming units (CFU) or more of bacteria per milliliter, even when paired bladder aspirates were sterile.[15,16] These so-called contaminants usually consist of fewer than 10^4 CFU/ml. Direct-needle aspiration and bladder catheterization are obviously impractical screening techniques for identifying UTIs.

Significant bacteriuria, i.e., acutal bacterial multiplication in the bladder urine, is best and most practically identified by collecting a clean, freshly voided urine specimen for a quantitative bacterial culture. Significant bacteriuria generally requires 10^5 or more CFU/ml. This most useful cutoff point was established by the pioneering work of Marple, Kass, and Sanford et al.[17-20] Actually, significant bacteriuria is usually characterized by counts well in excess of 10^6 CFU/ml. This principle of the quantitative bacterial count for defining significance is based on the fact that most urinary infections are caused by enteric gram-negative bacteria and enterococci, which grow well in urine.

Colony counts less than 10^5 CFU/ml need to be considered significant in the following settings: when bacteria are introduced into the bladder shortly after placement of an indwelling urinary catheter[21]; when urine is aspirated aseptically from a catheter; when slow-growing organisms such as coagulase-negative staphylococci are present; and when fastidious organisms such as *Hemophilus* or *Gardnerella* species, and tubercle bacilli or fungi causing deep mycoses are causative.

It must be emphasized that the criterion of 10^5 CFU or more bacteria per milliliter is not an absolute requirement but rather is a statistical effort to differentiate the large bulk of specimens containing contaminants from most true infections. Although attempts have been made to lower the cutoff figure, true UTIs with quantitative bacterial colony counts less than 10^5/ml account for only 5 percent of patients. This will be dealt with again in the section entitled Minimal Diagnostic Criteria.

Timing of Specimen Collections

Early-morning specimens should be obtained whenever possible. This ensures the highest urinary bacterial counts because the bacteria have multiplied overnight in the bladder. It is often necessary, however, to compromise and accept the second specimen of the day. This will usually provide excellent results. Similar principles apply to children.

Collection and Handling of Specimens

The objective is to collect a specimen that reflects the character of the bladder urine as closely as possible. It is, of course, obvious that this mission can be accomplished by either direct-needle aspiration of the bladder or bladder catheterization, but the clean-voided method should be used whenever possible to avoid any unnecessary instrumentation or discomfort to the patient. There are, however, times when these more invasive methods are particularly useful and may indeed be the only technique for collecting meaningful specimens. These situations may include impaired spontaneous voiding; patients who are too ill, immobilized, or obese to obtain a reliable clean-voided sample; or when a catheter is required to relieve obstruction or for diagnostic purposes. Reliable clean-voided specimens are also difficult to obtain from the newborn and from infants, rendering suprapubic aspiration a popular and extremely useful technique.

It should be noted that the reliability of cultures from females is about 80 percent. This increases to approximately 90 percent when two consecutive specimens are positive and virtually 100 percent when three consecutive specimens are positive and when each has the same organism. A single clean-voided specimen should be considered diagnostic in the adult male provided that he is circumcised or has used care in retraction of the foreskin and cleaning of the glans.

In the asymptomatic individual, two or three consecutive specimens are highly desirable to avoid overdiagnosis and to prevent unwarranted therapy and further diagnostic studies. Symptomatic patients often require early treatment, so that one specimen usually must suffice.

Detailed step by step instructions with illustrations on how to obtain diagnostically useful urine specimens by various methods have been very well described previously.[12] A reliable method of obtaining urine specimens for culture in men with external catheters has previously been described.[22] It should be noted that a concurrent antibiotic therapy[23] or the use of a cleansing solution containing chlorhexidine[24] may lower the bacterial count, and providone-iodine may give a false-positive test for occult blood.[25]

Once the urine specimens are obtained, they should be processed for quantitative microbiologic and biochemical studies without undue delay, or they should be refrigerated (4 to 10° C). Delays of greater than 2 hours may allow sufficient growth to raise bacterial counts in contaminated specimens to greater than 1×10^5/ml.[26] Prolonged storage will also alter formed elements in the urine.

To overcome the problems associated with delays in transport and processing of specimens, two general options may be used when refrigeration is not available. These include immediate inoculation on an agar surface or directly into a transport medium. Dip-slide methods that will be discussed further, are very convenient and fulfill the requirement for immediate inoculation. Transport media, used to preserve specimens for up to 24 hours, are reported to be quite reasonable. They contain boric acid (1.8 percent), sodium chloride-polyvinyl pyrrolidone or a mixture of boric acid-glycerol-sodium formate. The solutions may be toxic when insufficient urine (less than 3.0 ml) is added and may result in lowering the bacterial counts below the standard cutoff points.[27] Because various dip-slides are readily available as is refrigeration, the need for transport media would be unusual.

Examination of the Specimens: General Versus Microscopic

Normal urine has a clear amber color. A cloudy appearance of the urine can be caused by bacteria but more often is due to crystals or leukocytes. Many solutes remain in solution at body temperature but often precipitate as insoluble crystals in the urine as the ambient temperature falls. Acidic urine, often found with first-morning specimens or in patients on acid-ash diets, characteristically contain yellow-orange urate salts whereas alkaline urine may contain cloudy phosphate crystals. Specific gravity and urine pH are usually of no value in detecting bacteriuria, except that a pH of 8.0 suggests the possibility of urea-splitting organisms. Although *Proteus* species are best known for this property, a number of strains of *Pseudomonas, Klebsiella, Serratia, Ureaplasma, Bacteroides, Staphylococcus, Helicabcter* and *Cryptococcus* also produce the enzyme urease.[28] But this high pH could also be due to an alkaline ash diet or as an artifact from a poorly stored specimen. Urinary carbon dioxide will escape from uncapped containers, causing the pH to progressively rise.

Parameters commonly analyzed in the urine, including the presence of glucose or protein, are of little aid in the diagnosis of UTI. Hematuria, when complicating an infection, can be seen in acute cystitis, but it is more often associated with stones or tumor, or occasionally with tuberculosis or fungal infections of the urinary tract.

Microscopic examination of the urine specimen can be useful in detecting infection. A Gram stain prepared from an uncentrifuged sample should be examined with an oil immersion lens. Finding at least one organism per oil immersion field correlates with quantitative cultures 80 to 90 percent of the time.

The centrifuged sediment is examined with the high–dry objective, under reduced light, with or without the addition of methylene blue. This test can be performed in conjuction with the routine study for formed elements. This procedure is particularly well suited for detecting UTI in an office practice and for rapidly assessing the effectiveness of therapy, thereby obviating the delays in waiting for culture reports. A positive sediment should contain many bacteria, preferably more than 20 per high power field (hpf). Marked pyuria may obscure the presence of bacteria in the sediment. If crystals are formed and interfere with microscopy, the urine should be warmed until they dissolve.

The major advantages of these microscopic methods are that physicians can ask for a sensitivity test immediately based on the microscopic findings, and therapeutic responses can be followed quite reliably. When patients are placed on appropriate antimicrobial therapy, bacteria should vanish from the urine by 24 to 48 hours.

Chemical Tests for Bacteriuria

The microscopic methods described here directly demonstrate the presence of bacteria by actual visualization. Chemical tests indirectly demonstrate the presence of bacteria by tracing specific metabolic products generated by uropathogens. The ideal chemical test should have the following characteristics: (1) It should be an office procedure. (2) Patients should not require special preparation for specimen collections. (3) Results should be obtained rapidly (within 1 hour). (4) It should be inexpensive. (5) Its sensitivity and specificity should be high. Currently, no chemical test meets all these criteria, making microscopic and culture methods the best diagnostic techniques.

The four most thoroughly evaluated chemical tests are summarized in Table 11-1. The *nitrite method* is the chemical test with the greatest potential for mass screening and for following treated patients. The method is available either as part of the culture pad test (described below) or as individual test strips (Micro-Stix-Nitrite, Ames Laboratory, Elkhart, IN, or Bac-U-Dip, Warner-Chilcott Laboratories, Morris Plains, NJ, and B M Test-Nitrite, Boerhinger, Mannheim, Germany). The test is carried out by immersing the test strip into freshly passed, first-morning urine and by recording the immediate appearance of a pink color. The bacteria convert nitrate to nitrite, which in turn causes the aromatic amines present in the test strip to undergo a diazotization reaction to form a diazo dye, which is pink. The same specimen is then brought to the laboratory, and the test is repeated together with a quantitative culture. This test has been used in a large field study with no false-positives in the almost 1,000 women tested.[29] Of the 40 cases of infected urine detected, two-thirds were positive on the nitrite screening. When tests were done on three serial first-morning specimens, the nitrite test was positive in almost all patients (90 percent) with significant bacteriuria. The method was similarly used on 3 consecutive days each month to screen preschool girls. Mothers tested their child's first-voided specimen, and 82 percent of recurrent episodes of significant bacteriuria were detected, again with no false-positives.[30,31]

Another test, still considered primarily as a research tool, is the *Limulus gelation test.* This is a remarkably sensitive test for endotoxin and is based on the finding that minute amounts of endotoxin cause gelation of lysates of amebocytes, the erythrocytes of the horseshoe crab *(Limulus polyphemus).* The test, when properly conducted, detects significant bacteriuria in about 1 hour.[32,33] This method will not detect gram-positive organisms or yeasts.

A *colorimetric method* has been developed to detect bacteriuria.[34] Passage of 1 ml of urine through a small filter (10 mm in diameter) traps the bacteria. The organisms on the filter are stained by passing 3 ml of safranin O dye through the filter followed by differential decolorization with 3 ml of 2.4 percent acetic acid. This decolorizer removes the dye from the filter without affecting the stained organisms. The color intensity is coded 0 to 4+ with the color guide provided. A positive test gives a pink color recorded as 1+ or greater, representing 1×10^5 or greater CFU/ml. The entire procedure takes less than 2 minutes. The test is rapid and relatively inexpensive. Interpretation of test results may be interfered with by the urinary pigments, and the filter becomes clogged by urinary debris in 3 to 17 percent.[12,35] An unacceptably high number of false-negative tests have been reported.[36] When the

Table 11-1. Chemical Methods Available for Bacteriuria Screening

Method	Principle	Sensitivity	Specificity	Comments
Nitrite (Griess's test)	Nitrate is reduced to nitrite by bacteria (i.e., *E coli*). Nitrite is detected by colorimetric methods.	Fair	Good	A prolonged bladder incubation time (first morning urine) is needed for adequate accumulation of the reduction product (nitrite). Excellent method for gram-negative bacteria but poor for gram-positive organisms.
Glucose oxidase	The trace amount of glucose present in normal urine (2 to 10 mg/100 ml) is metabolized by bacteria; the absence of glucose is tested evidence of bacteriuria.	Good	Fair	Bladder incubation is again necessary and a first-morning specimen is required. Abnormal sugar metabolism interferes with interpretation of test results; a significant number of false-positives occur; requires confirmation with urine culture.
Tetrazolium reduction	Triphenyltetrazolium is reduced by bacteria to become bright red-colored triphenyl formzan.	Good	Poor	Testing solutions are best prepared daily, and the test takes several hours for completion. Requires confirmation with urine culture.
Catalase	The enzyme catalase, present in most bacteria, hydrolyzes hydrogen peroxide to generate bubbles of oxygen.	Good	Poor	Catalase is also found in mammalian cells such as renal tubular cells, erythrocytes, and leukocytes; other inflammatory renal disease must be excluded.

nitrite dip-slide for bacteriuria and the leukocyte esterase test (see below) for pyuria are used together, the reliability may approach the value of the microscopic method.[37]

URINE CULTURE METHODS

Standard Culture Methods

Two major methods, the pour plate and streak plate techniques, are briefly reviewed.

Pour Plate

In the pour plate method, 0.1 ml of urine is added to 10 ml of diluent (broth or buffer solution), followed by vigorous mixing, and 0.1 ml of the mixture is transferred to a sterile Petri dish using a fresh pipet. Approximately 10 ml of liquid agar, maintained at 45° C in a water bath, are poured into the dish. The plate is gently swirled while the agar is allowed to harden. The inverted plate is incubated at 37° C for 24 hours. One colony on this plate represents, on the average, 1,000 living organisms from the original specimen. Addition of 0.1 ml of the diluted urine into an additional 10 ml of diluent followed by addition of 0.1 ml to the plate will permit more accurate counts. One colony on this plate represents 100,000 living organisms. Similar further dilutional steps can be used if the colony counts are higher.

Streak Plate

The streak plate method uses a bacteriologic loop, which delivers a fixed amount of urine (0.001 ml) to an agar plate. One technique uses one loopful of urine for an eosin-methylene blue (EMB) plate and another loopful for a blood agar plate. The EMB is a nonselective but differential medium for enterobacteriaceae whereas blood agar will foster growth of most bacteria. The plate may be streaked by following the method of Hirsch and Bray[37] or maybe placed on a turntable and spun. With the turntable method, the inoculum is spread from the center to the periphery four times with a large flamed loop. One hundred colonies are equivalent to 100,000 colonies per milliliter of urine.

Streak methods are used more commonly because of their simplicity and low cost. The pour plate method is still considered the standard against which all other methods are compared. One advantage of pour plates over streak plates is that highly motile strains of *Proteus* migrate less well and give more accurate colony counts.[12]

Simple Culture Techniques

Culture by traditional methods in the hospital is both costly and time-consuming, requiring several days for the results to become available. Currently a wide variety of screening culture techniques is commercially available. All require the placement of a measured amount of urine on an agar surface and subsequent counting of the number of bacterial colonies. Several representative techniques are described following.

Filter Paper

In one filter paper method (Testuria R), an inoculum is spread on a small trypticase soy agar plate with a filter paper strip, which has been dipped in the urine. The paper delivers the same quantity of urine to each plate. The culture is then incubated at 37° C for 10 to 24 hours. More than 25 colonies on the plate are equivalent to greater than 100,000 bacteria per milliliter of the original urine specimen. Because most aerobic bacteria grow on the nutrient agar, identification can only be done by subculture on to appropriate diagnostic media. False-positive and false-negative results are less than 5 percent.

Dip-Slide

The dip-slide method uses a glass slide or plastic template coated with an agar medium on each side. The slide is dipped into the urine specimen and then incubated. The two sides of the slide may have the same or different agar media. For example, one side can be coated with nutrient agar, and the other side with a differential media such as EMB or cystine-lactose-electrolyte deficient (CLED). Most bacteria grow on the nutrient agar side, while only gram-negative organisms grow on both sides. If the organism grows only on nutrient agar, it is probably gram-positive and likely to be a contaminant, particularly if present in small numbers. It must be recalled, however, that 5 to 15 percent of UTIs are caused by gram-positive organisms. Growths on both sides in high concentration are more likely to represent true infection.

The dip-slide method has been shown to correlate well with standard streak and pour plate methods.[38-40] Results are easily quantitated by comparison with the interpretation guides provided. The major commercial dip-slides and related devices include Uricult (Orion Laboratories, Helsinki, Finland, distributed by Medical Technology Corporation, Hackensack, NJ); the Oxoid dip-slide (Flow Laboratories, Rockville, MD); Dipinoc (Stayne Diagnostics, East Rutherford, NJ); Bacteriuria Screening Test (BST) (BBL Division of Becton, Dickinson and Company, Cockeysville, MD); and Clinicult (Smith Kline and French Laboratories, Philadelphia, PA).

Cup

Cup method devices are based on the same principles as the dip-slide method but use a tube, the sides of which are internally coated with the indicator culture medium, Bacturcult (Wampole Diagnostics, Stanford, CT).

These methods provide about the same information as dip-slide but are limited by use of one culture method. Inoculation is accomplished by filling the cup with urine and pouring it off.

Droplet

Mixing of the sample is first accomplished with a low-power sonic oscillation bath to break apart bacterial clumps. The sonically treated urine is diluted 1:1,000 and 0.1 ml, in four drops, is applied to the CLED plate to prevent overgrowth by *Proteus* species, using a standard disposable glass pipet. Colonies are counted after 18 hours of incubation and multiplied by the dilution factor (1×10^5).

Pad Culture

The pad culture method device consists of a clear plastic strip at the end of which is a row of three separate pads, i.e., a chemical pad and two media pads. The device is dipped into the urine and placed into a plastic envelope from which air is expressed before incubating overnight at $37°$ C. The chemical reagent pad, designed to detect traces of nitrite in the urine, turns bright pink within a few seconds of contacting the chemical. The proximal media pad contains an inhibitor of gram-positive organisms while the distal pad supports growth of both gram-positive and gram-negative bacteria. The media pads also contain the colorless dye tetrazolium, which when reduced in the presence of bacterial multiplication, produces discrete red spots on the pad. The density of the spots indicates the number of bacteria inoculated into the pad. (This device, Microstix, is manufactured by Ames Laboratories, Elkhart, IN.)

The method has been compared to pour plates in 1,000 consecutive specimens sent to the routine diagnostic laboratory. It has been shown to have a sensitivity of 91 percent and a specificity of 99 percent in detecting a colony count of 100,000 or more bacteria per milliliter of urine.[41] Similar results have also been reported by other investigators.[37,42] Antibiotics tend to interfere with this test more than with the other methods, and the method will not detect *Candida* species.

Almost all the simple culture techniques described here are inexpensive (approximately $1.00 per test), and costs should be lowered even further as use increases and competition becomes greater. Additional advantages of these devices include the elimination of the delays involved in transporting samples and a significant reduction in the time required for reporting urine culture results. A particularly attractive use for screening tests would be in hospitalized patients. This has already been successfully done both in the United Kingdom[40] and the United States.[38]

The dip-slide culture method can be performed by patients and has also been useful in epidemiologic studies.[43] This method is clearly as reliable as other quantitative culture methods, and colonies can be readily subcultured for identification and sensitivity testing. The key to management of recurrent urinary tract infections is frequent follow-up. The self-administered dip-slide, nitrite test, or culture pad-nitrite methods may prove to be as common and useful in some patients as a urine test for glucose in the diabetic.

METHODS FOR DETECTING PYURIA: MICROSCOPIC AND BIOCHEMICAL

Pyuria, i.e., urinary pus, indicates the presence of an inflammatory process somewhere in the urinary tract. Although UTIs are undoubtedly the most common cause of pyuria, other important causes must also be considered. Conditions that may be associated with pyuria without immediate evidence of bacterial involvement are multiple and may include both infectious and noninfectious causes. Examples of noninfectious, "sterile pyuria" include tubulointerstitial nephritis, stones and foreign bodies, genitourinary trauma and neoplasms, renal transplant rejection, glomerulonephritis, vaginal contamination, and appendicitis. Successful antibiotic therapy causes bacteria to disappear faster than leukocytes, thus sterile pyuria is a frequent but transient finding during this reparative phase. In addition, infections that are due to fastidious or slow-growing organisms such as mycobacteria, fungi, chlamydia, various viruses, leptospira, *Haemophilus* species, and anaerobes may all cause a spurious sterile pyuria.

The most commonly used method for determining pyuria is direct microscopic examination of the centrifuged urine sediment. This technique is affected by many variables that are difficult to control. For example, the survival of leukocytes in urine is reduced by a high pH, low osmolality, and increased temperature.[44] The most rapid disappearance of leukocytes was observed in hypotonic, alkaline suspensions at 37° C, while little change was seen in hypertonic or acid urine. The resuspension volume also has profound effects on the final counts, resulting in as much as a tenfold difference.[45]

Excretion of 400,000 or more leukocytes per hour (equivalent to 10 cells per mm³) correlates well with the presence of a UTI.[46,47] Ten or more cells per cubic millimeter were found in the urine of 281/291 (97 percent) symptomatic, bacteriuric patients, whereas only 5/313 (1.6 percent) asymptomatic, abacteriuric subjects had a similar finding.[46] In actual practice, the excretion rate or concentration of leukocytes in bacteriuric urines is usually considerably higher than 400,000/h or 10/mm³, rendering the need for minimal criteria less important. A useful guideline is that one white blood cell (WBC) per low-power ($\times$ 10 objective) microscopic field reflects the presence of three WBC/mm³.[48] Urine specimens from patients with UTIs usually contain more than 30 WBCs per low- or 1 to 2 WBCs per high-power field (HPF).

The significance of pyuria in otherwise healthy individuals cannot easily be defined. For example, the medical records of 1,000 healthy young men who had persistent pyuria (four to six or more WBC/HPF) on reported annual examinations failed to reveal any evidence of systemic or local disease.[49] The authors concluded that routine screening of young adults for pyuria was unrewarding. Their conclusion may be premature; rather, we may simply need more precise definitions of what constitutes significant pyuria.

Neutrophils contain several esterases that are not present in serum, urine, or renal tissue. Detection of esterase activity in the urine, therefore, indicates the presence of neutrophils. A dip-stick test, Chemstrip-L (Biodynamics Division, Boehringer Mannheim, Indianapolis), for this enzyme, is now available. The test consists of a filter paper pad containing indoxyl carboxylic acid ester. Leukocyte esterase(s) convert(s) this substrate into an indoxyl moiety, which undergoes oxidation in room air to an indigo color. The currently available test is read at 1 minute, and the degree of positivity is proportional to the intensity of the blue color.

The test was compared to the chamber count method using a leukocyte cutoff of $10/mm^3$ or more, and the results revealed 90 percent agreement between the two tests with 6.5 percent false-negatives and 4 percent false-positives.[50] This has been confirmed by other investigators.[51–53] Commonly used drugs, proteinuria and the pH of the urine do not influence the test. The presence of colored substances such as rifampin, nitrofurantoin, and bilirubin may, however, interfere with the interpretation of the results. False-positive tests have been reported with trichomonads. Ascorbic acid may inhibit the oxidation of indoxyl. These minor problems aside, the leukocyte esterase test is sensitive and specific enough to be a useful clinical tool in detecting the presence of leukocytes. It must be emphasized that positive leukocyte esterase test is not synonymous with bacteriuria. Bacteriuria should be assessed independently by the appropriate microbiologic methods described previously.

Minimal Diagnostic Criteria

As discussed previously, the vast majority (95 percent) of UTIs manifest 100,000/ml or more of bacteria in urine. However, such factors as forced fluid intake, and use of antibiotics for co-existing conditions may reduce this number despite the presence of infection. It is also true that some UTIs, e.g., those due to *Staphylococcus epidermidis,* may be present despite the finding of less than 100,000 CFU/ml. The totality of the clinical and laboratory findings therefore must be taken into consideration when assessing the urinary findings.

In general, it is wise to use the most rigid quantitative criteria when evaluating asymptomatic patients and so guard against unnecessary therapies and diagnostic procedures. Clean-voided specimens are more reliably obtained from males, making fewer cultures necessary for a diagnosis. Commonly, the clinical situation demands initiation of therapy for symptomatic patients when only the results of a microscopic examination are available. Confirmatory culture reports and the clinical response to antibiotics determine whether initial therapy will continue unchanged or will be modified.

Chemical Methods

The nitrite test is so highly specific that a positive test provides strong evidence of infection. A negative test, however, by no means rules out infection.

Culture Methods

The culture techniques used and their interpretation are influenced by the clinical setting and by a variety of host factors. These issues are sumarized in Table 11-2.

LOCALIZATION OF URINARY TRACT INFECTIONS

Bacterial colonization of the urine or hematogenous delivery to the renal parenchyma are the two key routes for initiating UTIs. Although initially restricted to one part of the urinary tract, the infection often spreads to other parts of the system via urinary spread. UTIs have been traditionally classified into lower (bladder) and upper (kidney) tract infections. They are often erroneously labeled "insignificant" and "important" infections, respectively, in clinical practice.

The clinical management of patients with UTIs rarely requires that the exact location of the infection be identified. It again needs to be emphasized that the prognosis of UTIs depends not on the location but rather on whether the patient has an uncomplicated or a complicated infection. Uncomplicated infection is referred to as UTI in which no underlying structural or neurologic lesions are present, whereas complicated infections are defined as situations in which the urinary tract has been invaded by bacteria repeatedly, leaving residual inflammatory changes, or when obstruction, stones, or neurologic lesions interfere with drainage of urine in some part of the tract. Localization studies, however, have proved useful in studies of the natural history of UTIs and in evaluating chemotherapeutic agents. As such, these tests are largely used as research tools. The approaches to localization are reviewed below.

Clinical Features

Analysis of the medical history and the outcome of a given therapeutic regimen are somewhat helpful in localizing the site of the UTI. Patients with complicated UTIs, recurrent infections, or delay of medical management tend to have upper UTIs.[54] The majority of patients with infections restricted to the lower tract respond favorably to short or single-dose therapy, while those who relapse early after treatment are more likely to have upper

UTIs.[54,55] When elderly institutionalized women with asymptomatic bacteriuria were analyzed by the Fairley bladder washout method (see below), the majority (67 percent) had upper UTI.[56] This observation underscores the fact that clinical features alone are not reliable markers for the localization of the infection.

The presence of WBC casts and bits of renal papillary tissue in the urine specimen are obvious indicators of upper UTI.

Differential Culture Methods

Differential culture methods are used primarily by urologists in distinguishing whether an infected male's disease is localized to the urethra or prostate. A description of these methods follows.

Ureteral Catheterization and Bladder Washout

The technique of ureteral catheterization and bladder washout is based on the supposition that if bacteria are found in the renal pelvis or ureters, using the Stamey, Govan, and Palmer catheterization method,[16] the kidney must be infected. Although there is some correlation between the presence of bacteria in the renal pelvis or ureteral urine and the presence of high antibody titers and urinary concentration defects on the affected side (i.e., more definitive evidence of renal infection), these correlations often break down in individual cases. In fact, it has been shown that many patients whose infection was apparently localized to the lower urinary tract had evidence of upper UTI as well.[57]

Segmented Cultures of the Lower Urinary Tract in the Male (Method of Meares and Stamey)

For bacteriologic localization, the voided urine and expressed prostatic secretions are labeled as follows: the first voided 5 to 10 ml (VB_1, i.e., voided bladder 1); the midstream aliquot, VB_2; the pure prostratic secretion expressed by prostatic massage (EPS, i.e., expressed prostatic secretions); and first voided 5 to 10 ml immediately after prostatic massage, VB_3. These aliquots are illustrated in Figure 11-1.

To properly execute the test, the patient must be hydrated and have a full bladder. The foreskin must be fully retracted and maintained in this position throughout the study to prevent contamination. The glans is cleansed with a detergent soap. All of the soap is removed with a wet sponge, and the glans is then dried carefully with a sterile sponge. The VB_1 is collected by holding a sterile culture tube directly in front of the urethral meatus. As the patient continues to void, the physician quickly removes the VB_1 culture tube from the stream of urine. When the patient has voided approximately 200 ml (about one-half of the bladder urine), a second sterile culture tube (VB_2) is inserted into the stream of urine for a 5- to 10-ml sample. The patient is

Table 11-2. Culture Methods for Diagnosis of Urinary Tract Infection

Patient Category	Recommended Methods for Diagnosis	Discussion and Comments
1. Asymptomatic females, in-field screening programs	A. Three consecutive clean-voided specimens revealing 10^5/ml or more colonies in urine, with same organisms in all three cultures.	Cultures should preferably be obtained on 3 separate days; the initial field screening should be followed up with two more cultures done under direct supervision.
	B. Three consecutive clean-voided specimens revealing 5×10^4/ml or more colonies in urine, with the same organisms in all three.	In this case, all *E. coli* should be of the same serotype; all *Proteus* are of the same species; all *Staphylococci* are of the same phage type, etc.
2. Asymptomatic females in office practice or the hospital where collections are closely supervised	C. Two consecutive positive clean-voided specimens with the same organisms using the same criteria as A or B.	
	D. Single urethral catheter specimens revealing 10^5/ml or more colonies in urine; lower counts require repeat collection.	Catheterization should not be done routinely. It is indicated for relief of obstruction, in marked obesity, or in debility.
	E. Single suprapubic bladder puncture revealing any number of colonies.	Counts will generally exceed 5×10^3 to 10^4/ml of urine and should be in pure culture unless complicated by stones or obstruction. Recovery of small numbers of skin contaminants such as *Staphylococcus epidermidis* or diphtheroids requires repeat study.

3. Symptomatic females	F. Preferably two consecutive clean-voided specimens. However, symptoms may require therapy before more than one culture can be taken. In this case, the urinary sediment should reveal numerous inflammatory cells and abundant bacteria. Single catheter or suprapubic collections may be used if collection of a clean-voided specimen is impractical. The bacteriologic criteria for "significant" bacteriuria is the same as for females with asymptomatic bacteriuria.	Treatment should not be begun until a carefully collected fresh specimen has been examined microscopically. Physicians managing young women with the pyuria-dysuria syndrome with low-count bacteriuria on repeated examination should request the laboratory to report the total count and to identify the putative organism rather than for the laboratory to alter the standard criteria for "significant bacteriuria."
4. Follow-up of females under treatment; failures and recurrences	G. Single clean-voided specimen revealing 10^5/ml or more colonies in urine or two consecutive clean-voided specimens with the same organism if counts range between 10^4 and 10^5/ml. Same criteria as above for catheterized specimens.	Recurrences in asymptomatic patients will often reveal numerous bacteria without pyuria. Persistence of pyuria without bacteriuria is commonly seen after 2 or 3 days of successful treatment. The pus cells clear from the urine much more slowly than do the bacteria.
5. Asymptomatic males	H. Two consecutive clean-voided specimens revealing 10^5/ml or more colonies in urine, with the same organisms in both. If counts are lower than 10^5, three consecutive specimens should reveal the same organisms, preferably in pure culture.	Low bacterial colony counts in clean-voided specimens from males may reflect true bladder colonization, particularly when the patient is undergoing diuresis or is being treated with antibacterial suppressive agents.
6. Symptomatic males	I. Single urethral catheter or suprapubic specimens as in D and E. J. Same as F for symptomatic females.	

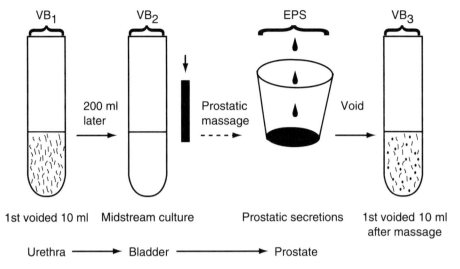

Fig. 11-1. Partition of voided urine in the male into four aliquot parts to localize infection to urethra, bladder, or prostate. See text for details. (*Abbreviations:* VB, voided bladder urine; EPS, expressed prostatic secretions.) (From Mears and Stamey,[58] with permission.)

immediately instructed to stop voiding. He then bends forward, maintains the foreskin in a retracted state with one hand, and holds a wide-mouth sterile container near the meatus with the other hand. As the physician massages the prostate gland, drops of prostatic fluid (EPS), when obtainable, fall directly into the specimen container held by the patient. Immediately after massage, the patient voids again and the VB_3 is collected in manner similar to that for the VB_1. Throughout the collections, contamination of the specimens must be prevented in uncircumcised males. If the foreskin slips over the meatus during the collections, the glans must be cleansed again. It is equally important to remove all the detergent before collecting any of these cultures, especially the VB_1; if the 5 to 10 ml of urine for cultures are contaminated by even a small amount of detergent, the quantitative colony counts will not be valid. If the patient is circumcised, it is not necessary to cleanse the glans before collecting the cultures.

Other methods have been described for localizing infections to the prostate. Mobley has described the use of semen cultures to diagnose prostatitis. The glans is washed after the foreskin is retracted. The ejaculate is cultured quantitatively in the same manner as the expressed prostatic secretions described previously.[59] The test is valid only in patients with sterile urine. This method is comparable to the method of Meares and Stamey and is an alternative in patients from whom prostatic secretions cannot be obtained by massage or those who do not tolerate the procedure.

Riedasch and co-workers carried the Stamey method one step further by examining the specimens for presence of antibody-coated bacteria (ACB) (see below). These workers report that antibody-coated bacteria were present in 25 of 51 patients with prostatic symptoms including 8 of whom had negative cultures. They also detected ACB in all 5 of their patients with bacterial epididymitis.[60]

Cystoscopic Differentiation Between Bladder Bacteriuria and Renal Bacteriuria (Method of Stamey, Govan, and Palmer)

This cystoscopic technique distinguishes between bladder and renal pelvic bacteriuria and was developed by Stamey and Pfau.[61]

The technical problem that Stamey and Pfau had to overcome was identifying how to pass ureteral catheters through infected bladder urine while ensuring that subsequent ureteral cultures were uncontaminated by downstream bladder urine.

The cystoscope is introduced into the bladder of a patient who has been previously well hydrated and given the appropriate local (or occasionally general) anesthesia. A culture is obtained through the open stopcock of the cystoscope. This sample is labeled CB (i.e., catheterized bladder). The bladder is then washed repeatedly with 2 or 3 L of sterile irrigating fluid and then emptied. Number 5 French polyethylene ureteral catheters are introduced with the catheterizing element into the cystoscope, but passed only as far as the bladder. At this time, a few ounces of irrigating fluid are allowed to enter the bladder to facilitate catheterization of the ureteral orifices; the stopcock controlling the inflow of irrigating fluid is then turned off. The irrigating fluid passing from the bladder out through the ureteral catheters is collected for culture by holding the ends of both catheters over the open end of a sterile culture tube. This culture (labeled WB, i.e., washed bladder) indicates the number of bacteria per milliliter carried within the lumina of the catheters as they are advanced to the midureter. These bacteria represent the maximal contamination possible in the first kidney culture if the total volume of urine collected from the kidney is equal to the volume of irrigating fluid displaced from the ureteral catheter (approximately 1.0 ml for #5 Fr. polyethylene catheter). Since, in actual practice, the first 5 to 10 ml from each catheter are never cultured, and since cultured aliquots are always several times (5 to 10 ml) the volume of the ureteral catheter lumen, the bacterial count in this WB culture represents a theoretic maximum. Nonetheless, if the bladder wash leaves many bacteria in the irrigating water within the ureteral catheter, and if the patient has an antidiuresis (0.2 ml/min/kidney) rather than a water diuresis, large numbers of bacteria may be recovered from the ureteral catheter when the kidney urine is sterile.

The ureteral catheters are then quickly passed to the midportion of each ureter, and consecutive urine cultures are obtained in paired, simultaneous samples (5 to 10 ml) from each kidney. The first 5 to 10 ml of urine from each of the ureteral catheters are discarded. These subsequent ureter specimens are labeled LK1, RK1, LK2, RK2, and so on. If the urine flow is too slow, mannitol can be given intravenously to produce a diuresis. Renal urines are collected for microscopic study before removing the ureteral catheters. If the diuresis is brisk, the sediment from each "renal urinary aliquot" (5 to 10 ml) may be examined microscopically to lateralize the pyuria to one or both kidneys. This technique usually agrees quite well with the bacteriologic cultures. The specific gravity, urine creatinine concentration, and osmolality are determined on several pairs of "renal samples" because the major functional defect in pyelonephritis is a failure to reabsorb water in the renal medulla. Because a water diuresis tends to mask this functional defect in concentrating ability, some patients have one or two urine samples collected before initiating their water diuresis. These concentrated aliquots are never used for culture.

Bladder Washout Method in Differentiating the Site of Urinary Tract Infection (Method of Fairley)

The bladder washout method of Fairley, originally developed in 1967[62] and modified in 1971,[57] is considered to be the gold standard by which all other localization methods are measured. It is relatively simple and does not require the more invasive ureteral catheterization technique. The test is based on the concept that if bacteria are present only in bladder urine or are lightly adherent to the bladder mucosa, they can be washed away with water and the residual organisms can be killed by neomycin.

In this method, a catheter is inserted into the bladder through the urethra and left in place. After collecting the initial specimen, the bladder is emptied, and 40 ml of 0.2 percent neomycin and one ampule of Elase (mostly DNAse, Parke-Davis), is introduced into the bladder. After 10 minutes, the bladder is distended with 0.2 percent neomycin to reduce the folds in the mucosa and the catheter is occluded for 20 minutes. The bladder is then emptied and washed out with two liters of sterile saline solution. Some of the saline from the final washout is collected for culture, and after the bladder is empty, three more timed specimens are collected at 10-minute intervals. Bacterial counts are done on all specimens.

Patients with infection localized to the bladder will have sterile urine during all collection periods following the washout. Patients with renal (upper tract) infection will have bacteria (usually in excess of 1,000 and often more than 10,000 per ml) in each of the post-washout samples.

This method compares favorably with that of Stamey, Govan and Palmer[16] in localizing infection to the upper or lower tracts. It has the advantage of not requiring that the urologist have extensive experience with the technique. This test will not lateralize the infection to an individual kidney. One remarkable feature is that patients with only bladder bacteriuria may be cured simply by the washout procedure.

Serologic Methods

Pyelonephritis resembles other infectious diseases in that a prompt serologic response occurs when the tissue is invaded. The principal tests for detecting the specific antibody response use whole bacteria agglutination methods similar to those used for serologic typing and indirect hemagglutination tests in which the antigen is coated onto erythrocytes. Latex particles may be substituted for erythrocytes, thereby adding a measure of stability to the test. Several other more sophisticated methods, such as the enzyme linked immunosorbent assay (ELISA), have also been employed. Most of the tests measure the antibody response to the O antigens of enterobacteriaceae. The K and H antigens are often much less helpful.

As is the case with other infectious diseases, the initial immunologic response to UTIs is the production of immunoglobulin M (IgM) antibody followed later by IgG antibody. The latter antibodies are also characteristic of chronic UTIs. The hemagglutination test is more sensitive to IgM, whereas the IgG response is more readily detected by bacterial agglutination. High bacterial agglutination titers have been shown to correlate well with other tests of upper UTI.[63,64] Significant increments in titer (usually fourfold or greater) in any of the tests are strong evidence of tissue invasion. Most authors equate a serologic rise with pyelonephritis or upper tract infection. This is probably correct in most instances, but it also seems more reasonable that invasion of the prostate or bladder could also elicit an antibody response (see below).

The tests are most effective when the O antigen is used from an organism recovered from the urine. More recently, a new ELISA method using the major outer membrane protein (MOMP) complex of one *Escherichia coli* strain as the antigen, has been described by Nicolle and co-workers.[65] With a convalescent specimen with an antibody titer 3 standard deviations (SD) or more above the acute, the sensitivity of the assay method for identifying invasive infection was 74 percent, the specificity 86 percent, the positive predictive value 82 percent, and the negative predictive value 79 percent.

So-called "nonspecific-phase reactants" may also be detected in the presence of inflammation, regardless of their type or location in the body. The erythrocyte sedimentation rate (ESR) and C-reactive protein (CRP) are known to be elevated in children with acute pyelonephritis.[66] The ESR tended to fall more slowly than the CRP in response to adequate treatment. The observation that some children who did not respond bacteriologically, but in whom fever had resolved, still maintained a high serum level of CRP. This response may be a useful sign of therapeutic efficacy and may be of potential value in localizing infection to the upper tract. According to Mundt and Polk, the tests most likely to be abnormal in children with symptomatic pyelonephritis line up in the following order: CRP, followed by antibody titers, ESR, and renal concentrating ability.[67] These tests will probably have their greatest value in establishing baselines for longitudinal studies of the natural history of UTIs.

Tamm-Horsfall and Cross-Reactive Antigens in Kidney

Tamm-Horsfall mucoprotein is the most prevalent of the urine proteins and is produced by the cells of the ascending limb of the loop of Henle. It is normally excreted in small amounts and elicits an antibody response at low levels in healthy individuals.

Hanson and co-workers observed that significantly elevated titers of IgG class antibodies to Tamm-Horsfall protein occurred in girls with acute pyelonephritis but not in those with cystitis. They suggest that this may be an additional test to distinguish upper from lower UTIs.[68]

Antibody-Coated Bacteria in Urine

A novel approach to the localization of infections of the urinary tract was devised by Thomas et al. in 1974,[69] revealing a high correlation between the presence of ACB in the sediment of urine and upper UTI. This has since been confirmed by other studies in adult patient populations.[70,71] In children, however, the correlation has been shown to be rather poor.[72–74]

The test is based on the concept that bacteria invading tissue elicit a local antibody response, which then reacts with the surface antigens of the bacteria. The presence of antibody coating of the bacteria can then be detected by fluorescein-conjugated immunoglobulins raised against human antibodies in the horse or goat. Specific immunoglobulin doses may be detected on the bacteria by use of nonspecific sera directed against human IgG, IgA, and IgM. It has been demonstrated that, although these immunoglobulins are present in the urine of patients with cystitis, they do not react with bacteria in urine.[75] This further supports their thesis that coating of bacteria with antibody occurs only in infected tissue.

It should be pointed out, however, that various workers employ somewhat different criteria for a positive test. Thomas et al., for example, define a positive test as one in which 25 percent or more of the bacterial cells fluoresce.[76] On the other hand, Jones considers a test positive if at least two uniformly fluorescent bacteria are observed in 200 defined microscopic fields.[77] Several conditions that are reported to give false-positive test include funguria, pseudomonads[78] proteinuria,[79] bladder tumors, and bladder stones.[80] The test is often positive in bacterial prostatitis also, so that a positive test for ACB should be used as evidence of tissue invasion rather than of upper UTI alone. This in no way detracts from the significance of the observation, because patients with tissue invasion may be at greater risk of disease than those whose urine is simply colonized with bacteria. Of course, false-negative ACBs also have been reported.[70]

It appears that the most important application of the test may be in attempting to differentiate individuals at highest risk of developing renal damage from those who will have a benign course. Another potential use of the ACB test is to identify individuals who have uncomplicated bladder bacteriuria and may respond to a single dose of an effective antimicrobial agent.[55]

The correlation of a positive ACB test with various clinical syndromes was studied in 350 consecutive patients by Rumans and Vosti.[81] The test was positive in asymptomatic bacteriuria (15 percent), cystitis (8.6 percent), acute hemorrhagic cystitis (67 percent), prostatitis (67 percent), and acute pyelonephritis (62 percent). These results reinforce the caution expressed here that the test probably more clearly reflects tissue invasion than anatomic localization of infection. To assess the applicability of the test further, Mundt and Polk reviewed the literature up to 1979.[67] When compared to acceptable standards (bilateral ureteral catheterization or bladder washout), the overall sensitivity of the ACB method was 83 percent, the specificity 76 percent, the predictive value of a positive test 81 percent, and the predictive negative value 79 percent. Unfortunately, they concluded that the ACB test had no role in the management of patients with UTI. A similar negative analysis on the value of ACB test as a guide to treatment of UTIs has recently been reported.[82] In contrast, there is considerable evidence that the ACB test is a reasonably good predictor of which patients will require prolonged courses of antimicrobial therapy. In a multicenter trial of single-dose therapy with amoxicillin for bacteriuria, a cure rate of 90 percent obtained in ACB-negative patients and fell to 33 percent in those with a positive ACB test.[54] Similarly, in bacteriuric patients receiving 7 days of appropriate therapy, the cure rate of ACB-negative patients was 85 percent but was only 36 percent in those in whom more than 1 percent of bacteria were ACB-positive.[83]

Diagnostic Imaging and Radionuclide Methods

Diagnostic imaging or radionuclide methods are rarely necessary in the management of uncomplicated UTIs. In some complicated infections, however, results of these diagnostic procedures can modify the management plan. *Intravenous pyelography (IVP)* has been the standard diagnostic imaging technique to which all the imaging methods have been compared. It allows accurate visualization of the renal parenchyma and collecting system. Adequate assessment of excretory function can also be accomplished by the method. This procedure should be performed in a well-hydrated patient who is adequately prepared. Relative contraindications include proteinuria, azotemia, and allergy to the contrast dye material. In a typical case of pyelonephritis, one observes a localized scar over a deformed calyx with calyceal distortion. Diffuse irregularity of the renal contour and multiple cortical scars are seen in advanced cases. Other conditions that may reveal similar findings include renal stones, obstruction, tuberculosis, and papillary necrosis caused by analgesic nephropathy.[80] The yield has been reported to be higher if the procedure is performed on patients who respond slowly to therapy with fever lasting more than 72 hours.[84]

Renal ultrasonography provides a safe and noninvasive assessment of the general renal morphology and perirenal structures. When combined with a plain abdominal radiograph, ultrasonography compares favorably with the IVP.[85] The IVP, however, is the more definitive procedure, especially in cases where corrective surgery is contemplated.

Radionuclide renal scans (see Ch. 10) involve the use of injectable radio-pharmaceutical agents such as [131]I Hippuran and gallium citrate Ga 67 (^{67}Ga) and a γ-radiation detector. Scans have been used to evaluate active infections in the kidney. In an animal model, Janson and Roberts demonstrated a close correlation between the appearance of ACB in the urine and poor perfusion and delayed excretion of [131] hippuran as well as accumulation of ^{67}Ga over the kidney that contained abscesses.[86] Gallium scanning is useful in localizing neoplasms and detecting occult inflammatory and psoas abscesses and serves as a useful guide to the presence of active bacterial pyelonephritis.

Computed tomography (CT) and magnetic resonance imaging (MRI) are two new advanced radiographic imaging techniques. Their use in the localization of infection in the urinary tract is limited.

Enzymuria

The kidney contains numerous enzymes that are continously shed into the urine in small amounts. Particular attention has been given to high-molecular-weight enzymes, which when excreted in large amounts, may indicate renal damage. Among these enzymes, the most extensively studied are the glycosidases (β-glucuronidase and N-acetyl-β-glucosaminidase) and the isoenzymes of lactic dehydrogenase (LDH).

Because virtually any cause of renal damage—including ischemia, nephrotoxic drugs, neoplasms, and transplant rejection—produces enzymuria, attempts to make reliable and specific correlations between enzymuria and upper UTI have been without success. LDH isoenzyme 5 correlates well, when found in elevated levels in the urine, with bladder washout localization and the ACB method. However, there is considerable controversy concerning the relative value of LDH isoenzyme 5 as a marker of upper UTI. LDH isoenzyme 5 is also found in leukocytes.[87] Its excretion may simple reflect the presence of pyuria, unless the leukocytes are removed while the cells are still fresh. The current methods of determining enzymuria add little to the localization of infection within the urinary tract.

Tests of Renal Function in Urinary Tract Infection

Uncomplicated UTIs, particularly those localized to the lower tract, are not ordinarily associated with abnormalities of renal function unless there is preexistent damage to the kidney. Patients with overt pyelonephritis or silent active renal infection, however, often have an abnormality in renal concentrating ability. The two most useful tests of renal function in pyelonephritis are the maximum concentrating test and the creatinine clearance.

Maximum Urinary Concentrating Test

Before proceeding with the maximum urinary concentrating test, one should first screen patients for their ability to produce a concentrated urine in a first-morning voided sample. The urine will be almost maximally concentrated if the subject did not take fluids after the evening meal on the proceeding day. Finding a specific gravity of more than 1.020 or an osmolality of more than 600 mosm obviates the need for more complicated testing. Failure to achieve these concentrations may require more rigid protocols for ensuring dehydration.

A protocol similar to that used in evaluating patients for diabetes insipidus also works well in this setting.[88] Following an overnight (12-hour) fast, the bladder is emptied and the osmolality is measured in the voided urine. Urine osmolality is reevaluated every 1 to 2 hours thereafter until it plateaus. The end point is taken as 2 to 3 hourly specimens that agree to within 5 percent. This response occurs within 12 to 16 hours of thirsting, with loss of 3 to 5 percent of body weight.

REFERENCES

1. Kass EH, Savage W, Santamarina BA: The significance of bacteriuria in preventive medicine. p. 3. In Kass EH (ed): Progress in Pyelonephritis. FA Davis, Philadelphia, 1965
2. Cypress BK: Patients' reasons for visiting physicians: National Ambulatory Medical Care Survey. United States, 1977–78. In: Vital and Health Statistics. Data from the National Health Survey, Series 13, no. 56 [DHHS Pub., no. (PHS) 82-1717]. National Center for Health Statistics, Hyattsville, MD, 1981
3. Kunin CM: An overview of urinary tract infections. p. 1. In Kunin CM (ed): Detection, Prevention and Management of Urinary Tract Infections. 4th Ed. Lea & Febiger, Philadelphia, 1987
4. Myerowitz RL, Medeioros AA, O'Brien TF: Bacterial infection in renal homotransplant recipients; a study of fifty three bacteremic episodes. AM J Med 53:308, 1972
5. Rubin RH, Fang LS, Cosimi AB et al: Usefulness of the antibody-coated bacteria assay in the management of urinary tract infection in the renal transplant patient. Transplantation 27:18, 1979
6. Ramsey DE, Finch WT, Birtch AG: Urinary tract infections in kidney transplant recipients. Arch Surg 114:1022, 1979
7. Krieger JN, Kaiser DL, Wenzel RP: Urinary tract etiology of bloodstream infections in hospitalized patients. J Infect Dis 148:57, 1983
8. Strand CL, Bryant JK, Sutton KH: Septicemia secondary to urinary tract infection with colony counts less than 10^5 CFU/ml. Am J Clin Pathol 83:619, 1985
9. Warren JW, Muncie HL, Jr, Berqquist EJ, Hoopes JM: Sequelae and management of urinary tract infection in the patient requiring chronic catheterization. J Urol 125:1, 1981
10. Dontas AS, Kasviki-Charvati P, Papanayiotou PC, Marketos SG: Bacteriuria and survival in old age. N Engl J Med 304:939, 1981
11. Platt R, Polk BF, Murdock B, Rosner B: Mortality associated with nosocomial urinary-tract infection. N Engl J Med 307:637, 1982

12. Kunin CM: Diagnostic methods. p. 195. In Kunin CM (ed): Detection, Prevention and Management of Urinary Tract Infections. 4th Ed. Lea & Febiger, Philadelphia, 1987

13. Monzon OT, Ory EM, Dobson HL et al: A comparison of the urine obtained by needle aspiration of the bladder, catheterization and midstream voided methods. N Engl J Med 259:764, 1958

14. Platt R: Quantitative definition of bacteriuria. Am J Med 75:44, 1983

15. Pfau A, Sacks TG: An evaluation of midstream urine cultures in the diagnosis of urinary tract infections in females. Urol Intern 25:326, 1970

16. Stamey TA, Govan DE, Palmer JM: The localization and treatment of urinary tract infections: the role of bactericidal urine levels as opposed to serum levels. Medicine 44:1, 1965

17. Kass EH: Asymptomatic infections of the urinary tract. Trans Assoc Am Phys 69:56, 1956

18. Kass EH: Bacteriuria and the diagnosis of infections of the urinary tract. Arch Intern Med 100:709, 1957

19. Marple CD: The frequency and character of urinary tract infections in an unselected group of women. Ann Intern Med 14:2220, 1941

20. Sanford JP, Favour CB, Mao FG, Harrison JH: Evaluation of the positive urine culture. Am J Med 20:88, 1956

21. Stark R, Maki D: Bacteriuria in the catheterized patient. What quantitative level of bacteriuria is relevant? N Engl J Med 311:560, 1984

22. Ouslander JG, Greengold BA, Silverblatt FJ, Garcia JP: An accurate method to obtain urine for culture in men with external catheters. Arch Intern Med 147:286, 1987

23. Hyams KC: Inappropriate urine cultures in hospitalized patients receiving antibiotic therapy. Arch Intern Med 147:48, 1987

24. Roberts AP, Robinson RE, Beard RW: Some factors affecting bacterial counts in urinary infection. Br Med J 1:40, 1967

25. Said R: Contamination of urine with providone-iodine: cause of false positive test for occult blood in urine. JAMA 242:748, 1979

26. Hindman R, Tronic B, Bartlett R: Effect of delay on culture of urine. J Clin Microbiol 4:102, 1976

27. Nickander KK, Shanholtzer CJ, Peterson LR: Urine culture transport tubes: effect of sample volume on bacterial toxicity of the preservative. J Clin Microbiol 15:593, 1982

28. Griffith DP: Infection-induced stones. p. 203. In Coe FL (ed): Nephrolithiasis: Pathogenesis and Treatment. Year Book Medical Publishers, Chicago, 1978

29. Kunin CM, DeGroot JE: Self-screening for significant bacteriuria. JAMA 231:1349, 1975

30. Kunin CM, DeGroot JE, Uehling D, Ramgopal V: Detection of urinary tract infections in 3- to 5- year-old girls by mothers using a nitrite indicator strip. Pediatrics 57:829, 1976

31. Kunin CM, DeGroot JE: Sensitivity of a nitrite indicator strip method in detecting bacteriuria in preschool girls. Pediatrics 60:244, 1977

32. Garibaldi RA, Allman GW, Larsen DH et al: Detection of endotoxemia by the limulus test in patients with indwelling urinary catheters. J Infect Dis 128:551, 1973

33. Jorgensen JH, Carvajel HF, Chipps BE, Smith RF: Rapid detection of gram-negative bacteriuria by use of the Limulus endotoxin assay. Appl Microbiol 26:38, 1973

34. Wallis C, Melnick JL, Longoria CJ: Colorimetric method for rapid determination of bacteriuria. J Clin Microbiol 14:342, 1981

35. Pfaller MA, Koontz FP: Use of rapid screening tests in processing urine specimens by conventional culture and the automicrobic system. J Clin Microbiol 21:783, 1985

36. Wu TC, Williams EC, Koo SY, MacLowry JD: Evaluation of three bacteriuria screening methods in a clinical research hospital. J Clin Microbiol 21:796, 1985

37. Moffat CM, Britt MR, Burke JP: Evaluation of miniature test for bacteriuria using dehydrated media and nitrite pads. Appl Microbiol 28:95, 1974

38. Ellner PD, Papchristos T: Detection of bacteriuria by dip-slide. Am J Clin Pathol 63:516, 1975

39. Guttmann D, Naylor GRE: Dip-slide: an aid to quantitative urine culture in general practice. Br Med J 3:343,1967

40. Jackaman FR, Darrell JH, Shackman R: The dip-slide in urology. Br Med J 1:207, 1973

41. Craig WA, Kunin CM: Quantitative urine culture method using a plastic paddle containing dual media. Appl Microbiol 23:919, 1972

42. Bailey R, Dann E: Bactercult in the diagnosis of urinary tract infection. N Zealand Med J 81:517, 1975

43. Brundtland GH, Hovig B: Screening for bacteriuria in school girls. An evaluation of a dip-slide culture method and the urinary glucose method. Am J Epidemiol 97:246, 1973

44. Triger DR, Smith WG: Survival of urinary leukocytes. J Clin Pathol 19:443, 1966

45. Gadeholt H: Quantitative estimation of urinary sediment, with special regard to sources of error. Br Med J 1:1547, 1964

46. Little PJ: Urinary white-cell excretion. Lancet 1:1149, 1962

47. Mabeck CE: Studies in urinary tract infections: IV. Urinary leukocyte excretion in bacteriuria. Acta Med Scand 186:193, 1969

48. Musher DM, Thorsteinsson SB, Airola VM: Quantitative urinalysis. JAMA 236:2069, 1976

49. Benbassat J, Froom P, Feldman M, Margaliot S: The importance of leukocyturia in young adults. Arch Intern Med 145:79, 1985

50. Banauch D: Leukozyten-Nachweis in Urin mit einem Testreifen. Eine Kooperative Studie on elf Zentrum. Deutsche Medizinische Wochenschrift. 104:1236, 1979

51. Gillenwater JY: Detection of urinalysis leukocytes by chemstrip-1. J Urol 125:383, 1981

52. Kusumi RK, Grover PJ, Kunin CM: Rapid detection of pyuria by leukocyte esterase activity. JAMA 245:1653, 1981

53. Pfaller M, Ringenberg B, Rames L et al: The usefulness of screening tests for pyuria in combination with culture in the diagnosis of urinary tract infection. Diagn Microbiol Infect Dis 6:207, 1987

54. Rubin RH, Fang LST, Jones ST: Single-dose amoxicillin therapy for urinary tract infection. J Am Med Assoc 244:561, 1980

55. Fang LST, Tolkoff-Rubin NE, Rubin RH: Efficacy of single-dose and conventional amoxicillin therapy in urinary-tract infection localized by the antibody-coated bacteria technic. N Engl J Med 298:413, 1978

56. Nicolle LE, Muir P, Harding GKM, Norris M: Localization of urinary tract infection in elderly, institutionalized women with asymptomatic bacteriuria. J Infect Dis 157:65, 1987

57. Fairley KF, Grounds AD, Carson NE et al: Site of infection in acute urinary-tract infection in general practice. Lancet 2:615, 1971
58. Meares EM, Stamey TA: Bacteriologic localization patterns in bacterial prostatitis and urethritis. Invest Urol 5:492, 1968
59. Mobley DR: Semen cultures in the diagnosis of bacterial prostatitis. J Urol 114:83, 1975
60. Riedasch G, Ritz E, Mohring K, Ikinger U: Antibody-coated bacteria in the ejaculate: a possible test for prostatitis. J Urol 118:787, 1977
61. Stamey TA, Pfau A: Some functional, pathologic, bacteriologic, and chemotherapeutic characteristics of unilateral pyelonephritis in man. II. Bacteriologic and chemotherapeutic characteristics. Invest Urol 1:162, 1963
62. Fairley KF, Bond AG, Brown RB, Habersberger P: Simple test to determine the site of urinary tract infection. Lancet 2:427, 1967
63. Clark H, Ronald AR, Turck M: Serum antibody response in renal versus bladder bacteriuria. J Infect Dis 123:539, 1971
64. Norden CW, Levy PS, Kass EH: Predictive effect of urinary concentrating ability and hemagglutinating antibody titer upon response to antimicrobial therapy in bacteriuria in pregnancy. J Infect Dis 121:588, 1970
65. Nicolle LE, Brunka J, Ujack E, Bryan L: Antibodies to major outer membrane proteins of *Escherichia coli* in urinary tract infection in the elderly. J Infect Dis 160:627, 1989
66. Jodal U, Hanson LA: Sequential determination of C-reactive protein in acute childhood pyelonephritis. Acta Paediatr Scand 65:319, 1976
67. Mundt KA, Polk BP: Identification of site of urinary-tract infections by antibody-coated bacteria assay. Lancet 2:1172, 1979
68. Hanson LA, Fasth A, Jodal U: Autoantibodies to Tamm-Horsfall protein, a tool for diagnosing the level of urinary-tract infection. Lancet 1:226, 1976
69. Thomas V, Shelokov A, Forland M: Antibody-coated bacteria in the urine and the site of urinary tract infection. N Engl J Med 290:588, 1974
70. Harding GKM, Marrie TJ, Ronald AR et al: Urinary tract localization in women. JAMA 240:1147, 1978
71. Jones SR, Smith JW, Sanford JP: Localization of urinary tract infections by detection of antibody-coated bacteria in urine sediment. N Engl J Med 290:591, 1979
72. Forsum U, Hjelm E, Jonsell G: Antibody-coated bacteria in the urine of children with urinary tract infections. Acta Paediatr Scand 65:639, 1976
73. Hellerstein S, Kennedy E, Nussbaum L, Rice K: Localization of the site of urinary tract infections by means of antibody-coated bacteria in the urinary sediments. J Pediatr 92:188, 1978
74. Hawthorne NJ, Kurtz SB, Anhalt JP, Sequra JW: Accuracy of antibody-coated bacteria test in recurrent urinary tract infections. Mayo Clin Proc 53:651, 1978
75. Ratner JJ, Thomas VL, Sanford BA, Forland M: Bacteria-specific antibody in the urine of patients with acute pyelonephritis and cystitis. J Infect Dis 143:404, 1981
76. Thomas VL, Forland M, Shelokov A: Antibody-coated bacteria in urinary tract infection. Kidney Int 8:S20, 1975
77. Jones SR: Antibody-coated bacteria in urine, letter. N Engl J Med 295:1380, 1976
78. Harding SA, Merz WG: Evaluation of antibody coating of yeasts in urine as an indicator of the site of urinary tract infection. J Clin Microbiol 2:222, 1975
79. Thomas VL, Forland M, LeStourgeon D, Shelokov A: Antibody-coated bacteria in persistent and recurrent urinary tract infections. Kidney Int 14:607, 1978

80. Stamey TA: Diagnosis, localization and classification of urinary infections. p. 1. In Stamey TA (ed): Pathogenesis and Treatment of Urinary Tract Infections. Williams & Wilkins, Baltimore, 1980

81. Rumans LW, Vosti KL: The relationship of antibody-coated bacteria to clinical syndromes. Arch Intern Med 138:1077, 1978

82. Leibovici L, Wysenbeck AJ: Single-dose treatment of urinary tract infections with and without antibody-coated bacteria: A metaanalysis of controlled trials. J Infect Dis 163:928, 1991

83. Gargan RA, Brumfit W, Hamilton-Miller JMT: Antibody-coated bacteria in urine: criterion for a positive test and its value in defining a higher risk of treatment failure. Lancet 2:704, 1983

84. Kanal KT, Korboth FJ, Schwentker FN, Lecky JW: The intravenous pyelogram in acute pyelonephritis. Arch Intern Med 148:2144, 1988

85. Spencer J, Lindsell D, Mastoraku I: Ultrasonography compared with intravenous urography in investigation of urinary tract infection in adults. Br Med J 301:221, 1990

86. Janson KL, Roberts JA: Non-invasive localization of urinary-tract infection. J Urol 117:624, 1977

87. Malik GM, Canawati HN, Keyser AJ et al: Correlation of urinary lactic dehydrogenase with polymorphonuclear leukocytes in urinary tract infections in patients with spinal cord injury. J Infect Dis 147:161, 1983

88. Miller M, Dalakos T, Moses M et al: Recognition of partial defects in antidiuretic hormone secretion. Ann Intern Med 73:721, 1970

Index

Page numbers followed by f indicate figures; those followed by t indicate tables.